Teen Health Series

Cancer Information For Teens, Third Edition

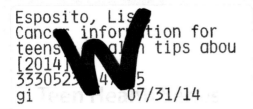

Cancer Information For Teens, Third Edition

Health Tips About Cancer Prevention, Risks, Diagnosis, And Treatment

Including Facts About Cancers Of Most Concern To Teens And Young Adults, Coping Strategies, Survivorship, And Dealing With Cancer In Loved Ones

Edited by Lisa Esposito

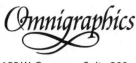

155 W. Congress, Suite 200
Detroit, MI 48226

Bibliographic Note

Because this page cannot legibly accommodate all the copyright notices, the Bibliographic Note portion of the Preface constitutes an extension of the copyright notice.

Edited by Lisa Esposito

Teen Health Series

Karen Bellenir, *Managing Editor*
David A. Cooke, M.D., *Medical Consultant*
Elizabeth Collins, *Research and Permissions Coordinator*
EdIndex, *Services for Publishers, Indexers*

* * *

Omnigraphics, Inc.
Matthew P. Barbour, *Senior Vice President*
Kevin M. Hayes, *Operations Manager*

* * *

Peter E. Ruffner, *Publisher*
Copyright © 2014 Omnigraphics, Inc.
ISBN 978-0-7808-1319-9
E-ISBN 978-0-7808-1320-5

Library of Congress Cataloging-in-Publication Data

Cancer information for teens : health tips about cancer prevention, risks, diagnosis, and treatment including facts about cancers of most concern to teens and young adults, coping strategies, survivorship, and dealing with cancer in loved ones / edited by Lisa Esposito. -- Third edition.
    pages cm. -- (Teen health series)
 Audience: Grade 9 to 12.
 Summary: "Provides basic consumer health information for teens about cancer risk factors, prevention, and treatment, along with tips for coping with cancer at home and school, and helping a friend or family member who has cancer. Includes index, resource information, and recommendations for further reading"-- Provided by publisher.
 Includes bibliographical references and index.
 ISBN 978-0-7808-1319-9 (hardcover : alk. paper) -- ISBN 978-0-7808-1320-5 (ebook) 1. Cancer--Juvenile literature. I. Esposito, Lisa, editor.
 RC264.C36 2013
 616.99'4--dc23
                                                                          2013026651

Table of Contents

Preface

Part One: Cancer Facts And Risk Factors

Chapter 1—What Is Cancer?..3

Chapter 2—Cancer In Young People: An Overview 7

Chapter 3—Cancer Facts, Myths, And Unknowns..........................11

Chapter 4—Genes, Genetic Disorders, And Cancer......................15

Chapter 5—Cancer And The Environment...21

Chapter 6—Tanning And Cancer Risk..27

Chapter 7—Is Some Sun Good?...35

Chapter 8—Cancer Risks Associated With Smoking
And Other Tobacco Use 39

Chapter 9—Safer Grilling To Reduce Cancer Risk 45

Chapter 10—Obesity And Cancer Risk...49

Chapter 11—Human Papillomavirus And Cancer Risk 53

Chapter 12—Hormonal Drugs And Cancer Risk:
Oral Contraceptives And Anabolic Steroids 59

Chapter 13—Cancer Prevention For Girls:
Why See A Gynecologist?...................................65

Chapter 14—How To Perform A Breast Self-Exam...........................73

Part Two: Cancers Of Most Concern To Teens And Young Adults

Chapter 15—Bone Cancer 79

Chapter 16—Brain Tumors 85

Chapter 17—Breast Cancer 93

Chapter 18—Cervical Cancer 101

Chapter 19—Colorectal Cancer 111

Chapter 20—Germ Cell Tumors.. 123

Chapter 21—Leukemia... 131

Chapter 22—Lymphoma 145

Chapter 23—Melanoma And Other Skin Cancers 155

Chapter 24—Neuroblastoma: Cancer Of The Nervous System.... 171

Chapter 25—Soft Tissue Sarcomas 173

Chapter 26—Testicular Cancer... 181

Chapter 27—Thyroid Cancer 187

Part Three: Cancer Awareness, Diagnosis, And Treatment

Chapter 28—Bumps And Lumps: When Do They Require
              Medical Attention? 197

Chapter 29—Questions To Ask Your Doctor About Cancer 201

Chapter 30—Specialized Children's Cancer Centers 207

Chapter 31—Your Cancer Care Hospital Team 213

Chapter 32—Cancer Staging.. 217

Chapter 33—Chemotherapy And Side Effects................................ 223

Chapter 34—Steroids And Cancer Treatment 235

Chapter 35—Radiation Therapy For Cancer.................................... 239

Chapter 36—What To Expect If You Need Surgery 251

Chapter 37—Bone Marrow And Peripheral Blood
              Stem Cell Transplantation 257

Chapter 38—Cancer And Complementary Health Therapies 265

Chapter 39—Cancer Clinical Trials.. 273

Part Four: Cancer Survivorship

Chapter 40—Cancer Fatigue 283

Chapter 41—Cancer Pain..291

Chapter 42—What Will Happen To My Body
During Cancer Treatment?..301

Chapter 43—After Cancer Treatment Ends 305

Chapter 44—Cancer And Your Friendships..........................319

Chapter 45—Cancer And Your Education..............................323

Chapter 46—Late Effects: Chronic Problems That
Can Result After Cancer And Treatment 329

Chapter 47—Can I Have Children After Cancer Treatment?..........343

Part Five: When A Loved One Has Cancer

Chapter 48—When Your Parent Has Cancer 349

Chapter 49—When Your Brother Or Sister Is Seriously Ill...............363

Chapter 50—How Can I Help If My Friend Has Cancer?.................367

Part Six: If You Need More Information

Chapter 51—Additional Reading About Cancer 373

Chapter 52—Web-Based Resources And Support Groups............377

Chapter 53—How To Find Clinical Cancer Trials 383

Index **389**

Preface

About This Book

Most often, teens with cancer overcome the disease. In fact, five years after diagnosis, 80 percent of teens and children who have experienced cancer are cancer survivors. Treatment has improved and more is known about what causes cancer and how to prevent it. However, cancer is still a formidable diagnosis, and it remains the leading cause of death by disease among teens.

Cancer affects adolescents differently than older adults or young children. Additionally, teens face environmental factors and make lifestyle choices that may influence their disease risk. For instance, research shows that indoor tanning raises cancer risk although cell phone use likely does not. Decisions about other issues, such as sun exposure, tobacco use, and sexual practices, may all have implications for teens' health now and as adults.

Cancer Information For Teens, Third Edition presents updated facts about cancer causes, prevention, diagnosis, and treatment. It explains how cancer occurs in the body and describes some warning signs. A chapter focused on cancer myths helps teens sort fact from fiction. For teens who do have cancer, the book gives practical advice about important topics, such as which questions to ask health care providers and how to cope with treatment side effects and changes in body image. Social worries at school and among friends are addressed, and cancer survivorship issues, including fertility concerns, are discussed frankly. A separate section focuses on teens with friends or family members who have cancer. Finally, a resource section provides suggestions for additional reading, a directory of web-based support sources, and list of websites for finding cancer trials.

How To Use This Book

This book is divided into parts and chapters. Parts focus on broad areas of interest; chapters are devoted to single topics within a part.

Part One: Cancer Facts And Risk Factors explains that cancer is a variety of diseases that begin the same way: cells divide in an uncontrolled manner with the ability to attack the body's tissues. This part also discusses risk factors for cancer. These include familial or genetic predisposition, outdoor and indoor tanning, tobacco use, obesity, chemicals in the environment, and human papillomavirus infection. Ways to reduce modifiable risks are suggested.

Part Two: Cancers Of Most Concern To Teens And Young Adults gives facts on the cancer types most often diagnosed in adolescents and young adults. Among these are bone cancer, brain and spinal cord tumors, leukemia, lymphoma, and testicular cancer.

Part Three: Cancer Awareness, Diagnosis, And Treatment explains the signs and symptoms that may indicate the presence of cancer, and it describes how doctors diagnose the disease and determine how advanced it is. Chapters in this part discuss commonly used cancer treatments, including surgery, chemotherapy, radiation, and bone marrow and stem cell transplantation. The part also offers information on supportive care and cancer clinical research.

Part Four: Cancer Survivorship acknowledges the wide-ranging and sometimes long-term impact that cancer can have on teens' lives. It describes temporary effects of treatment on appearance and how to deal with friendships and school challenges during recovery. The part includes a straightforward summary of chronic health problems that can result after cancer, including fertility issues.

Part Five: When A Loved One Has Cancer gives guidance for teens with a parent, sibling, or friend who has cancer. It explains how to cope with the sometimes-confusing emotions that can arise and how teens can help others while still taking of themselves.

Part Six: If You Need More Information includes suggestions for additional reading about cancers, a directory of web-based resources including teen-focused support groups, and guidance for people who want to learn more about specific clinical trials.

Bibliographic Note

This volume contains documents and excerpts from publications issued by the following government agencies: Centers for Disease Control and Prevention (CDC); National Cancer Institute (NCI); National Center for Complementary and Alternative Medicine (NCCAM); National Institute on Drug Abuse; and the Office of Women's Health.

In addition, this volume contains copyrighted documents, articles, and images produced by the following individuals and organizations: American Society of Clinical Oncology; American Thyroid Association; California Environmental Health Tracking Program; Cancer Research UK; Center for Young Women's Health/Boston Children's Hospital; CureSearch; Jeanne Kelly; MD Anderson Cancer Center; Melissa's Living Legacy Teen Cancer Foundation; National Children's Cancer Society; Nemours Foundation; Obesity Society; Palo Alto Medical Foundation; Seattle Cancer Care Alliance; Seattle Children's Hospital, Research and Foundation; Skin Cancer Foundation; Sun Safety for Kids; Teenage Cancer Trust; the Testicular Cancer Resource Center; and Terese Winslow.

The photograph on the front cover is © CleoMiu/Bigstock Photo.

Full citation information is provided on the first page of each chapter. Every effort has been made to secure all necessary rights to reprint the copyrighted material. If any omissions have been made, please contact Omnigraphics to make corrections for future editions.

Acknowledgements

In addition to the organizations listed above, special thanks are due to Liz Collins, research and permissions coordinator; Karen Bellenir, managing editor; and WhimsyInk, prepress services provider.

About The *Teen Health Series*

At the request of librarians serving today's young adults, the *Teen Health Series* was developed as a specially focused set of volumes within Omnigraphics' *Health Reference Series*. Each volume deals comprehensively with a topic selected according to the needs and interests of people in middle school and high school.

Teens seeking preventive guidance, information about disease warning signs, medical statistics, and risk factors for health problems will find answers to their questions in the *Teen Health Series*. The *Series*, however, is not intended to serve as a tool for diagnosing illness, in prescribing treatments, or as a substitute for the physician/patient relationship. All people concerned about medical symptoms or the possibility of disease are encouraged to seek professional care from an appropriate health care provider.

If there is a topic you would like to see addressed in a future volume of the *Teen Health Series*, please write to:

Editor, *Teen Health Series*
Omnigraphics, Inc.
155 W. Congress, Suite 200
Detroit, MI 48226

A Note About Spelling And Style

Teen Health Series editors use *Stedman's Medical Dictionary* as an authority for questions related to the spelling of medical terms and the *Chicago Manual of Style* for questions related to grammatical structures, punctuation, and other editorial concerns. Consistent adherence is not always possible, however, because the individual volumes within the *Series* include many documents from a wide variety of different producers and copyright holders, and the editor's primary goal is to present material from each source as accurately as is possible following the terms specified by each document's producer. This sometimes means that information in different chapters or sections may follow other guidelines and alternate spelling authorities. For example, occasionally a copyright holder may require that eponymous terms be shown in possessive forms (Crohn's disease *vs.* Crohn disease) or that British spelling norms be retained (leukaemia *vs.* leukemia).

Locating Information Within The *Teen Health Series*

The *Teen Health Series* contains a wealth of information about a wide variety of medical topics. As the *Series* continues to grow in size and scope, locating the precise information needed by a specific student may become more challenging. To address this concern, information about books within the *Teen Health Series* is included in *A Contents Guide to the Health Reference Series*. The *Contents Guide* presents an extensive list of more than 16,000 diseases, treatments, and other topics of general interest compiled from the Tables of Contents and major index headings from the books of the *Teen Health Series* and *Health Reference Series*. To access *A Contents Guide to the Health Reference Series*, visit www.healthreferenceseries.com.

Our Advisory Board

We would like to thank the following advisory board members for providing guidance to the development of this *Series*:

> Dr. Lynda Baker, Associate Professor of Library and Information Science, Wayne State University, Detroit, MI
>
> Nancy Bulgarelli, William Beaumont Hospital Library, Royal Oak, MI
>
> Karen Imarisio, Bloomfield Township Public Library, Bloomfield Township, MI
>
> Karen Morgan, Mardigian Library, University of Michigan-Dearborn, Dearborn, MI
>
> Rosemary Orlando, St. Clair Shores Public Library, St. Clair Shores, MI

Medical Consultant

Medical consultation services are provided to the *Teen Health Series* editors by David A. Cooke, M.D. Dr. Cooke is a graduate of Brandeis University, and he received his M.D. degree from the University of Michigan. He completed residency training at the University of Wisconsin Hospital and Clinics. He is board-certified in internal medicine. Dr. Cooke currently works as part of the University of Michigan Health System and practices in Ann Arbor, MI. In his free time, he enjoys writing, science fiction, and spending time with his family.

Part One
Cancer Facts And Risk Factors

Chapter 1

What Is Cancer?

Defining Cancer

Cancer is a term used for diseases in which abnormal cells divide without control and are able to invade other tissues. Cancer cells can spread to other parts of the body through the blood and lymph systems.

Cancer is not just one disease but many diseases. There are more than 100 different types of cancer. Most cancers are named for the organ or type of cell in which they start—for example, cancer that begins in the colon is called colon cancer; cancer that begins in melanocytes of the skin is called melanoma.

Origins Of Cancer

All cancers begin in cells, the body's basic unit of life. To understand cancer, it's helpful to know what happens when normal cells become cancer cells.

The body is made up of many types of cells. These cells grow and divide in a controlled way to produce more cells as they are needed to keep the body healthy. When cells become old or damaged, they die and are replaced with new cells.

However, sometimes this orderly process goes wrong. The genetic material (DNA) of a cell can become damaged or changed, producing mutations that affect normal cell growth and division. When this happens, cells do not die when they should and new cells form when the body does not need them. The extra cells may form a mass of tissue called a tumor.

About This Chapter: Text in this chapter is from "What Is Cancer?" National Cancer Institute (NCI), February 8, 2013.

Types Of Cancer

Cancer types can be grouped into broader categories. The main categories of cancer include the following:

- **Carcinoma:** Cancer that begins in the skin or in tissues that line or cover internal organs. There are a number of subtypes of carcinoma, including adenocarcinoma, basal cell carcinoma, squamous cell carcinoma, and transitional cell carcinoma.

- **Sarcoma:** Cancer that begins in bone, cartilage, fat, muscle, blood vessels, or other connective or supportive tissue.

- **Leukemia:** Cancer that starts in blood-forming tissue such as the bone marrow and causes large numbers of abnormal blood cells to be produced and enter the blood.

- **Lymphoma And Myeloma:** Cancers that begin in the cells of the immune system.

- **Central Nervous System Cancers:** Cancers that begin in the tissues of the brain and spinal cord.

Source: NCI, February 8, 2013.

Not all tumors are cancerous; tumors can be benign or malignant.

- **Benign tumors** aren't cancerous. They can often be removed, and, in most cases, they do not come back. Cells in benign tumors do not spread to other parts of the body.

- **Malignant tumors** are cancerous. Cells in these tumors can invade nearby tissues and spread to other parts of the body. The spread of cancer from one part of the body to another is called metastasis.

Some cancers do not form tumors. For example, leukemia is a cancer of the bone marrow and blood.

Cancer Statistics

A report from the nation's leading cancer organizations shows that rates of death in the United States from all cancers for men and women continued to fall between 2005 and 2009, the most recent reporting period available.

Estimated new cases and deaths from cancer in the United States in 2013 are as follows:

- New cases: 1,660,290 (does not include nonmelanoma skin cancers)

- Deaths: 580,350

Additional Information

Cancers that are diagnosed with the greatest frequency in the United States are listed below:

- Bladder cancer
- Breast cancer
- Colon and rectal cancer
- Endometrial cancer
- Kidney (renal cell) cancer
- Leukemia
- Lung cancer
- Melanoma
- Non-Hodgkin lymphoma
- Pancreatic cancer
- Prostate cancer
- Thyroid cancer

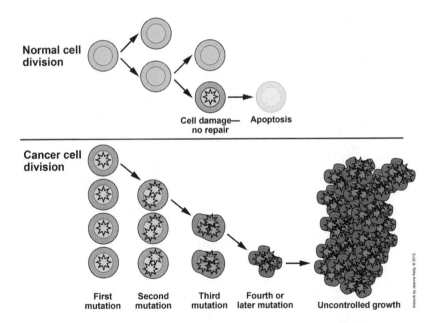

Figure 1.1. Loss of normal growth control. Artwork originally created for the National Cancer Institute. Reprinted with permission of the artist, Jeanne Kelly. Copyright 2012.

The risk of developing many types of cancer can be reduced by practicing healthy lifestyle habits, such as eating a healthy diet, getting regular exercise, and not smoking. Also, the sooner a cancer is found and treatment begins, the better the chances are that the treatment will be successful.

Contact NCI For Help

National Cancer Institute (NCI) cancer information specialists can answer your questions about cancer and help you with quitting smoking. They can also help you with using this website and can tell you about NCI's printed and electronic materials. Contact information for the NCI can be found on their website at http://www.cancer.gov/global/contact.

Chapter 2

Cancer In Young People: An Overview

Every bodily cell is tightly regulated with respect to growth, interaction with other cells, and even its life span. Cancer occurs when a type of cell has lost these normal control mechanisms and grows in a way that the body can no longer regulate.

Different kinds of cancer have different signs, symptoms, treatments, and outcomes, depending on the type of cell involved and the degree of uncontrolled cell growth.

About Cancer

All kinds of cancer, including childhood cancer, have a common disease process—cells grow out of control, develop abnormal sizes and shapes, ignore their typical boundaries inside the body, destroy their neighbor cells, and ultimately can spread (or metastasize) to other organs and tissues.

As cancer cells grow, they demand more and more of the body's nutrition. Cancer takes a child's strength, destroys organs and bones, and weakens the body's defenses against other illnesses.

Typically, factors that trigger cancer in kids usually differ from those that cause cancer in adults, such as smoking or exposure to environmental toxins. Rarely, there may be an increased risk of childhood cancer in kids who have a genetic condition, such as Down syndrome. Those who have had chemotherapy or radiation treatment for a prior cancer episode may also have an increased risk of cancer.

About This Chapter: "Childhood Cancer," September 2010, reprinted with permission from www.kidshealth .org. This information was provided by KidsHealth®, one of the largest resources online for medically reviewed health information written for parents, kids, and teens. For more articles like this, visit www.KidsHealth.org, or www.TeensHealth.org. Copyright © 1995-2013 The Nemours Foundation. All rights reserved.

In most cases, however, childhood cancers arise from noninherited mutations (or changes) in the genes of growing cells. Because these errors occur randomly and unpredictably, there's no effective way to prevent them.

Sometimes, a doctor might spot early symptoms of cancer at regular checkups. However, some of these symptoms (such as fever, swollen glands, frequent infections, anemia, or bruises) are also associated with other infections or conditions that are much more common than cancer. Because of this, both doctors and parents might suspect other childhood illnesses when cancer symptoms first appear.

Once cancer has been diagnosed, it's important for parents to seek help from a medical center that specializes in pediatric oncology (treatment of childhood cancer).

Cancer Treatment

The treatment of cancer in children can include chemotherapy (the use of medical drugs to kill cancer cells), radiation (the use of radiant energy to kill cancer cells), and surgery (to remove cancerous cells or tumors). The type of treatment needed depends on the type and severity of cancer and the child's age.

Surgery

For children with leukemia or lymphoma, surgery generally plays a minor role. This is because leukemia and lymphoma involve the circulatory system and lymphatics, two systems that are located all throughout the body, making it difficult to treat by operating on one specific area.

In children with solid tumors that haven't spread to other parts of the body, however, surgery can often effectively remove cancer when used in combination with chemotherapy and/or radiation.

It's A Fact!

Cancer affects only about 14 of every 100,000 children in the United States each year. Among all age groups, the most common childhood cancers are leukemia, lymphoma, and brain cancer. As kids enter the teen years, there is an increase in the incidence of osteosarcoma (bone cancer).

The sites of cancer are different for each type, as are treatment and cure rates.

Chemotherapy

Chemotherapy is medication which is used as a tool to eliminate cancer cells in the body. Kids with cancer can be given the chemotherapy medications *intravenously* (through a vein) or *orally* (by mouth). Some forms of chemotherapy can be given *intrathecally,* or into the spinal fluid. The drugs enter the bloodstream and work to kill cancer in all parts of the body.

The duration of chemotherapy treatment and type and number of different of drugs used depends on the type of cancer and the child's response to the drugs. Every child's treatment differs, so a child may receive daily, weekly, or monthly chemotherapy treatments. The doctor may also recommend cycles of treatment, which allow the body to rest and recover between periods of chemo.

All of the medications used as chemotherapy also carry the risk of both short-term and long-term problems. Short-term side effects may include nausea, vomiting, hair loss, fatigue, anemia, abnormal bleeding, and increased risk of infection due to destruction of the bone marrow, as well as kidney damage and menstrual irregularities. Some drugs carry a risk of bladder inflammation and bleeding into the urine, hearing loss, and liver damage. Others may cause heart and skin problems. Longer-term effects can include infertility, growth problems, organ damage, or increased risk of other cancers.

Your doctor will use precautions as well as other medications to counteract as many of the side effects as possible.

Bone Marrow Transplants

Kids with certain types of cancer may receive bone marrow transplants. Bone marrow is a spongy tissue inside certain bones of the body that produces blood cells. If a child has a type of cancer that affects the function of blood cells, a bone marrow transplant (along with chemotherapy to kill the defective cells) may allow new, healthy cells to grow. Bone marrow transplant is also sometimes used to treat cancer that does not involve blood cells because it lets doctors use higher doses of chemo than would otherwise be tolerated.

Radiation

Radiation is one of the most common treatments for cancer. A child who receives radiation therapy is treated with a stream of high-energy particles or waves that destroy or damage cancer cells. Many types of childhood cancer are treated with radiation along with chemotherapy or surgery.

Radiation has many potential side effects (such as increased risk of future malignancy and infertility), which you should discuss with the doctor.

The primary goal when treating kids with cancer is to cure them; this takes priority over all other aspects of care. However, many medications and therapies can make kids more comfortable while undergoing treatment for cancer.

Coping With Cancer

When possible, older kids should be involved with their own cancer treatment. Facts about the specific type of cancer and its effects should be explained in language suitable for the child's age. However, when cancer affects younger children—toddlers and those under age four—simply telling them that they are "sick" and need "medicine" to get better is often enough explanation. For all age groups, the goal is to prevent fear and misunderstanding.

Many kids might feel guilty, as if the cancer is somehow their fault. Psychologists, social workers, and other members of the cancer treatment team can be a great help in reassuring and helping them with their feelings.

The cancer treatment team can guide patients and families through the pain, uncertainty, and disruptions caused by cancer. If necessary, team can also contact or visit the child's school to explain the diagnosis to teachers and classmates. Replacing fear and misunderstanding with compassion and information is a goal in helping kids with cancer cope with the illness.

The diagnosis and treatment of childhood cancers takes time, and there are both short-term and long-term side effects. But thanks to medical advances, more and more kids with cancer are finishing successful treatment, leaving hospitals, and growing up just like everybody else. Today, up to 70 percent of all children with cancer can be cured.

Chapter 3

Cancer Facts, Myths, And Unknowns

Myth Buster

A survey was conducted with 13 to 24 year olds to reveal the top 20 cancer myths believed by teenagers and young adults throughout the United Kingdom (U.K.).

The Top 20 Cancer Myths

The top 20 cancer myths believed by teenagers and young adults in the U.K., answered:

We are all born with the cancer gene.

False. Some people are born with genetic mutations but there needs to be a number of these within a cell before it becomes cancerous. Although a mutation at the start of your life can mean it is more likely statistically that a person will develop cancer during their lifetime which doctors call a "genetic predisposition" at the same time it doesn't always mean they will definitely be diagnosed with cancer.

You are never really cured of cancer.

False. If you have been in remission for 10 years then you are considered cured of cancer.

Mobile phones give you brain tumors.

False. There is currently no firm evidence that using a mobile phone will increase your risk of developing a brain tumor or any other type of cancer. There is also no evidence of an increase in cancer incidences of cancer in the bone or tissue in the hands from holding mobile phones while in use.

Living near electricity pylons causes cancer.

False. Currently there is insufficient evidence that magnetic fields from power lines have the capacity to cause cancer. This is not to suggest there is absolutely no possibility of a causal link between the two but research cannot yet scientifically link the two as cause and effect.

Skin color is a factor in getting cancer.

False. However having a fair complexion and skin that burns easily or does not tan can increase your risk of developing skin cancer.

Cancer makes your hair fall out.

False. It is chemotherapy treatment that can make your hair fall out, not the cancer itself. Chemotherapy is toxic and acts by killing cells that divide rapidly, one of the main properties of most cancer cells. This means that as well as killing the bad cells it also kills the good cells, which results in the most commonly known side effects of chemotherapy—hair loss.

Eating red meat gives you cancer.

False. Generally speaking red meat does not give you cancer, however eating high amounts of red or processed meat on a very regular basis can increase your risk. Bowel and stomach cancer are more common in people who eat lots of red and processed meat. Red meat includes all fresh, minced and frozen beef, pork, lamb, or veal. Processed meats have been preserved in some way other than freezing and include bacon, ham, salami, sausages, spam, corned beef, black pudding, pâté, and tinned meat. The way you cook meat may increase cancer risk. Certain chemicals are made when red and processed meats are cooked at high temperatures, such as on a barbeque. These chemicals can damage our cells, making them more likely to become cancerous.

If you have cancer when you're pregnant your baby will get it.

False. A barrier between the mother's and the baby's body blocks any cancer cells from entering the baby or its blood supply.

Keeping your mobile phone in your bra gives you breast cancer.

False. Currently, there is no firm evidence that keeping a mobile phone in your bra will increase your risk of developing breast cancer. However we would always recommend that it is more comfortable keeping your phone in your bag or in a pocket.

Getting kicked in the testicles gives you testicular cancer.

False. Although this will undoubtedly hurt, it doesn't cause cancer. Typically, testicular cancer produces a painless swelling of one testicle, a swelling which cannot be distinguished from the testicle itself by examination. Testicular cancer is the most common cancer in young men aged between 18 and 35 and because it can prove serious if neglected and left untreated, any lump in the scrotum that is new and abnormal should always be reported urgently to the doctor. Testicular cancer is often diagnosed while being examined for sports injuries.

If you don't inhale when you smoke you won't get cancer.

False. Smoking is a major risk factor for lung cancer, but also increases the risk of mouth cancer, pharyngeal cancer, and cancer of the larynx as smoke passes over these areas as it is breathed in. Smoking also increases the risk of cancer of the esophagus and stomach cancer. The amount you smoke, the age you started and the longer you keep on smoking, are all factors in your risk of getting cancer.

You can catch cancer from toilet seats.

False. Cancer cannot be transmitted through sitting on a toilet seat. Cancer is not contagious and cannot be caught from somebody else. However, the human papillomavirus (HPV virus), which is linked to cervical cancer, can be passed between people through sexual activity.

You can get cancer from eating colored Jelly Babies sweets.

False. All food colorings have to pass strict food regulations so it is unlikely that they can cause cancer. However, although strict food regulations such as those in U.K. and European Union (E.U.), and Australia pass these colors as safe for use with food, there is a growing minority who believe the effects of colorings have not been well enough researched and consider their use an unnecessary risk.

Being fat gives you cancer.

False. However, cancer experts estimate that maintaining a healthy bodyweight, making changes to our diet and taking regular physical activity could prevent about one in three deaths from cancer in the U.K. In the western world, many of us eat too much red and processed meat and not enough fresh fruit and vegetables. This type of diet is known to increase the risk of cancer. Drinking alcohol can also increase the risk of developing some types of cancer. Overweight or obese people have an increased risk of bowel cancer and pancreatic cancer and this could be because they tend to have higher insulin levels.

You can catch cancer from kissing.

False. You cannot catch cancer through kissing. Cancer is not contagious and cannot be caught from somebody else. However, the HPV virus which is linked to cervical cancer, can be passed between people through sexual activity.

You always die from cancer.

False. As with all cancers, if it is diagnosed quickly and treatment begins quickly, then it may be easier to treat.

You can get cancer from eating too much tomato ketchup.

False. In fact, there has been a lot of interest in whether eating certain foods might reduce the risk of certain types of cancer. There is some evidence that eating plenty of fruit and vegetables, such as tomatoes, can protect against cancer. Fruit and vegetables contain a wide variety of nutrients and are high in fiber and scientists are fairly sure that vitamins A and C and folate play an important role in protecting against cancer.

Only babies get leukemia.

False. Although leukemia is the most common childhood cancer, teenagers and adults are also diagnosed with it. Different cancers predominate at different ages in young people and leukemia is one of the most common in 13- to 18-year-olds.

Only old people get cancer.

False. It doesn't matter what age you are, we are all at risk of cancer. Every day in the U.K., six young people aged between 13 to 24 are diagnosed with cancer and the numbers are rising. However, it is true that most types of cancer become more common as we get older, as cells take a long time to develop and there has to be a number of changes to the genes within a cell before it turns into a cancer cell. The longer we live, the more time there is for genetic mistakes to happen in our cells.

Masturbation causes cancer.

False. Masturbation does not cause cancer to grow.

Chapter 4

Genes, Genetic Disorders, And Cancer

Have people ever said to you, "It's in your genes?" They were probably talking about a physical characteristic, personality trait, or talent that you share with other members of your family. We know that genes play an important role in shaping how we look and act and even whether we get sick. Now scientists are trying to use that knowledge in exciting new ways, such as preventing and treating health problems.

What Is A Gene?

To understand how genes (pronounced: jeens) work, let's review some biology basics. Most living organisms are made up of cells that contain a substance called deoxyribonucleic (pronounced: dee-ahk-see-rye-bow-noo-klee-ik) acid (DNA). DNA is wrapped together to form structures called chromosomes (pronounced: krow-muh-soams).

Most cells in the human body have 23 pairs of chromosomes, making a total of 46. Individual sperm and egg cells, however, have just 23 unpaired chromosomes. You received half of your chromosomes from your mother's egg and the other half from your father's sperm cell. A male child receives an X chromosome from his mother and a Y chromosome from his father; females get an X chromosome from each parent.

So where do genes come in? Genes are sections or segments of DNA that are carried on the chromosomes and determine specific human characteristics, such as height or hair color. Because

About This Chapter: "The Basics On Genes And Genetic Disorders," April 2009, reprinted with permission from www.kidshealth.org. This information was provided by KidsHealth®, one of the largest resources online for medically reviewed health information written for parents, kids, and teens. For more articles like this, visit www.KidsHealth.org, or www.TeensHealth.org. Copyright © 1995-2013 The Nemours Foundation. All rights reserved.

each parent gives you one chromosome in each pair, you have two of every gene (except for some of the genes on the X and Y chromosomes in boys because boys have only one of each).

Some characteristics come from a single gene, whereas others come from gene combinations. Because every person has about 25,000 per cell, there is an almost endless number of possible combinations.

Genes And Heredity

Heredity is the passing of genes from one generation to the next. You inherit your parents' genes. Heredity helps to make you the person you are today: short or tall, with black hair or blond, with green eyes or blue.

Can your genes determine whether you'll be a straight-A student or a great athlete? Heredity plays an important role, but your environment (including things like the foods you eat and the people you interact with) also influences your abilities and interests.

How Do Genes Work?

DNA contains four chemicals (adenine, thymine, cytosine, and guanine—called A, T, C, and G for short) that are strung in patterns on extremely thin, coiled strands in the cell. How thin? Cells are tiny—invisible to the naked eye—and each cell in your body contains about six feet of DNA thread, for a total of about three billion miles (if all your DNA threads were stretched out straight) of DNA inside you. The DNA patterns are the codes for manufacturing proteins, chemicals that enable the body to work and grow.

Genes hold the instructions for making protein products (like the enzymes to digest food or the pigment that gives your eyes their color). As your cells duplicate, they pass this genetic information to the new cells. Genes can be dominant or recessive. Dominant genes show their effect even if there is only one copy of that gene in the pair. For a person to have a recessive disease or characteristic, the person must have the gene on both chromosomes of the pair.

What Are Genetic Disorders?

Cells can sometimes contain changes or variants in the information in their genes. This is called gene mutation, and it often occurs when cells are aging or have been exposed to certain chemicals or radiation. Fortunately, cells usually recognize these mutations and repair them by themselves. Other times, however, they can cause illnesses, such as some types of cancer. And if the gene mutation exists in egg or sperm cells, children can inherit the mutated gene from their parents.

Researchers have identified more than 4,000 diseases that are caused by genetic variants. But having a genetic mutation that may cause disease doesn't always mean that a person will actually get that disease. Because you inherit a gene from each parent, having one disease gene usually does not cause any problems because the normal gene can allow your body to make the normal protein it needs.

On average, people probably carry from five to ten variant or disease genes in their cells. Problems arise when the disease gene is dominant or when the same recessive disease gene is present on both chromosomes in a pair. Problems can also occur when several variant genes interact with each other—or with the environment—to increase susceptibility to diseases.

If a person carries the dominant gene for a disease, he or she will usually have the disease and each of the person's children will have a one in two (50 percent) chance of inheriting the gene and getting the disease. Diseases caused by a dominant gene include achondroplasia (pronounced: ay-kon-druh-play-zhuh, a form of dwarfism), Marfan syndrome (a connective tissue disorder), and Huntington disease (a degenerative disease of the nervous system).

People who have one recessive gene for a disease are called carriers, and they don't usually have the disease because they have a normal gene of that pair that can do the job. When two carriers have a child together, however, the child has a one in four (25 percent) chance of getting the disease gene from both parents, which results in the child having the disease. Cystic fibrosis (a lung disease), sickle cell anemia (a blood disease), and Tay-Sachs disease (which causes nervous system problems) are caused by recessive disease genes from both parents coming together in a child.

Some recessive genetic variants are carried only on the X chromosome, which means that usually only guys can develop the disease because they have only one X chromosome. Girls have two X chromosomes, so they would need to inherit two copies of the recessive gene to get the disease. X-linked disorders include the bleeding disorder hemophilia (pronounced: hee-muh-fih-lee-uh) and color blindness.

Sometimes when an egg and sperm unite, the new cell gets too many or too few chromosomes. Most children born with Down syndrome, which is associated with mental retardation, have an extra chromosome number 21.

In some cases, people who are concerned that they might carry certain variant genes can have genetic testing so they can learn their children's risk of having a disease. Pregnant women can also have tests done to see if the fetus they are carrying might have certain genetic illnesses. Genetic testing usually involves taking a sample of someone's blood, skin, or amniotic fluid, and checking it for signs of genetic diseases or disorders.

Who Needs Genetic Testing For Cancer?

Some of your relatives have had cancer. And, you've heard that people with a family history of the disease may be more likely to get cancer.

So, should you consider genetic testing to find out if cancer runs in your family?

Here's what you need to know to make a more informed decision.

Most cancer cases aren't related to family history.

"Only about 5 to 10 percent of cancer cases are due to an inherited cause," says Karen Lu, M.D., co-medical director of the Clinical Cancer Genetics Program at MD Anderson Cancer Center. "Genetic testing is a powerful tool to identify those individuals who are at especially increased risk for developing certain cancers."

You can inherit abnormal genes from a parent. And, if you inherit one of these genes, you're much more likely to develop cancer—and at a younger age.

Breast, colorectal, ovarian, prostate, pancreatic, and endometrial cancers sometimes run in the family.

But most cancers are related to lifestyle choices like smoking, not exercising, and eating unhealthy foods.

Map your family's cancer history.

You can begin to gauge your risk for an inherited cancer by mapping your family's cancer history.

Start by downloading MD Anderson's family history form. [Available at http://www.mdanderson.org/publications/focused-on-health/issues/2010-november/ccg-genriskassqx-eng.pdf]. Then, speak with relatives to fill in as much information as possible.

Pay special attention to the cancer histories of first- and second-degree blood relatives. First-degree relatives include siblings, parents, and children. Second-degree relatives include grandparents, aunts, uncles, nieces, and nephews.

In general, people at risk for an inherited cancer have one or more first- or second-degree members who were diagnosed with:

- Cancer at a young age (before age 50)
- The same type of cancer
- Two or more different cancers in the same person
- A rare cancer, such as male breast cancer or sarcoma
- A BRCA1 or BRCA2 mutation

Discuss your family history with your doctor.

Does your family history raise some red flags? Use your completed form to talk to your doctor about your cancer risks.

Based on your family history, your doctor may refer you to a genetic counselor, who will review your family medical history, discuss the role of genetics in cancer, and perform a hereditary cancer risk assessment. This assessment covers:

- Your odds of having a genetic mutation
- An estimate of your cancer risks
- Personalized genetic testing recommendations
- Individualized cancer screening and prevention recommendations

Based on your cancer risk assessment, the genetic counselor may recommend genetic testing. This simply involves having blood drawn.

The best person to test is usually the person with cancer. "After we identify the mutation that caused cancer to occur, we can test first-degree relatives—mother, sisters, daughters—to see if they also carry it," Lu says.

Carefully weigh the pros and cons of testing.

One of the benefits of knowing if you have a genetic mutation is that you can work with your doctor to monitor and address your cancer risks. This can help prevent cancer or find it early, when it's most treatable.

But your decision won't just affect you. It will also impact your family since your test results may forecast their cancer risks, too.

Some people worry that their results will make it harder for them to get insurance coverage. But group plans are prohibited by law from using genetic information to discriminate against you.

No matter what you decide, remember: finding out that you have a gene mutation doesn't mean you'll definitely get cancer. And, learning that you don't have a gene mutation doesn't guarantee that you won't get cancer.

Source: "Who Needs Genetic Testing for Cancer?" by Laura Nathan-Garner, Focused on Health, www.mdanderson.org/focused, October 2011. © 2011 The University of Texas MD Anderson Cancer Center. All rights reserved. Reprinted with permission.

Changing Genes

Sometimes scientists alter genes on purpose. For many years, researchers have altered the genes in microbes and plants to produce offspring with special characteristics, such as an increased resistance to disease or pests, or the ability to grow in difficult environments. We call this genetic engineering.

Gene therapy is a promising new field of medical research. In gene therapy, researchers try to supply copies of healthy genes to cells with variant or missing genes so that the "good" genes will take over. Viruses are often used to carry the healthy genes into the targeted cells because many viruses can insert their own DNA into targeted cells.

But there are problems with gene therapy. Scientists haven't yet identified every gene in the human body or what each one does. Huge scientific efforts like The Human Genome (pronounced: jee-nome) Project and related projects have recently completed a map of the entire human genome (all of the genetic material on a living thing's chromosomes), but it will take many more years to find out what each gene does and how they interact with one another. For most diseases, scientists don't know if and how genes play a role. Plus, there are major difficulties inserting the normal genes into the proper cells without causing problems for the rest of the body.

There are also concerns that people might try changing genes for ethically troubling reasons, such as to make smarter or more athletic children. No one knows what the long-term effects of that kind of change would be.

Still, for many people who have genetic diseases, gene therapy holds the hope that they—or their children—will be able to live better, healthier lives.

Chapter 5

Cancer And The Environment

How could the environment be related to cancer?

Cancers are a diverse collection of diseases, each with a different clinical appearance, set of symptoms, and range of severity. What they have in common is the process occurring at the cellular level that brings these diseases about. Although this cellular process may not be the main concern among cancer patients and their families, it allows us to group cancers together, particularly when considering compounds in the environment that may be related to cancer.

All cancers are a result of a single type of cell, somewhere in the body, reproducing in a disordered way, usually at an abnormally fast pace. Knowing this helps us understand what kinds of environmental factors might be associated with cancer. Possibilities include:

- Chemicals known to damage DNA, which contains the information cells use to reproduce normally.

- Chemicals that alter how a cell regulates its own reproduction, which may have to do with its DNA or with cellular proteins that interact with DNA.

- Chemicals that induce epigenetic modifications. Epigenetic modifications are reversible, heritable changes that impact how genes are expressed without actually changing DNA. In particular, they may play a role in cancers thought to be associated with infectious agents.[1]

- Infectious agents (particularly viruses) that take over cellular functions and may rearrange pieces of DNA as part of their infectious process.

About This Chapter: From "Cancer and the Environment," © 2013 California Environmental Health Tracking Program (http://cehtp.org). All rights reserved. Reprinted with permission.

- Agents that harm the immune system. A person's immune system is believed to play a role in clearing the body of at least some types of cancerous cells, so damage to the immune system may encourage some forms of cancer.

Table 5.1 Possible Environmental Causes Of Cancer

Cancer Type	Reasons For Concern[2]
Breast	Breast cancer is the most commonly diagnosed cancer among women. Some breast cancers are known to respond to hormone levels in women's bodies, and a variety of persistent chemicals such as DDT, PCBs, and dioxin have the potential to alter hormone activities in people.
Lung And Bronchus	Lung cancer is the leading cause of cancer death in the United States. Occupational exposure to certain metals, polycyclic aromatic compounds, and vinyl chloride has been associated with lung cancer. Certain types of air pollution have also been associated with this disease.
Bladder	Occupational exposures to truck exhaust and compounds used in the textile and leather dye industries have been associated with bladder cancer.
Brain And Other Nervous System	Occupational exposures to radiation and a variety of metallic, petrochemical, and organic compounds have been associated with brain cancer. There is some concern that children may be at risk when their parents are exposed to these substances, particularly during pregnancy.
Thyroid	Increases in risk for thyroid cancer have been observed with exposure to ionizing radiation.
Non-Hodgkin Lymphoma	Rates of this disease have increased dramatically over the last few decades, although no reasons for this increase have yet been found.
Leukemia	Rates of various forms of leukemia are increasing among children, although the reasons for this are not known. Exposure to ionizing radiation, benzene, and some agricultural chemicals has been associated with increased risk.
Mesothelioma	Mesothelioma is a rare cancer affecting the linings of internal organs, most often the lungs. It is most often caused by exposure to asbestos.
Skin	Ultraviolet light (UV) radiation from prolonged sun exposure or tanning beds has been associated with this cancer. Exposures to environmental pollutants such as arsenic or dioxins may also contribute to increased risk.
Liver And Bile Duct	Exposures to environmental pollutants such as solvents and persistent organic compounds may contribute to increased risk of these cancers.
Kidney And Renal Pelvis	In addition to smoking and long-term use of certain pain medications, there is also concern that exposure to cadmium, arsenic, and disinfection by-products in drinking water may increase risk for these cancers.

Scientists have found at least one example for each of these scenarios, but it's generally agreed that there may be others yet to be observed. In its 2008–2009 report entitled *Reducing Environmental Cancer Risk*, the President's Cancer Panel notes that environmental sources of cancer have been largely underestimated and understudied, particularly in light of the growing incidence of a number of cancer types.

To what degree is cancer an environmental disease?

This question has received increasing attention among scientists, policy makers, and the public. It is not easy to answer for several reasons, the most prominent of which is that the majority of cancers take years, or even decades, to develop.

Scientists rarely have the opportunity to take a large number of people, measure the amount of a specific pollutant they are exposed to, and then follow them over time to see if they develop cancer.

There are two exceptions to this problem, however, and they form the foundation of much of what we do know about the environment and cancer:

- **Behavioral Risk Factors:** Behaviors such as cigarette smoking or diet frequently persist over many years, so it can be relatively simple for people to quantify exposures they have experienced, even decades after the fact.

- **Occupational Risk Factors:** People are frequently able to recall their work histories during the course of their lives, and in some cases records of the types and quantities of chemicals to which they may have been exposed have been kept.

In spite of how little we know, there is concern that environmental factors play a larger role in cancer than has previously been thought. Much of this concern stems from the fact that the incidence rates of a large variety of cancers have been increasing over the last several decades. Most traditional explanations for this increase fail to explain why this is happening. For example:

- Rates of alcohol and tobacco consumption, the behaviors most consistently linked to cancer, have been declining during the same period.

- It is unlikely that genetic susceptibility to cancer has changed at a rate rapid enough to account for the increase.

- Cancer rates have increased even among young and middle-aged people, so increased life expectancy cannot account for the shift.[2]

- Obesity has been increasing to alarming rates in the United States and abroad, and obesity may be related to some—but not all—of the cancer types for which rates have been increasing. Recent meta-analyses have linked increased body weight with esophageal cancer, thyroid, colon, and kidney cancers in men and with endometrial, gallbladder, and esophageal cancers in women.

Meanwhile, the number and quantities of compounds that could cause cancer—at least in theory—in the global environment have been increasing.

Table 5.2. Specific Environmental Causes of Concern

Environmental Factors Associated With Cancers	Description And Potential Sources
Arsenic[3,4]	A metal that is naturally occurring but becomes available to humans through industrial processes and mining. Exposure most commonly occurs through contaminated water, foods, or medications.
Benzene[5]	A chemical that is both synthetic (i.e., human-made) and from natural sources (i.e. emissions from volcanoes and forest fires). Commonly used in industries to make other chemicals and products, and is a component of crude oil, gasoline, and cigarette smoke. Exposure most commonly occurs through breathing contaminated air; gases from products (i.e., glues, paints, wax); or working in industries that make or use benzene.
DDT[5]	A synthetic insecticide that was banned for use in the U.S. in 1972, but remains persistent in the environment. Exposure most commonly occurs through eating contaminated foods, breathing contaminated air, or drinking contaminated water near landfills and waste sites.
Dioxin[5]	A synthetic chemical that is a byproduct of incineration and chemical manufacturing. Exposure most commonly occurs through eating contaminated foods (responsible for 90 percent of intake); living near contaminated sites; or working in paper mills, incinerators, or occupations that produce dioxins as a byproduct.
Ionizing Radiation[5]	Energy in the form of particles or rays that is emitted from radioactive material, high-voltage equipment, and nuclear reactions. Exposure most commonly occurs through low levels in the environment; working as a pilot, flight attendant, astronaut, nuclear power plant worker, or x-ray technician; or receiving an x-ray exam.
Metallic Compounds[5]	A group of chemical compounds that are metals, including lead, tungsten, and mercury. Exposure can occur through eating fish, from lead paint in older buildings, or through contaminated water passing through aging pipes.

Specific Environmental Concerns

Exposure to cigarette smoke, either through smoking or second-hand, is associated with a large number of cancers. Besides this, specific environmental concerns include those listed in Table 5.2.

For more information on toxic substances, including those listed, see the Agency for Toxic Substances and Disease Registry website at http://www.atsdr.cdc.gov/toxfaqs/index.asp.

Table 5.2. Specific Environmental Causes of Concern (*continued*)

Environmental Factors Associated With Cancers	Description And Potential Sources
Nitrates[6,7]	A group of nitrogen compounds; the greatest use of nitrates is as fertilizer. Exposure most commonly occurs through contaminated drinking water.
Organic Compounds[5]	A large group of chemical compounds that contain carbon, including benzene and DDT, and can be both synthetic and naturally forming. Exposure can occur in many ways including use of household chemicals, vehicle exhaust, and from pesticides.
Petrochemical Compounds[8]	A group of chemical compounds that are made from petroleum or natural gas. Exposure most commonly occurs through use of gasoline pumps, spilled oil on pavement, and chemicals used at home or work.
Polychlorinated Biphenyls (PCBs)[9]	A synthetic chemical that was used prior to 1977 in electrical equipment; manufacturing was stopped in the U.S. in 1977 due to health concerns. Exposure can occur through: use of old fluorescent lights and appliances made 30 or more years ago; eating contaminated food; breathing air or drinking water near contaminated waste sites; or working to repair, maintain, clean up, or dispose of products that contain PCBs (e.g., transformers, fluorescent lights, electrical devices.
Polycyclic Aromatic Compounds[5]	A group of chemicals formed from the incomplete burning of coal, oil and gas, garbage, or other organic materials like tobacco or charbroiled meat, emitted from volcanoes and forest fires. Exposure can occur through: working in industries such as coal-tar and asphalt production and incinerators; breathing air contaminated with cigarette smoke, wood smoke, or vehicle exhaust; eating grilled or contaminated foods; or drinking contaminated water.
Trihalomethanes[10]	Trihaloamines (THM) form when chlorine used to disinfect water supplies react with organic and inorganic material in water to form disinfection by products (DBPs). Exposure most commonly occurs through drinking water.
Vinyl Chloride[5]	A synthetic substance used in the production of certain plastics. Exposure most commonly occurs through breathing air that is contaminated from plastics industries, hazardous waste sites, and landfills; working in an industry that uses vinyl chloride; or drinking contaminated water.

References

1. Stein RA, Epigenetics—the link between Infectious Diseases and Cancer. *Journal of the American Medical Association,* April 13, 2011. Vol. 305, No. 14. 1484–1485.

2. Irigaray P, Newby JA, Clapp R, Hardell L, Howard V, Montagnier L, Epstein S, Belpomme D. Lifestyle-related factors and environmental agents causing cancer: An overview. *Biomedicine & Pharmacotherapy.* 2007. 61;640–658.

3. Lewis DR, Southwich JW, Ouellet-Hellstrom R, Rench J, and Calderon RL. Drinking Water Arsenic in Utah: A Cohort Mortality Study. *Environmental Health Perspectives.* 1999. 107:359–365

4. Ferreccio C, González C, Milosavjlevic V, Marshall G, Sancha AM, Smith AH. Lung cancer and arsenic concentrations in drinking water in Chile. *Epidemiology.* 2000 Nov;11(6):673–9

5. US Department of Health and Human Services, National Cancer Institute and the National Institute of Environmental Health Sciences. *Cancer and the Environment.* NIH Publication No. 03–2039. 2003. http://www.niehs.nih.gov/health/docs/canceren-viro.pdf

6. Barrett JH, Parslow RC, McKinney PA, Law GR, and Forman D. Nitrate in Drinking Water and the Incidence of Gastric, Esophageal, and Brain Cancer in Yorkshire, England. *Cancer Causes Control.* 1998. 9(2):153–9.

7. Gulis G, Czomployova M, Cerhan JR. An Ecologic Study of Nitrate in Municipal Drinking Water and Cancer Incidence in Trnava District, Slovakia. *Environ Res.* 2002. 88(3):182–7.

8. Agency for Toxic Substances and Disease Registry (ATSDR). 1999. *Toxicological Profile for total petroleum hydrocarbons (TPH).* Atlanta, GA: U.S. Department of Health and Human Services, Public Health Service. http://www.atsdr.cdc.gov/tfacts123.html

9. Agency for Toxic Substances and Disease Registry (ATSDR). 2000. *Toxicological Profile for Polychlorinated Biphenyls (PCBs).* Atlanta, GA: U.S. Department of Health and Human Services, Public Health Service. http://www.atsdr.cdc.gov/tfacts17.pdf.

10. King WD, Marrett LD. Case-control study of bladder cancer and chlorination byproducts in treated water (Ontario, Canada). *Cancer Causes Control.* 1996. 7(6):596–604.

Chapter 6

Tanning And Cancer Risk

Basic Information About Skin Cancer

Skin cancer is the most common form of cancer in the United States. The two most common types of skin cancer—basal cell and squamous cell carcinomas—are highly curable. However, melanoma, the third most common skin cancer, is more dangerous. About 65 percent to 90 percent of melanomas are caused by exposure to ultraviolet (UV) light.

Ultraviolet (UV) Light

Ultraviolet (UV) rays are an invisible kind of radiation that comes from the sun, tanning beds, and sunlamps. UV rays can penetrate and change skin cells.

The three types of UV rays are ultraviolet A (UVA), ultraviolet B (UVB), and ultraviolet C (UVC). They differ in the following ways:

- UVA is the most common kind of sunlight at the earth's surface, and reaches beyond the top layer of human skin. Scientists believe that UVA rays can damage connective tissue and increase a person's risk of skin cancer.

- Most UVB rays are absorbed by the ozone layer, so they are less common at the earth's surface than UVA rays. UVB rays don't reach as far into the skin as UVA rays, but they can still be damaging.

About This Chapter: Text in this chapter is from the following documents produced by the Centers for Disease Control and Prevention (CDC): "Basic Information About Skin Cancer" and "Prevention," April 23, 2013, "Risk Factors," March 27, 2013, and "Indoor Tanning," March 21, 2013.

- UVC rays are very dangerous, but they are absorbed by the ozone layer and do not reach the ground.

Too much exposure to UV rays can change skin texture, cause the skin to age prematurely, and can lead to skin cancer. UV rays also have been linked to eye conditions such as cataracts.

Risk Factors

People with certain risk factors are more likely than others to develop skin cancer. Risk factors vary for different types of skin cancer, but some general risk factors include having the following:

- A lighter natural skin color
- Family history of skin cancer
- A personal history of skin cancer
- Exposure to the sun through work and play
- A history of sunburns early in life
- A history of indoor tanning
- Skin that burns, freckles, reddens easily, or becomes painful in the sun
- Blue or green eyes
- Blond or red hair
- Certain types and a large number of moles

The UV Index

The National Weather Service and the Environmental Protection Agency developed the UV Index to forecast the risk of overexposure to ultraviolet rays at http://www.epa.gov/sunwise/uvindex.html. It lets you know how much caution you should take when working, playing, or exercising outdoors.

The UV Index predicts exposure levels on a 1 to 15 scale. Higher levels indicate a higher risk of overexposure. Calculated on a next-day basis for dozens of cities across the United States, the UV Index takes into account clouds and other local conditions that affect the amount of UV rays reaching the ground.

Source: "Basic Information About Skin Cancer," CDC, April 23, 2013.

Sunscreen And SPF

The sun's UV rays can damage your skin in as little as 15 minutes. Put on sunscreen before you go outside, even on slightly cloudy or cool days. Don't forget to put a thick layer on all parts of exposed skin. Get help for hard-to-reach places like your back.

How Sunscreen Works: Most sun protection products work by absorbing, reflecting, or scattering sunlight. They contain chemicals that interact with the skin to protect it from UV rays. All products do not have the same ingredients; if your skin reacts badly to one product, try another one or call a doctor.

SPF: Sunscreens are assigned a sun protection factor (SPF) number that rates their effectiveness in blocking UV rays. Higher numbers indicate more protection. You should use a sunscreen with at least SPF 15.

Reapplication: Sunscreen wears off. Put it on again if you stay out in the sun for more than two hours, and after you swim or do things that make you sweat.

Expiration Date: Check the sunscreen's expiration date. Sunscreen without an expiration date has a shelf life of no more than three years, but its shelf life is shorter if it has been exposed to high temperatures.

Cosmetics: Some make-up and lip balms contain some of the same chemicals used in sunscreens. If they do not have at least SPF 15, don't use them by themselves.

Source: "Prevention," CDC, April 23, 2013.

Tanning And Burning

UV rays come from the sun or from indoor tanning (using a tanning bed, booth, or sunlamp to get tan). When UV rays reach the skin's inner layer, the skin makes more melanin. Melanin is the pigment that colors the skin. It moves toward the outer layers of the skin and becomes visible as a tan.

A tan does not indicate good health. A tan is a response to injury, because skin cells signal that they have been hurt by UV rays by producing more pigment.

People burn or tan depending on their skin type, the time of year, and how long they are exposed to UV rays. The six types of skin, based on how likely it is to tan or burn, are as follows:

- **Type I:** Always burns, never tans, sensitive to UV exposure

- **Type II:** Burns easily, tans minimally

- **Type III:** Burns moderately, tans gradually to light brown

- **Type IV:** Burns minimally, always tans well to moderately brown
- **Type V:** Rarely burns, tans profusely to dark
- **Type VI:** Never burns, deeply pigmented, least sensitive

Although everyone's skin can be damaged by UV exposure, people with skin types I and II are at the highest risk.

Prevention

Protection from ultraviolet radiation is important all year round, not just during the summer or at the beach. UV rays from the sun can reach you on cloudy and hazy days, as well as bright and sunny days. UV rays also reflect off of surfaces like water, cement, sand, and snow. Indoor tanning (using a tanning bed, booth, or sunlamp to get tan) exposes users to UV radiation.

The hours between 10 a.m. and 4 p.m. daylight savings time (9 a.m. to 3 p.m. standard time) are the most hazardous for UV exposure outdoors in the continental United States. UV rays from sunlight are the greatest during the late spring and early summer in North America.

The Centers for Disease Control and Prevention (CDC) recommends the following easy options for protection from UV radiation:

- Seek shade, especially during midday hours.
- Wear clothing to protect exposed skin.
- Wear a hat with a wide brim to shade the face, head, ears, and neck.
- Wear sunglasses that wrap around and block as close to 100 percent of both UVA and UVB rays as possible.
- Use sunscreen with sun protective factor (SPF) 15 or higher, and both UVA and UVB protection.
- Avoid indoor tanning.

Shade

You can reduce your risk of skin damage and skin cancer by seeking shade under an umbrella, tree, or other shelter before you need relief from the sun. Your best bet to protect your skin is to use sunscreen or wear protective clothing when you're outside—even when you're in the shade.

Clothing

Loose-fitting long-sleeved shirts and long pants made from tightly woven fabric offer the best protection from the sun's UV rays. A wet T-shirt offers much less UV protection than a dry one. Darker colors may offer more protection than lighter colors.

If wearing this type of clothing isn't practical, at least try to wear a T-shirt or a beach cover-up. Keep in mind that a typical T-shirt has an SPF rating lower than 15, so use other types of protection as well.

Hats

For the most protection, wear a hat with a brim all the way around that shades your face, ears, and the back of your neck. A tightly woven fabric, such as canvas, works best to protect your skin from UV rays. Avoid straw hats with holes that let sunlight through. A darker hat may offer more UV protection.

If you wear a baseball cap, you should also protect your ears and the back of your neck by wearing clothing that covers those areas, using sunscreen with at least SPF 15, or by staying in the shade.

Sunglasses

Sunglasses protect your eyes from UV rays and reduce the risk of cataracts. They also protect the tender skin around your eyes from sun exposure.

Sunglasses that block both UVA and UVB rays offer the best protection. Most sunglasses sold in the United States, regardless of cost, meet this standard. Wrap-around sunglasses work best because they block UV rays from sneaking in from the side.

Avoid Indoor Tanning

Using a tanning bed, booth, or sunlamp to get tan is called "indoor tanning." Indoor tanning has been linked with skin cancers including melanoma (the deadliest type of skin cancer), squamous cell carcinoma, and cancers of the eye (ocular melanoma).

Indoor Tanning

Dangers Of Indoor Tanning

Indoor tanning exposes users to both UV-A and UV-B rays, which damage the skin and can lead to cancer. Using a tanning bed is particularly dangerous for younger users;

people who begin tanning younger than age 35 have a 75 percent higher risk of melanoma. Using tanning beds also increases the risk of wrinkles and eye damage, and changes skin texture.

Myths About Indoor Tanning

"Tanning indoors is safer than tanning in the sun."

Indoor tanning and tanning outside are both dangerous. Although tanning beds operate on a timer, the exposure to ultraviolet (UV) rays can vary based on the age and type of light bulbs. You can still get a burn from tanning indoors, and even a tan indicates damage to your skin.

Congressional Report Exposes Tanning Industry's Misleading Message To Teens

A new report released by leaders of the House Committee on Energy and Commerce reveals that tanning salons are routinely not providing accurate information about skin cancer and other risks to teens seeking their services. The alarming results show that the vast majority of tanning salons contacted by Committee investigators provided false information about the serious risks of indoor tanning and made erroneous claims about the health benefits that indoor tanning provides.

Committee investigators representing themselves as fair-skinned teenage girls contacted 300 tanning salons nationwide, including at least three in each state and the District of Columbia. The investigators asked each salon a series of questions about its policies and the risks and benefits of tanning. Committee investigators also reviewed the print and online advertising of tanning salons.

Specifically, Committee investigators found:

- **Nearly all salons denied the known risks of indoor tanning.** When asked whether tanning posed any health risks for fair-skinned teenage girls, 90 percent of the salons stated that indoor tanning did not pose a health risk. When asked about the specific risk of skin cancer, over half (51 percent) of the salons denied that indoor tanning would increase a fair-skinned teenager's risk of developing skin cancer. Salons described the suggestion of a link between indoor tanning and skin cancer as "a big myth," "rumor," and "hype."

- **Four out of five salons falsely claimed that indoor tanning is beneficial to a young person's health.** Four out of five (78 percent) of the tanning salons claimed that indoor tanning would be beneficial to the health of a fair-skinned teenage girl. Several salons even said that tanning would prevent cancer. Other health benefits claimed by tanning salons included vitamin D production, treatment of depression and low self-esteem,

"I can use a tanning bed to get a base tan, which will protect me from getting a sunburn."

A tan is a response to injury: Skin cells respond to damage from UV rays by producing more pigment. The best way to protect your skin from the sun is by using these tips for skin cancer prevention.

"Indoor tanning is a safe way to get vitamin D, which prevents many health problems."

Vitamin D is important for bone health, but studies showing links between vitamin D and other health conditions are inconsistent. Although it is important to get enough vitamin D,

prevention of and treatment for arthritis, weight loss, prevention of osteoporosis, reduction of cellulite, "boost[ing] the immune system," sleeping better, treating lupus, and improving symptoms of fibromyalgia.

- **Salons used many approaches to minimize the health risks of indoor tanning.** During their calls, Committee investigators representing themselves as fair-skinned teenage girls were told that young people are not at risk for developing skin cancer; that rising rates of skin cancer are linked to increased use of sunscreen; that government regulators had certified the safety of indoor tanning; and that "it's got to be safe, or else they wouldn't let us do it." Salons also frequently referred the investigators to industry websites that downplay indoor tanning's health risks and tout the practice's alleged health benefits.

- **Tanning salons fail to follow FDA recommendations on tanning frequency.** The U.S. Food and Drug Administration recommends that indoor tanning be limited to no more than three visits in the first week. Despite this recommendation, three quarters of tanning salons reported that they would permit first-time customers to tan daily; several salon employees volunteered that their salons did not even require 24-hour intervals between tanning sessions.

- **Tanning salons target teenage girls in their advertisements.** The print and online advertising for tanning salons frequently target teenage and college-aged girls with student discounts and "prom," "homecoming," and "back-to-school" specials. These youth-oriented specials often feature "unlimited" tanning packages, allowing frequent—even daily—tanning, despite research showing that frequent indoor tanning significantly increases the likelihood that a woman will develop melanoma, the deadliest form of skin cancer, before she reaches 30 years of age.

Source: Excerpted from "Congressional Report Exposes Tanning Industry's Misleading Message to Teens," February 1, 2012. © Skin Cancer Foundation (www.skincancer.org). All rights reserved. Reprinted with permission.

the safest way is through diet or supplements. Tanning harms your skin, and the amount of time spent tanning to get enough vitamin D varies from person to person.

Indoor Tanning Policies

Indoor tanning is restricted in some areas, especially for minors.

United States

- California and Vermont have banned the use of tanning beds by minors.

- Some local jurisdictions also have banned the use of tanning beds by minors.

International

- Brazil and one state in Australia (New South Wales) have banned the use of tanning beds.

- The United Kingdom, Germany, Scotland, France, several Australian states, and several Canadian provinces have banned indoor tanning for people younger than age 18.

It's A Fact!

According to the 2011 Youth Risk Behavior Surveillance System, the following proportions of youth report indoor tanning:

- 13 percent of all high school students
- 32 percent of girls in the 12th grade
- 21 percent of high school girls
- 29 percent of white high school girls

According to the 2010 National Health Interview Survey, indoor tanners tended to be young, non-Hispanic white women.

Healthy People 2020 Goals For Indoor Tanning

Healthy People provides science-based, 10-year national objectives for improving the health of all Americans. Healthy People 2020 has 20 cancer objectives, including the following:

- Reduce the proportion of adolescents in grades 9 through 12 who report using artificial sources of ultraviolet light for tanning to 14 percent.

- Reduce the proportion of adults aged 18 years and older who report using artificial sources of ultraviolet light for tanning to 13.7 percent.

Source: CDC, March 21, 2013.

Chapter 7

Is Some Sun Good?

Vitamin D

The one health benefit that sunlight has on human skin is the production of vitamin D. Unfortunately, the ultraviolet rays that stimulate vitamin D production (UVB rays) are the same ones that cause sunburn and skin cancer.

There isn't very much vitamin D in the typical American's diet. Some is present in oily fish (such as salmon, mackerel, sardines), milk, and fortified cereal or orange juice, but dietary sources alone are usually not sufficient for a healthy blood level without the addition of substantial sun exposure or a vitamin supplement.

Vitamin D deficiency can cause rickets in children, and osteoporosis in adults. An increased risk of other ills, such as cancer of the colon, breast, or prostate, as well as multiple sclerosis and type 1 diabetes might be linked to vitamin D deficiency. More research is needed before all of these associations can be considered certain but in the meantime it seems reasonable for everyone to take prudent measures to maintain an adequate blood level of vitamin D.

During summer months, particularly in the southern latitudes, some individuals acquire enough sun exposure to achieve an adequate vitamin D level. However, while sun exposure is an effective source of vitamin D, it can simultaneously increase the risk of skin cancer. When sunscreen is applied to the skin, it not only reduces sun damage, but unfortunately it also blocks vitamin D production.

About This Chapter: This information is reprinted with permission from Sun Safety for Kids, © 2013. All rights reserved. For additional information, visit www.sunsafetyforkids.org.

Darkly pigmented skin, advanced age, and low UV index (for example, winter months in northern latitudes) are some of the factors that decrease the amount of vitamin D produced by the skin in response to sun exposure. Because of the dual impact of the sun's UV rays (skin cancer induction and vitamin D production) those with the lightest skin pigment are at the highest risk of sun damage resulting in skin cancer, while people with darker skin pigment are at lower risk of skin cancer but higher risk for vitamin D deficiency.

Some authorities recommend routine limited or "sensible" sun exposure for vitamin D. However, too many variables affect the amount of exposure time needed (for example, season, time of day, weather conditions, skin color, age) making it impossible to give a simple recommendation such as "[X] minutes of sun per day" that would be assured to provide sufficient vitamin D for all people. This introduces the risk that people will unintentionally over-expose (fall asleep while sunning) and increase their risk of skin cancer in the process.

Sun Safety for Kids agrees with the American Academy of Dermatology which "does not recommend getting vitamin D from sun exposure (natural) or indoor tanning (artificial) because ultraviolet (UV) radiation from the sun and tanning beds can lead to the development of skin cancer."

The amount of Vitamin D in food or in a supplement is commonly listed in international units (IU). Evidence is still emerging to determine the ideal safe and effective amount of vitamin D that average healthy people should ingest. At present, the National Institutes of Health recommends an intake of 600 IU per day for Americans 1 to 70 years of age. Some experts

---

Quick Tip

Vitamin D Blood Test

A simple blood test called "25-hydroxy vitamin D" measures circulating vitamin D and provides a fair assessment of the body's vitamin D status. The NIH recommends that the level should be 21 nanograms/milliliter (ng/ml) or higher, but some experts suggest that blood levels in the range of 30 to 50 ng/ml are preferred. There is no evidence that levels above 50 provide any added benefit and vitamin D toxicity becomes a concern with higher levels. Levels tend to fluctuate with the seasons (lower in winter/higher in summer) due to incidental sun exposure. A doctor might order the blood test to help in determining the amount of vitamin D supplementation that will provide optimum vitamin D status year round.

Source: Sun Safety for Kids, 2013.

recommend a higher intake, in the range of 1,000 to 2,000 IU/day but the NIH warns that intakes in excess of 4,000 IU/day might lead to vitamin D toxicity. The NIH also discourages intentional sun exposure as a source of vitamin D, saying "it is prudent to limit exposure of skin to sunlight."

Because vitamin D is fat soluble, vitamin D supplements are most effective if taken with food.

The directors of Sun Safety for Kids believe that optimum health will be achieved if people practice careful sun protection year round and compensate by ingesting a sufficient daily amount of vitamin D.

Chapter 8

Cancer Risks Associated With Smoking And Other Tobacco Use

This chapter contains highlights from the 2012 Surgeon General's report on tobacco use among youth and teens ages 12 through 17 and young adults ages 18 through 25.

The Problem

Today's teens and young adults can access information on millions of subjects almost instantly. But many of the same media that warn of the dangers of tobacco use also carry messages that smoking is cool—edgy—adult. That's one reason nearly 4,000 kids under age18 try their first cigarette every day. That's almost 1.5 million youth a year.

In fact, nearly nine out of ten smokers start smoking by age 18, and 99 percent start by age 26.

On any given day, more than 2,500 youth and young adults who have been occasional smokers will become regular smokers. And at least a third of these replacement smokers will die early from smoking.

The percentage of youth who smoke went down every year between 1997 and 2003.

But since then, the decrease in teen smoking has slowed and the use of some forms of tobacco by youth has leveled out. Today, one out of four high school seniors and one out of three young adults under age 26 are smokers.

About This Chapter: Text is excerpted from "Preventing Tobacco Use Among Youth And Young Adults: We Can Make the Next Generation Tobacco Free," from the U.S. Surgeon General's report, and published by the Centers for Disease Control and Prevention (CDC)'s Office on Smoking and Health, 2012.

Smoking Causes Disease And Death

People who smoke don't have to wait for tobacco use to damage their health. There are more than 7,000 chemicals and chemical compounds in cigarette smoke, many of which are toxic. These chemicals can cause immediate damage to the human body. Even young adults under age 30 who started smoking in their teens and early twenties can develop smoking-related health problems, such as the following:

- Early cardiovascular disease
- Smaller lungs that don't function normally
- Wheezing that can lead to a diagnosis of asthma
- DNA damage that can cause cancer almost anywhere in the body

On average, lifelong smokers get sicker and die younger than nonsmokers. These smokers die an average of 13 years sooner.

Source: Surgeon General's Report, 2012.

The Causes

Young people start using tobacco for many reasons. These are some of the most important:

The Tobacco Industry

Fewer adults are smoking today, both because many have quit and because about half of long-term smokers die from diseases caused by their tobacco use. So, cigarette companies look to young people as replacement smokers. They use a variety of marketing strategies to encourage new consumers to try their products, and to continue using them.

Susceptibility Of Youth And Young Adults

Adolescence and young adulthood are the times when people are most susceptible to starting tobacco use. Young people are more vulnerable and more influenced by marketing than adults. They are also more willing to take risks, even with their health. When smoking is portrayed as a social norm among others who are seen as cool, sophisticated, rebellious, or fun loving, teens often respond by copying the behavior and trying cigarettes themselves. If their friends smoke, or their siblings smoke, they are even more likely to smoke themselves.

And young people are sensitive to nicotine. The younger they are when they start using tobacco, the more likely they are to become addicted to nicotine and the more heavily addicted they will become.

Young people sometimes believe nothing can hurt them. Facts about health problems that could happen in middle age—or even right away—may mean little to them now. Many teens and young adults don't realize how addictive nicotine is. Some may have a tough time making healthy choices or sorting out tobacco myths from facts. Others may want to fit in with a group or seem older, edgier, or more socially grounded. And images that encourage tobacco use are everywhere—from the Internet to the movies to big, bright advertisements at convenience stores. All of these factors make youth a prime market for tobacco products.

Social Norms

Many norms in our society influence young people to try tobacco products. People smoke in public in half of U.S. states because there are no comprehensive smoke-free laws that prohibit smoking at work sites, restaurants, and bars. Even states that prohibit smoking inside public buildings often have outdoor smoking areas, some near schools and day care centers. Tobacco use is prominent in mass media, including in movies, social media, video games, and glossy magazines. And tobacco advertising both inside and outside retail stores is often the largest, most visible advertising for any product.

Tobacco Fact

If young people don't start using tobacco by age 26, they almost certainly will never start.

Source: Surgeon General's Report, 2012.

Smoking And Health: They Just Don't Mix

It's well known that smoking is bad for your health and causes many serious diseases later in life. In fact, one out of three adolescents who continues to smoke regularly will die prematurely from cigarette smoking. But did you know that smoking can also harm young smokers' health right away?

Early Smoking Can Cause Heart Disease

New research shows that smoking during adolescence and young adulthood causes early damage to the abdominal aorta, the large artery that carries oxygen-rich blood from the heart through the abdomen to major organs. Even young adults who have only been smoking for a few years can show signs of narrowing of this large artery. When a person breathes tobacco smoke, it causes immediate damage to blood vessels throughout the body.

Secondhand Smoke And Cancer

- Secondhand smoke (also called environmental tobacco smoke, involuntary smoke, and passive smoke) is the smoke given off by a burning tobacco product and the smoke exhaled by a smoker.
- At least 69 chemicals in secondhand smoke are known to cause cancer.
- Secondhand smoke causes lung cancer in nonsmokers.
- Secondhand smoke has also been associated with heart disease in adults and sudden infant death syndrome, ear infections, and asthma attacks in children.
- There is no safe level of exposure to secondhand smoke.

Source: Excerpted from "Secondhand Smoke and Cancer," National Cancer Institute, January 2011.

Repeatedly breathing tobacco smoke can cause a mixture of scar tissue and fats to build up inside blood vessels. This plaque makes blood vessels narrow and limits blood flow.

Early Smoking Can Harm Lungs Now

Young people are still growing. Their lungs don't reach full size until late teens for girls and after age 20 for boys. Adults who smoked during adolescence can have lungs that never grow to their potential size and never perform at full capacity.

The lungs of young smokers don't perform as well as those of nonsmokers. Because their lungs don't work as well, they are short of breath and may have more trouble participating in sports and other physical activities. Even though people who stop smoking will improve their health dramatically, early lung damage doesn't go away completely in most cases.

Why is early smoking so harmful?

People who start smoking as young teens are more likely to do the following:

- Get addicted to nicotine
- Become lifetime smokers
- Get diseases caused by tobacco use
- Die from a disease caused by tobacco use

Source: Surgeon General's Report, 2012.

Smoking Can Lead To Cancer

Tobacco smoke contains about 70 chemicals that can cause cancer. It's no surprise, then, that smoking causes about one in three of all cancer deaths in the United States. And it can cause cancer almost anywhere in the body by damaging DNA.

Young Tobacco Users

This is how many teens and young adults use tobacco today:

- Three million high school students and 600,000 middle school students smoke cigarettes.
- One in three young adults smokes cigarettes.
- One in four high school seniors smokes cigarettes.
- One in five male high school seniors smokes cigars and one in ten uses smokeless tobacco.
- Many young people use more than one type of tobacco. Among those who use tobacco, more than half of high school males and nearly a third of high school females use more than one tobacco product. These products include cigarettes, cigars, and smokeless tobacco, such as chew and snus, a dry snuff in a small teabag-like sachet.

Source: Surgeon General's Report, 2012.

Youth: A Great Time To Quit

The good news: Smokers who quit before age 30 will undo much of the health damage caused by tobacco use.

Why Is It So Hard To Quit?

Tobacco users often get hooked on nicotine—the drug in cigarettes, cigars, and smokeless tobacco (snuff and chewing tobacco). Many teens and young adults plan to quit using tobacco after a few years but find out too late how powerfully addictive nicotine can be. Like heroin and cocaine, nicotine acts on the brain and creates feelings of pleasure or satisfaction. Young brains are still developing. That may be one reason many teens feel dependent on tobacco after using it for only a short time.

Quitting isn't easy, but it can be done.

Better yet—don't start!

Not starting is even better than quitting. Learn what risk factors to look for and how to help yourself, your friends, or the young people in your life stay tobacco. Their health depends on it.

Pro Athlete On Why He Quit Using Smokeless Tobacco

After major league Hall of Famer Tony Gwynne of the San Diego Padres was diagnosed with parotid cancer, or cancer of the salivary gland, Washington Nationals' pitcher Stephen Strasburg announced his decision to give up smokeless tobacco, or "dip." Gwynne was Strasburg's hero growing up—and he made a conscious decision to copy his hero's every move as an aspiring professional baseball player, even the dip habit.

Just like cigarettes, smokeless tobacco contains nicotine, a highly addictive substance. Whether you smoke or chew it, tobacco has been proven to cause cancer.

Use of dip can lead to mouth cancer affecting the lips and gums, along with glands called the parotid glands, which pump saliva into your mouth. Juices produced from the dip contain heavy metals that, with repeated use, may lead to esophageal and pancreatic cancer—two very aggressive forms of the disease. Treatment can require several surgeries that leave the face and jaw disfigured, and in the most serious cases, it may even require removal of the jaw.

Sounds pretty scary, but not everyone is thinking of the consequences. The biggest appeal for young people to take up the habit is often through sports, kind of ironic since dip is definitely not healthy or good for athletic performance.

Strasburg's announcement that he wants to give quit the habit may help change this unhealthy part of baseball culture. He doesn't want young people who may admire his playing skills to think that this addictive habit has anything to do with his game. Strasburg admits that quitting is tough, and is taking things one step at a time. Now it's Major League Baseball's turn. Despite the fact that chewing tobacco has already been banned in Little League, high school, and college play, the MLB isn't banning use of dip, yet.

Sometimes, it takes a hero to throw the first pitch and help people understand that winners don't dip.

Source: From "With Announcement On Giving Up 'Dip,' Washington Nationals' Stephen Strasburg's Pitches Hit Home," National Institute on Drug Abuse (http://teens.drugabuse.gov/blog/announcement-giving-up-dip/), June 4, 2011.

Chapter 9

Safer Grilling To Reduce Cancer Risk

Warm weather. Family gatherings. Independence Day. Some things just call for a barbecue.

But before you fire up, beware.

Convincing research shows that many meats traditionally served at barbecues may increase your risk for colorectal cancer. And, even some "safer" meats can expose you to cancer-causing agents if they're cooked improperly.

Luckily, you don't have to cancel your grilling plans altogether. Make these changes at your next barbecue to keep your health from going up in flames.

1. Avoid Processed Meats

Skip processed meats like bacon, ham, pastrami, salami, sausage, hot dogs, and pepperoni.

Cancer-causing substances form when these meats are preserved, says the American Institute for Cancer Research. And, eating these meats can damage your DNA, upping your colorectal cancer risk.

2. Limit Red Meat

Eating too much red meat like pork, lamb, and beef (including hamburgers) can raise a person's cancer risk. Do your health a favor by grilling skinless chicken breasts and fish instead.

Insist on red meat? Curb your risk by limiting yourself to three, six-ounce (cooked) servings per week. One serving is the size of two decks of cards.

About This Chapter: "Healthier Ways to Grill Meat," by Laura Nathan-Garner, Focused on Health, www.mdanderson .org/focused, June 2011. © 2011 The University of Texas MD Anderson Cancer Center. All rights reserved. Reprinted with permission.

3. Don't Char Or Burn Meat, Poultry, Or Fish

The color black isn't chic at a barbecue. That's because meat, poultry, or fish that's charred or burned is covered with heterocyclic amines (HCAs). And, HCAs can damage your genes, raising your risk for stomach and colorectal cancers.

To keep HCAs off your guest list:

- **Stick With Fish:** Fish contains less fat and cooks faster than meat and poultry.

- **Lightly Oil The Grill:** This keeps charred materials from sticking to your food.

- **Pre-Cook Food:** Cook meat, poultry, or fish in the microwave or oven for two to five minutes, then finish them on the grill. Less grill time means less exposure to cancer-causing chemicals.

- **Lower The Temperature:** For a charcoal grill, spread the coals thin or prop the grill rack on bricks. This reduces the heat by increasing the distance between your food and the coals. And, use barbecue briquettes and hardwood products, such as hickory and maple. These burn at lower temperatures than softwood (pine) chips.

- **Scrub The Grill:** Cleaning the grill after each use prevents harmful chemicals from building up and transferring to your food at your next barbecue.

4. Use A Marinade

Meat, poultry and fish taste better when marinated in vinegar, lemon juice, seasonings, and herbs such as mint, rosemary, tarragon, or sage. But that's not the only reason marinade is a must.

Marinating meat also can reduce HCA formation. Just 30 minutes can help.

5. Trim The Fat

Cancer-causing polycyclic aromatic hydrocarbons (PAHs) form in the smoke when fat from meat, poultry, or fish drips onto the heat source, then the smoke coats your food.

Curb exposure to PAHs by trimming fat from meat before grilling. Or, choose cuts labeled "lean."

6. Showcase Fruits And Veggies

Don't make your barbecue a meat-only affair. Grilling your favorite fruits and veggies is a great way to load up on vitamins and nutrients that help your body fight off diseases like cancer.

To maximize your fruits' and veggies' flavor and nutrients:

- Add a dash of pepper, salt, and vinegar.

- Don't peel veggies—not even corn-on-the-cob. The peels provide more nutrients and a smokier flavor—and keep veggies from drying out.

- Sprinkle cinnamon or honey over fruit before grilling.

For some grilling fans, these changes might be a lot to stomach. But remember, giving your barbecue a healthy makeover may help ensure you continue to enjoy grilling for many summers to come.

Chapter 10

Obesity And Cancer Risk

Evidence For A Link Between Cancer And Obesity And Overweight

Considerable evidence suggests that obesity and overweight play an important role in cancer. Obesity and overweight have been clearly associated with increased risks for kidney cancer in both men and women (two-fold increased relative risk), and in women, endometrial cancer (one and a half-fold relative risk) and postmenopausal breast cancer (two-fold relative risk).

Building evidence suggests that obesity and overweight also are associated with an increased risk of colorectal cancer, gallbladder cancer, and perhaps more modestly, the risk of thyroid cancer in women. For colorectal cancer, the effect of obesity and overweight on risk may be due in part to low physical activity, as consistent evidence exists for a strong protective effect of physical activity against developing colorectal cancer.

Recent studies suggest that obesity and overweight may also play a role in the increasing incidence of some types of esophageal cancer, possibly through obesity's association with gastric reflux. For prostate cancer risk, inconsistent findings from studies evaluating obesity may result from limitations in the measurement of obesity, as more consistent results have come from recent studies of biological factors that are more directly associated with specific aspects of body composition (e.g., total fat).

For other types of cancer, in general, too few studies have been conducted to draw conclusions about the relationship between obesity and risk of disease development. However, strong experimental research in animal models of cancer development and disease progression have shown that maintenance of adequate and not overweight body size can delay development of cancer. Whether this can be achieved in humans has not been evaluated in prospective randomized trials.

Cancers With Lower Rates Among Obese

Obesity may also be somewhat protective against other forms of cancer. Among premenopausal women, heavier women appear to experience modest protection from breast cancer compared to leaner women (0.7-fold relative risk). Lung cancer is also less prevalent among the obese relative to leaner individuals (relative risk 0.7), possibly because of smoking-related effects on metabolism, although some investigators have argued that smoking or weight loss due to undetected disease may bias reported findings.

Cancer Death Rates And Obesity

Evaluating the influence of obesity on survival from cancer is complicated by a number of factors including variation in treatment regimens and completeness of vital status follow-up. For most types of cancer, little data exists on this topic, except for breast cancer. Most studies of obesity and breast cancer survival, but not all, suggest that obese women have poorer survival than leaner women. To date, little is known about the mechanisms that might contribute to this effect and no prospective randomized trials have been conducted.

Trends In Cancer Related To Obesity

Like obesity, cancer is a major health problem in the United States and in other countries as well. Based on the American Cancer Society's 2002 estimates for cancer incidence, cancers linked to obesity among women comprise approximately 51 percent of all new cancers diagnosed among women in 2002: 2 percent thyroid cancers (15,800 new cases), 6 percent uterine cancers (39,300 new cases), 12 percent colorectal cancers (75,700 new cases), and 31 percent breast cancers (203,500 new cases). Among men, cancers linked to obesity comprise approximately 14 percent of new cancers: 3 percent kidney cancers (19,100 new cases) and 11 percent colorectal cancers (72,600 new cases).

In terms of mortality, for women, obesity-related cancers are estimated to comprise 28 percent of cancer-related deaths in 2002: 15 percent breast cancers (39,600 deaths), 2 percent uterine cancers (6,600 deaths), and percent colorectal cancers (28,800 deaths). Among men, obesity-related cancers are estimated to comprise 13 percent of cancer-related deaths in 2002: 10 percent colorectal cancers (27,800 deaths) and 3 percent kidney cancers (7,200 deaths).

Overall, while the mechanisms underlying the obesity-carcinogenesis relationship are not fully understood, sufficient evidence exists to support recommendations that adults and children maintain reasonable weight for their height and ages for multiple health benefits, including decreasing their risk of cancer.

Chapter 11

Human Papillomavirus And Cancer Risk

Human Papillomavirus

Human papillomavirus (pronounced pap-ah-LO-mah-VYE-rus), also known as HPV, is a very common virus that is spread by skin-to-skin contact during any type of sexual activity with another person. HPV infection is common in people in their teens and early 20s.

Why are HPV vaccines needed?

Certain human papillomavirus (HPV) types cause cancer, including: cervical, vulvar, vaginal, penile, anal, and oropharyngeal (base of the tongue, tonsils, and back of throat) cancers. Certain HPV types also cause most cases of genital warts in men and women.

HPV is a common virus that is easily spread by skin-to-skin contact during sexual activity with another person. It is possible to have HPV without knowing it, so it is possible to unknowingly spread HPV to another person.

HPV vaccine is a strong weapon in prevention. These safe, effective vaccines are available to protect females and males against some of the most common HPV types and the health problems that the virus can cause.

How common are the health problems caused by HPV?

HPV is the main cause of cervical cancer in women. There are about 12,000 new cervical cancer cases each year in the United States. Cervical cancer causes about 4,000 deaths in

About This Chapter: From "HPV Vaccine––Questions and Answers," July 20, 2012, and "HPV Vaccine for Preteens and Teens," February 7, 2013, both documents produced by the Centers for Disease Control and Prevention (CDC).

women each year in the United States. There are about 15,000 HPV-associated cancers in the United States that may be prevented by vaccines each year in women, including cervical, anal, vaginal, vulvar, and oropharyngeal cancers.

About 7,000 HPV-associated cancers in the United States that may be prevented by vaccine each year in men, and oropharyngeal cancers are the most common.

About one in 100 sexually active adults in the United States has genital warts at any given time.

What HPV vaccines are available in the United States?

Two HPV vaccines are licensed by the FDA and recommended by the Centers for Disease Control and Prevention (CDC). These vaccines are Cervarix (made by GlaxoSmithKline) and Gardasil (made by Merck).

How are the two HPV vaccines similar?

- Both vaccines are very effective against diseases caused by HPV types 16 and 18; HPV 16 and 18 cause most cervical cancers, as well as other HPV associated cancers.

- Both vaccines have been shown to prevent cervical precancers in women.

- Both vaccines are very safe.

- Both vaccines are made with a very small part (in this case, the protein outer coat) of the human papillomavirus (HPV) that cannot cause infection.

- Both vaccines are given as shots and require three doses.

How are the two HPV vaccines different?

- Only one of the vaccines (Gardasil) protects against HPV types 6 and 11, the types that cause most genital warts in females and males.

- Only one of the vaccines (Gardasil) has been tested and licensed for use in males.

- While both vaccines protect against HPV16, which is the most common HPV type responsible for HPV associated cancers including cancers of cervix, vulva, vagina, penis, anus, and oropharynx, only one of the vaccines (Gardasil) has been tested and shown to protect against precancers of the vulva, vagina, and anus.

- The vaccines have different adjuvants—a substance that is added to the vaccine to increase the body's immune response.

Both Boys And Girls Can Get The HPV Vaccine

HPV vaccines protect against Human papillomavirus (HPV) infection and the diseases that are caused by HPV.

HPV vaccination is recommended for preteen girls and boys at age 11 or 12 years. If a teenager or young adult (age 13 through 26 years old) has not gotten any or all of the HPV shots when they were younger, they should ask their doctor about getting them now.

Preteens and teens should get all 3 doses of an HPV vaccine long before their first sexual contact, so they have time to develop protection from the vaccine. This is also the age when the vaccine will work the best since preteens have a better immune response from the vaccine than older teens.

There are two different HPV vaccines (Cervarix or Gardasil) that can be given to girls and young women. Only one HPV vaccine—Gardasil—can be given to boys and young men. Both Cervarix and Gardasil protects against HPV types that cause most cervical cancer and have been shown to prevent cervical cancer. Gardasil has been studied and shown to protect against cervical, anal, vaginal, and vulvar cancers. Gardasil also protects against HPV types that cause most genital warts and has been shown to prevent genital warts.

Source: Excerpted from "HPV Vaccine for Preteens and Teens," CDC, February 7, 2013.

Who should get HPV vaccine?

Cervarix and Gardasil are licensed, safe, and effective for females ages 9 through 26 years. CDC recommends that all 11- or 12-year-old girls get the three doses (shots) of either brand of HPV vaccine to protect against cervical cancer. Gardasil also protects against most genital warts, as well as some cancers of the vulva, vagina, and anus. Girls and young women ages 13 through 26 should get HPV vaccine if they have not received any or all doses when they were younger.

Gardasil is also licensed, safe, and effective for males ages 9 through 26 years. CDC recommends Gardasil for all boys aged 11 or 12 years, and for males aged 13 through 21 years, who did not get any or all of the three recommended doses when they were younger. All men may receive the vaccine through age 26, and should speak with their doctor to find out if getting vaccinated is right for them.

The vaccine is also recommended for gay and bisexual men (or any man who has sex with men) and men with compromised immune systems (including HIV) through age 26, if they did not get fully vaccinated when they were younger.

Why is HPV vaccine recommended at ages 11 or 12 years?

For the HPV vaccine to work best, it is very important for preteens to get all three doses (shots) long before any sexual activity with another person begins. It is possible to be infected with HPV the very first time they have sexual contact with another person. Also, the vaccine produces higher antibody that fights infection when given at this age compared to older ages.

How does getting HPV vaccine at ages 11 or 12 fit with other health recommendations?

Doctors recommend health check-ups for preteens and teens. The first dose of an HPV vaccine should be given to girls and boys aged 11 or 12 years during any visit to the doctor. Three other vaccines are recommended for preteens and teens. During one visit, HPV vaccine can be given safely with these other preteen and teen vaccines. Check-ups during the preteen and teen years are also times when older kids and their parents can talk to their providers about other ways to stay healthy and safe.

What is the recommended schedule (or timing) of the three HPV doses (shots)?

Three doses (shots) are recommended over six months. CDC recommends that the second dose be given one to two months after the first, and the third dose be given six months after the first dose.

Are the HPV vaccines safe and effective?

The Food and Drug Administration (FDA) has licensed the vaccines as safe and effective. Both vaccines were tested in thousands of people around the world. These studies showed no serious side effects. Common, mild side effects included pain where the shot was given, fever, headache, and nausea. As of July 2012, approximately 46 million doses of quadrivalent HPV vaccine were distributed in the United States. As with all vaccines, CDC and FDA continue to monitor the safety of these vaccines very carefully. These vaccine safety studies continue to show that HPV vaccines are safe.

Do people faint after getting HPV vaccines?

People faint for many reasons. Some preteens and teen may faint after any medical procedure, including receiving vaccines. It is possible for falls and injuries to occur after fainting. Sitting or lying down for about 15 minutes after a vaccination can help prevent fainting and related injuries.

Can HPV vaccines treat HPV infections, cancers, or warts?

HPV vaccines will not treat or get rid of existing HPV infections. Also, HPV vaccines do not treat or cure health problems (like cancer or warts) caused by an HPV infection that occurred before vaccination. It is important for adult women to still get cervical cancer screening even if they have completed the HPV vaccine series.

How important is it to get HPV vaccine?

The HPV vaccines are important tools to prevent cancer and genital warts.

Why aren't HPV vaccines recommended for people older than 26?

Both vaccines were studied in thousands of people from 9 through 26 years old and found to be safe and effective for these ages. The vaccine is not licensed in the United States for persons over age 26 years, as Gardasil has not been demonstrated to prevent HPV-related outcomes in a general population of women and men older than 26 years of age.

Should pregnant women be vaccinated?

Pregnant women are not included in the recommendations for HPV vaccines. Studies show neither vaccine caused problems for babies born to women who got the HPV vaccine while they were pregnant. Getting the HPV vaccine when pregnant is not a reason to consider ending a pregnancy. But, to be on the safe side until even more is known, a pregnant woman should not get any doses of either HPV vaccine until her pregnancy is completed.

Will HPV vaccination be covered by health insurance?

Most health insurance plans cover recommended vaccines. But there may be a lag time after a vaccine is recommended before it gets added to insurance plans. Some insurance plans may not cover any or all vaccines. Check with your insurance provider to see if the cost of the vaccine is covered before going to the doctor.

How can a child get an HPV vaccine if a family doesn't have insurance?

The Vaccines for Children (VFC) program helps families of eligible children who might not otherwise have access to vaccines. The program provides vaccines at no cost to doctors who serve eligible children. Children younger than 19 years of age are eligible for VFC vaccines if they are Medicaid-eligible, American Indian or Alaska Native, or have no health insurance.

"Underinsured" children who have health insurance that does not cover vaccination can receive VFC vaccines through Federally Qualified Health Centers or Rural Health Centers. Parents of uninsured or underinsured children who receive vaccines at no cost through the VFC Program should check with their health care providers about possible administration fees that might apply. These fees help providers cover the costs that result from important services like storing the vaccines and paying staff members to give vaccines to patients.

Chapter 12

Hormonal Drugs And Cancer Risk: Oral Contraceptives And Anabolic Steroids

Oral Contraceptives And Cancer Risk

What types of oral contraceptives are available in the United States today?

Two types of oral contraceptives (birth control pills) are currently available in the United States. The most commonly prescribed type of oral contraceptive contains man-made versions of the natural female hormones estrogen and progesterone. This type of birth control pill is often called a "combined oral contraceptive." The second type is called the minipill. It contains only progestin, which is the man-made version of progesterone that is used in oral contraceptives.

How could oral contraceptives influence cancer risk?

Naturally occurring estrogen and progesterone have been found to influence the development and growth of some cancers. Because birth control pills contain female hormones, researchers have been interested in determining whether there is any link between these widely used contraceptives and cancer risk.

The results of population studies to examine associations between oral contraceptive use and cancer risk have not always been consistent. Overall, however, the risks of endometrial and ovarian cancer appear to be reduced with the use of oral contraceptives, whereas the risks of breast, cervical, and liver cancer appear to be increased. A summary of research results for each type of cancer is given below.

About This Chapter: This chapter begins with information from "Oral Contraceptives and Cancer Risk," National Cancer Institute," March 21, 2012. Available at: www.cancer.gov. Accessed May 5, 2013. It continues with information from "Drug Facts: Anabolic Steroids," National Institute on Drug Abuse, July 2012.

How do oral contraceptives affect breast cancer risk?

A woman's risk of developing breast cancer depends on several factors, some of which are related to her natural hormones. Hormonal and reproductive history factors that increase the risk of breast cancer include factors that may allow breast tissue to be exposed to high levels of hormones for longer periods of time, such as the following:

- Beginning menstruation at an early age

- Experiencing menopause at a late age

- Later age at first pregnancy

- Not having children at all

A 1996 analysis of epidemiologic data from more than 50 studies worldwide by the Collaborative Group on Hormonal Factors in Breast Cancer found that women who were current or recent users of birth control pills had a slightly higher risk of developing breast cancer than women who had never used the pill. The risk was highest for women who started using oral contraceptives as teenagers. However, 10 or more years after women stopped using oral contraceptives, their risk of developing breast cancer had returned to the same level as if they had never used birth control pills, regardless of family history of breast cancer, reproductive history, geographic area of residence, ethnic background, differences in study design, dose and type of hormone(s) used, or duration of use. In addition, breast cancers diagnosed in women who had stopped using oral contraceptives for 10 or more years were less advanced than breast cancers diagnosed in women who had never used oral contraceptives.

A recent analysis of data from the Nurses' Health Study, which has been following more than 116,000 female nurses who were 24 to 43 years old when they enrolled in the study in 1989, found that the participants who used oral contraceptives had a slight increase in breast cancer risk. However, nearly all of the increased risk was seen among women who took a specific type of oral contraceptive, a "triphasic" pill, in which the dose of hormones is changed in three stages over the course of a woman's monthly cycle.

Because the association with the triphasic formulation was unexpected, more research will be needed to confirm the findings from the Nurses' Health Study.

How do oral contraceptives affect ovarian cancer risk?

Oral contraceptive use has consistently been found to be associated with a reduced risk of ovarian cancer. In a 1992 analysis of 20 studies, researchers found that the longer a woman used oral contraceptives the more her risk of ovarian cancer decreased. The risk decreased by 10 to 12 percent after one year of use and by approximately 50 percent after five years of use.

Researchers have studied how the amount or type of hormones in oral contraceptives affects ovarian cancer risk. One study, the Cancer and Steroid Hormone (CASH) study, found that the reduction in ovarian cancer risk was the same regardless of the type or amount of estrogen or progestin in the pill. A more recent analysis of data from the CASH study, however, indicated that oral contraceptive formulations with high levels of progestin were associated with a lower risk of ovarian cancer than formulations with low progestin levels. In another study, the Steroid Hormones and Reproductions (SHARE) Study, researchers investigated new, lower-dose progestins that have varying androgenic (testosterone-like) effects. They found no difference in ovarian cancer risk between androgenic and nonandrogenic pills.

Oral contraceptive use by women at increased risk of ovarian cancer due to a genetic mutation in the BRCA1 or BRCA2 gene has been studied. One study showed a reduction in risk among BRCA1- or BRCA2-mutation carriers who took oral contraceptives, whereas another study showed no effect. A third study, published in 2009, found that women with BRCA1 mutations who took oral contraceptives had about half the risk of ovarian cancer as those who did not.

How do oral contraceptives affect endometrial cancer risk?

Women who use oral contraceptives have been shown to have a reduced risk of endometrial cancer. This protective effect increases with the length of time oral contraceptives are used and continues for many years after a woman stops using oral contraceptives.

How do oral contraceptives affect cervical cancer risk?

Long-term use of oral contraceptives (five or more years) is associated with an increased risk of cervical cancer. An analysis of 24 epidemiologic studies found that the longer a woman used oral contraceptives, the higher her risk of cervical cancer. However, among women who stopped taking oral contraceptives, the risk tended to decline over time, regardless of how long they had used oral contraceptives before stopping.

In a 2002 report by the International Agency for Research on Cancer, which is part of the World Health Organization, data from eight studies were combined to assess the association between oral contraceptive use and cervical cancer risk among women infected with the human papillomavirus (HPV). Researchers found a nearly threefold increase in risk among women who had used oral contraceptives for five to nine years compared with women who had never used oral contraceptives. Among women who had used oral contraceptives for 10 years or longer, the risk of cervical cancer was four times higher.

Virtually all cervical cancers are caused by persistent infection with high-risk, or oncogenic, types of HPV, and the association of cervical cancer with oral contraceptive use is likely to be indirect. The hormones in oral contraceptives may change the susceptibility of cervical cells to HPV infection, affect their ability to clear the infection, or make it easier for HPV infection to cause changes that progress to cervical cancer. Questions about how oral contraceptives may increase the risk of cervical cancer will be addressed through ongoing research.

How do oral contraceptives affect liver cancer risk?

Oral contraceptive use is associated with an increase in the risk of benign liver tumors, such as hepatocellular adenomas. Benign tumors can form as lumps in different areas of the liver, and they have a high risk of bleeding or rupturing. However, these tumors rarely become malignant.

Whether oral contraceptive use increases the risk of malignant liver tumors, also known as hepatocellular carcinomas, is less clear. Some studies have found that women who take oral contraceptives for more than five years have an increased risk of hepatocellular carcinoma, but others have not.

Steroids And Health Risks

"Anabolic steroids" is the familiar name for synthetic variants of the male sex hormone testosterone. The proper term for these compounds is anabolic-androgenic steroids (abbreviated AAS)—"anabolic" referring to muscle-building and "androgenic" referring to increased male sexual characteristics.

Anabolic steroids can be legally prescribed to treat conditions resulting from steroid hormone deficiency, such as delayed puberty, as well as diseases that result in loss of lean muscle mass, such as cancer and AIDS. But some athletes, bodybuilders, and others abuse these drugs in an attempt to enhance performance and/or improve their physical appearance.

How are anabolic steroids abused?

Anabolic steroids are usually either taken orally or injected into the muscles, although some are applied to the skin as a cream or gel. Doses taken by abusers may be 10 to 100 times higher than doses prescribed to treat medical conditions.

Steroids are typically taken intermittently rather than continuously, both to avert unwanted side effects and to give the body's hormonal system a periodic chance to recuperate.

Continuous use of steroids can decrease the body's responsiveness to the drugs (tolerance) as well as cause the body to stop producing its own testosterone; breaks in steroid use are believed to redress these issues. "Cycling" thus refers to a pattern of use in which steroids are taken for periods of weeks or months, after which use is stopped for a period of time and then restarted.

What are some health effects of anabolic steroids?

Steroid abuse may lead to serious, even irreversible, health problems. Some of the most dangerous consequences that have been linked to steroid abuse include kidney impairment or failure; damage to the liver; and cardiovascular problems including enlargement of the heart, high blood pressure, and changes in blood cholesterol leading to an increased risk of stroke and heart attack (even in young people).

Steroid use commonly causes severe acne and fluid retention, as well as several effects that are gender- and age-specific:

- For men—shrinkage of the testicles (testicular atrophy), reduced sperm count or infertility, baldness, development of breasts (gynecomastia), increased risk for prostate cancer

- For women—growth of facial hair, male-pattern baldness, changes in or cessation of the menstrual cycle, enlargement of the clitoris, deepened voice

- For adolescents—stunted growth due to premature skeletal maturation and accelerated puberty changes, and risk of not reaching expected height if steroid use precedes the typical adolescent growth spurt

In addition, people who inject steroids run the added risk of contracting or transmitting HIV/AIDS or hepatitis.

Chapter 13

Cancer Prevention For Girls: Why See A Gynecologist?

Special Doctors For Women's Unique Health Needs

Going to see a gynecologist—a doctor who focuses on women's reproductive health—means you're taking responsibility for your body in new ways. It can be very exciting to know you're making sure all is going well with puberty, your reproductive system, and more. Keep in mind that other doctors also can help with gynecological issues. For example, an adolescent medicine specialist, family doctor, or pediatrician can answer questions and may be able to examine your vagina too.

Of course, it can be stressful to deal with a whole new type of doctor's visit (and nobody loves those paper gowns!), but learning more can help you know what to expect.

Why see a gynecologist?

Seeing a gynecologist can make the following things possible:

- Help you understand your body and how to care for it.

- Establish what is normal for you so you can notice any problem changes, like signs of a vaginal infection

- Allow the doctor to find problems early so they can be treated or kept from getting worse

- Explain what a normal vaginal discharge should look like and what could be a sign of a problem

About This Chapter: This chapter begins with information excerpted from "Cancer Prevention for Girls: Why See a Gynecologist," Office of Women's Health, October 13, 2010. Additional information from the Boston Children's Hospital is cited separately within the chapter.

- Teach you how to protect yourself if you have sex

Your gynecologist can answer any questions you have at what can be a time full of changes. It's great to build a relationship with your gynecologist over the years so he or she understands your health and what matters to you.

When do I need to go?

The American College of Obstetricians and Gynecologists recommends that teenage girls start seeing a gynecologist between the ages of 13 and 15. That way you can start forming a relationship with the doctor and learning about your body. If you don't go at that time, you should make sure to visit a gynecologist or other health professional who can take care of women's reproductive health if any of the following apply to you:

- You have ever had sex (vaginal, oral, or anal) or intimate sexual contact

- It has been three months or more since your last period and you haven't gotten it again

- You have stomach pain, fever, and fluid coming from your vagina that is yellow, gray, or green with a strong smell—all of which are possible signs of a serious condition called pelvic inflammatory disease (PID)

- You are having problems with your period, like a lot of pain, bleeding heavily, or bleeding for longer than usual

- You have not gotten your period by the age of 15 or within three years of when your breasts started to grow

- You've had your period for two years and it's still not regular or comes more than once a month

- If you are having sex and missed your period

What will happen at the visit?

It's understandable if you're nervous about your first visit. Keep in mind that part of the time will be spent just talking. Your doctor may ask questions about you and your family to learn if you have a history of illnesses. And you can ask the doctor any questions you might have. Don't worry—your doctor probably has already heard every question imaginable! You can talk about any concerns you have, including these below:

- Cramps and problem periods

- Acne

- Weight issues

- Feeling depressed

- Sexually transmitted infections

During your visit, your doctor will probably go through some of the usual items on a doctor's checkup checklist, like weighing you and measuring your blood pressure. He or she also may do a breast exam. It's common for young women to have some lumpiness in their breasts, but your doctor may want to make sure you don't have problem lumps or pain.

You may have heard of Pap tests and pelvic exams and wonder if you need them. Most likely you won't need either of these until you're 21. (The American College of Obstetricians and Gynecologists recommends Pap tests for women starting at 21.) If you are sexually active or have symptoms like an unusual vaginal fluid or a history of problems, there's a chance your doctor may choose to do one or both of these. It's helpful, then, to know what to expect.

A pelvic exam usually involves the doctor examining the outside of your genital area (the vulva). It may also involve the doctor using a tool called a speculum to look inside your vagina. Frequently, he or she also will feel inside to make sure organs like your ovaries and uterus feel okay. You probably will feel pressure, but it shouldn't hurt. Try to relax—breathing deeply can help.

A Pap test is done by gently taking some cells from your cervix. These cells are checked for changes that could be cancer or that could turn into cancer.

During the exam, if the doctor is male, a female nurse or assistant will also be in the room. Don't forget that you can ask for things that will make the visit more comfortable. For example, you usually can have your mom, sister, or a friend stay in the room with you during the visit. And you can ask questions about what's going to happen so you know what to expect.

Taking care of your health is a huge sign that you are growing up. Be proud of yourself for learning information that can protect your health.

Quick Tip

If you are sexually active, tell your doctor. You likely will need to be tested for sexually transmitted infections like HIV and chlamydia. STIs are common among young people, and you can have an STI without having any symptoms. Don't let any possible embarrassment put your health—or your life—at risk.

Source: Office of Women's Health, October 13, 2010.

Quick Tip

If you haven't already had the HPV vaccine, ask your doctor about it. It helps guard against the human papillomavirus, which is the major cause of cervical cancer.

Source: Office of Women's Health, October 13, 2010.

Abnormal Pap Tests

About This Section: Reprinted from "Abnormal Pap Tests," © 2010 Center for Young Women's Health (http://www.youngwomenshealth.org), Boston Children's Hospital. All rights reserved. Used with permission.

If you are reading this chapter, you probably have already had a Pap test and may have been told by your health care provider that your Pap test results were abnormal. Maybe you're worried and wondering what this means and how it will affect you. However, knowing the possible reasons for abnormal results will help. Read on to find out more about Pap test.

What is a Pap test?

A Pap test, also called a "Pap smear," is part of a pelvic exam. The word "Pap" is short for Papanicolaou, which is the last name of the doctor that studied changes in cervical cells. A Pap test is usually done at age 21 unless you have special risks such as immune problems, HIV disease, or early sexual activity or pregnancy. It is the only way to check the cells on your cervix for changes that can lead to cancer. Your HCP usually checks for STIs (sexually transmitted infections, such as chlamydia and gonorrhea) at the same time.

How is a Pap test done?

As part of your pelvic exam, your health care provider will take a thin plastic wand and a tiny brush and gently wipe away some of the cells from your cervix. Most girls don't feel anything at all. A few girls may feel a little cramping as their cervix is gently brushed. If you feel anything, it usually lasts less than one minute. These cells are placed in a bottle or on a glass slide and sent to a laboratory.

A trained technician then examines the sample of cells under a microscope to see if the cells are normal, or if there are any problems. The lab then gives the results to your health care provider, who will contact you if the results are *not* normal.

Does it mean that I have cancer if I've been told I have an abnormal Pap?

No. Cancer is usually *not* the reason why your Pap test is abnormal. The most common reason for an abnormal Pap test is a vaginal or cervical infection that causes changes in the cells of your cervix. Most of these changes can be followed closely until they return to normal.

Sometimes special treatments are needed. Regular Pap tests and treatment, if needed, can prevent most types of cervical cancer.

What does my Pap test result really mean?

Although most Pap tests come back as normal, it is not unusual for the test results to be abnormal if you are an adolescent.

The following words explain Pap test results:

- **Normal:** This means that your cervix is healthy. Your health care provider will tell you when you need your next Pap test.

- **Unsatisfactory:** For some reason the sample of cells was not a good sample and can't be read by the lab technician. Your health care provider will let you know when the Pap test needs to be repeated.

- **Benign Changes:** This means that your Pap test was basically normal. However, you may have an infection that is causing inflammation of the cervical cells. Your health care provider may do a pelvic exam to check for the cause of the infection and prescribe treatment if needed. Your health care provider will tell you when you need to have a follow-up Pap test.

- **ASCUS (Atypical Squamous Cells of Undetermined Significance):** This simply means there are some funny looking cells on the test and more tests may be done to figure out if the HPV (human papillomavirus) is the reason for the changes.

Remember
- A Pap test is usually done at age 21 unless you have special risk factors.
- Abnormal results usually mean you have an HPV infection, not cancer.
- Regular Pap tests and early treatment can prevent most types of cervical cancer.

Source: Center for Young Women's Health, June 10, 2010.

If you are healthy and your Pap shows ASCUS, you will need to have your Pap test repeated in one year. If the test (at the one year mark) is still abnormal you may need a colposcopy.

The following guidelines are for teens and young women who are 21 years of age or younger.

- **ASCUS-H:** This result means that the cervical cells are not the typical cells that are found on the cervix. They are most likely related to HPV. They are considered "atypical cells of undetermined significance." The "H" at the end of this abbreviation means that there is a possibility that "high-grade changes" may be the cause of the problem. If this is your Pap test result, you will need to have a colposcopy.

- **LSIL (Low Grade Squamous Intraepithelial Lesion):** This result usually means that you have been infected with the human papillomavirus (HPV). You will be asked to return in 12 months for a repeat Pap test. If the repeat Pap test comes back abnormal, you may be referred for colposcopy.

- **HSIL (High Grade Intraepithelial Lesion):** This result means that the cells on your cervix have changed. The results are more serious than low-grade changes. You likely do not have cancer now, but without treatment you are at risk for developing cervical cancer. Treatment can prevent this. Your health care provider will recommend that you have a colposcopy.

- **AGC (Atypical Glandular Cells):** This result means that there are changes in the glandular cells of the cervix. You will need a colposcopy.

- **Cancer:** Although this is very rare in young women, if your Pap test comes back showing cancer cells, you need to be seen by a gynecologist who specializes in patients with cancer (oncologist). Treatment is necessary right away and usually includes surgery. The earlier the treatment, the better your chances are of staying healthy.

If your doctor tells you that you have LSIL or HSIL on your colposcopy test, you will need to return to your health care provider for follow-up visits and have a Pap test every year for 20 years.

What if I need a repeat Pap test?

Your health care provider will decide if and when you need to have your Pap test repeated. If the Pap test is going to be repeated, you should:

- Schedule your appointment after any vaginal or cervical infection, yeast infection, or STI has been treated (wait two weeks after your last dose of medicine).

- Schedule your appointment after your period has completely stopped.

- Not place anything in your vagina for 48 hours before your Pap test. This includes tampons, douches, creams, and foams.

- Not have sexual intercourse for 48 hours before the test.

- Tell your health care provider if you think you might be pregnant.

- Tell your health care provider if you have any other health conditions or allergies.

What if my health care provider wants me to have a colposcopy?

After the nurse asks questions (for example; "When was your last period?"), and gives you information about what to expect, you will be given a gown to wear and be asked to remove your clothing from the waist down. The health care provider will then come in and speak with you, and have you sign a consent form for the procedure. You will then lie down on the exam table and place your feet in foot holders (the same position as a pelvic exam). Next, the health care provider will gently insert a speculum (just like when you have your Pap test) into your vagina in order to separate the vaginal walls so your cervix can be seen easily. The colposcope is a magnifying tool that is placed near the opening of your vagina. Your doctor will be able to see your cervix through the magnifying lens.

It might make you feel better to know that the colposcope is only placed at the outside of your vagina and does not touch you. It is similar to a large magnifying glass that helps your health care provider see the tiny cells on your cervix. Your health care provider will first swab your cervix and vagina with a vinegar solution. The solution temporarily causes the unhealthy cells to change color, so your health care provider can get a better look. If there are unhealthy cells, it is likely that your health care provider will do a biopsy. This is when your health care provider gently removes a tiny sample of tissue (much smaller than one-fourth of the size of a pencil eraser) with an instrument similar to a pair of tweezers. The tissue sample is then placed in a jar with a preservative liquid and is sent to the lab to be checked out.

Will the colposcopy procedure hurt?

The colposcopy itself usually isn't uncomfortable. It is really a long pelvic exam and a way for your health care provider to look at your cervix. A biopsy, sometimes done at the time of a colposcopy, may be a bit uncomfortable, but this part takes less than one minute. When the tiny tissue sample is removed, some young women feel nothing, while others describe a "pinching" feeling or "mild cramps." Your doctor may suggest taking an over the counter pain reliever such as ibuprofen or naproxen sodium before the procedure to help decrease any discomfort you may have. This is especially helpful if you tend to have menstrual cramps or if you have discomfort when you have a Pap test done. Ask about taking the medicine that you usually take for menstrual cramps. The entire colposcopy procedure takes about 15 to 20 minutes.

What happens after the colposcopy is over?

After the colposcopy, your health care provider will explain what he or she saw through the high-powered lens and if a sample of tissue was taken. It usually takes about two to three weeks for the results of the biopsy to be ready. Make sure to make a follow-up appointment. Be sure your health care provider has your correct phone number so he or she can contact you.

- It is common to have slight bleeding or spotting that lasts a few days after the biopsy.

- Use pads (not tampons) for any bleeding you might have.

- You may see brownish material or clumps along with blood on your underwear or pad. This is not tissue. This is from a certain kind of solution your doctor used, called "Monsel's." The brownish clumps will last about one to five days.

- It's even possible to have a "blackish discharge" if the health care provider used a solution called "silver nitrate" to control the bleeding. Again, this will not last long.

- Do not have sexual intercourse, douche, use tampons, or place anything in your vagina for at least two weeks.

What should I be concerned about after a colposcopy?

There are certain things your health care provider should be contacted about. Call immediately if you have:

- Any heavy bleeding (heavier than your normal menstrual period)

- Any bright red bleeding and you are not on your period

- A vaginal discharge that has an odor (other than blood)

- Severe abdominal/pelvic (belly) pain

Chapter 14

How To Perform A Breast Self-Exam

Breast development is usually a sign that a girl is entering puberty. Most girls' breasts start to develop before their first periods. During puberty, every girl's breasts go through regular changes. As you grow and develop, you may notice small lumps and other changes in your breasts, and during your period, you may find your breasts are sensitive and tender. Most of these developments are totally normal.

Getting into the habit of examining your breasts when you're still in your teens can help you get used to the way they normally look and feel. When you become familiar with them, it will be easier to recognize anything unusual.

Why do I need breast exams?

If you go for an annual checkup with a doctor, he or she will likely examine your breasts to evaluate your development and ensure that all changes are normal. Your doctor may recommend that you get into the practice of examining your breasts yourself—called a breast self-examination (BSE)—and can show you how to do this.

A BSE can help women detect cysts or other benign (noncancerous) breast problems between checkups. It can also help some women detect breast cancer—a disease that's extremely rare among teens.

About This Chapter: "How to Perform a Breast Self-Examination," May 2010, reprinted with permission from www.kidshealth.org. This information was provided by KidsHealth®, one of the largest resources online for medically reviewed health information written for parents, kids, and teens. For more articles like this, visit www .KidsHealth.org, or www.TeensHealth.org. Copyright © 1995-2012 The Nemours Foundation. All rights reserved.

It's easy to perform a breast self-examination, and it only takes a few minutes. Although it might seem strange or inconvenient at first, BSE is a skill you can use throughout your life to help ensure good breast health.

How do I examine my breasts?

It's a good idea to examine your breasts once a month, and it makes sense to choose the same time each month because breasts usually change with the menstrual cycle. The best time to do a BSE is about a week after your period starts.

There are two parts to a BSE:

• How your breasts look

• How they feel

The looking part is easy. Before you put on a bra, stand or sit in front of a mirror with your arms relaxed at your sides. Make sure you are in a place with good lighting. Look at your breasts carefully. Do you see anything unusual, like a change in the way your nipples look? Any dimples or changes in the skin?

Then look at yourself from different angles and arm positions. Keep your hands at your sides, raise your arms overhead, place your hands firmly on your hips (to tighten your chest wall muscles), and bend forward. Watch for dimples or changes in the skin. Everyone's breasts look different. Get to know what yours look like.

The next part is how your breasts feel. It may seem strange at first to handle your breasts. Some girls feel self-conscious about it, but there's no reason to feel guilty or awkward. BSE is a positive way to stay healthy.

Lie down flat on your back, with a pillow or towel under one shoulder. Put that arm under your head. Examine your breasts one at a time. If you're starting with your right breast, put a pillow under your right shoulder, raise your right arm, place your right hand behind your head, and use your left hand to feel your breast.

> ## Note On Breast Self-Exam
>
> Although breast self-exam can be a helpful method for teens to use in becoming familiar with their developing bodies, it is no longer recommended as a tool for cancer screening. The U.S. Preventive Services Task Force currently recommends against teaching breast self-examination as a cancer detection tool.
>
> —LE

Using the pads of your three middle fingers, move your fingers in in overlapping circular motions about the size of a dime. Move up and down from the outside of the breast (under your armpit) toward the middle of your chest, making sure to cover every area of the breast. Examine up to your collarbone and down to the bottom of the ribcage. Notice what feels normal and what may feel different from the last time you examined your breasts.

Use different levels of pressure—light, medium, and firm—to feel each part of your breast. This will allow you to feel the various layers of tissue in the breast. Start with light pressure, increase to medium pressure, and finish with firm pressure to feel the deepest tissue. When you have covered the entire breast, use your finger and thumb to gently squeeze your nipple, watching for any discharge. Then put your left arm behind your head and check your left breast the same way.

While you're doing the exam, it's a good idea not to take your hand off your breast so you don't miss a spot. You should also check your armpits for any lumps. Girls who have large breasts should also feel their breasts from the side, while lying on one side and then the other.

As you feel your breasts, you may notice lumps or bumps. This is usually normal—just like so many things about people, breasts are unique. Some girls' breasts are large, some are small; some are symmetrical, others are not. Some healthy breasts feel really bumpy, whereas others are less so. Most teens have healthy breasts no matter what they look or feel like. But if you're worried about the way your breasts look or feel, let your doctor know.

Warning Signs

If you feel an unusual lump in your breast, don't panic—*breast cancer is extremely rare in teens*. In fact, among teen girls, the most common type of breast lump is usually related to normal breast growth and development. Other common conditions can cause a breast lump, such as a noncancerous growth known as a fibroadenoma, and small, fluid-filled cysts that tend to vary in size with a girl's menstrual cycle and are called *fibrocystic breast change*s.

Fibrocystic breast changes are common. In fact more than half of all women have them. They're related to the normal cycling of hormones associated with menstruation. Fibrocystic breast changes are typically worse just before and at the start of a girl's period.

If you feel a lump in your breast, talk to your doctor to see if the cause is one of these common conditions. If you have fibrocystic breast changes or other breast problems that may make it difficult to perform a good BSE, your doctor can help.

Infections can also cause breast lumps, as can an injury to the breast.

If you have any of these problems, you should talk to your doctor:

- Pain in your breast that seems unrelated to your period

- A new lump, bump, or other change in your breast

- A red, hot, or swollen breast

- Fluid or bloody discharge from your nipple

- A lump in your armpit or near your collarbone

- Any questions or concerns about your breasts

The goal of a BSE is for you to get used to the way your breasts feel. The better you know your body, the healthier you can be.

I'm a Guy. Why Do I Have a Lump In My Breast?

When a guy goes through puberty, all kinds of changes take place in his body. One of these changes can be a condition called gynecomastia, when breast tissue enlarges. That small lump with tenderness beneath the nipple is a normal part of puberty. In fact, about half of all boys develop gynecomastia during puberty. It's usually temporary and can happen on just one side or both. Some guys also may feel tenderness in the breast area when they go through puberty.

Breast changes in teenage guys are part of puberty—and they're rarely serious. Some signs that it might be serious are if the lump gets a lot bigger, becomes hard, or if you notice any fluid coming from your nipple. If that happens, see your doctor just to make sure it isn't a sign of another problem—though, again, breast changes in teen guys are almost never serious.

Even if you're not worried, it's always a good idea to talk to your doctor about your changing body. Your doctor is your best resource when it comes to your health. Plus, getting used to talking to your doctor now will help you get more out of your medical care as you grow up.

Source: "I'm A Guy. Why Do I Have A Lump In My Breast?" January 2013, reprinted with permission from www.kids health.org. This information was provided by KidsHealth®, one of the largest resources online for medically reviewed health information written for parents, kids, and teens. For more articles like this, visit www.KidsHealth.org, or www.Teens Health.org. Copyright © 1995-2013 The Nemours Foundation. All rights reserved.

Part Two
Cancers Of Most Concern To Teens And Young Adults

Chapter 15

Bone Cancer

What is bone cancer?

Bone cancer is a malignant (cancerous) tumor of the bone that destroys normal bone tissue. Not all bone tumors are malignant. In fact, benign (noncancerous) bone tumors are more common than malignant ones. Both malignant and benign bone tumors may grow and compress healthy bone tissue, but benign tumors do not spread, do not destroy bone tissue, and are rarely a threat to life.

Malignant tumors that begin in bone tissue are called primary bone cancer. Cancer that metastasizes (spreads) to the bones from other parts of the body, such as the breast, lung, or prostate, is called metastatic cancer, and is named for the organ or tissue in which it began. Primary bone cancer is far less common than cancer that spreads to the bones.

Are there different types of primary bone cancer?

Yes. Cancer can begin in any type of bone tissue. Bones are made up of osteoid (hard or compact), cartilaginous (tough, flexible), and fibrous (threadlike) tissue, as well as elements of bone marrow (soft, spongy tissue in the center of most bones).

Common types of primary bone cancer include the following:

- Osteosarcoma, which arises from osteoid tissue in the bone. This tumor occurs most often in the knee and upper arm.

About This Chapter: From "Bone Cancer," National Cancer Institute, March 13, 2008. Reviewed by David A. Cooke, MD, FACP, May 2013.

- Chondrosarcoma, which begins in cartilaginous tissue. Cartilage pads the ends of bones and lines the joints. Chondrosarcoma occurs most often in the pelvis (located between the hip bones), upper leg, and shoulder. Sometimes a chondrosarcoma contains cancerous bone cells. In that case, doctors classify the tumor as an osteosarcoma.

- The Ewing sarcoma family of tumors (ESFTs), which usually occur in bone but may also arise in soft tissue (muscle, fat, fibrous tissue, blood vessels, or other supporting tissue). Scientists think that ESFTs arise from elements of primitive nerve tissue in the bone or soft tissue. ESFTs occur most commonly along the backbone and pelvis and in the legs and arms.

Other types of cancer that arise in soft tissue are called soft tissue sarcomas. They are not bone cancer and are not described in this chapter.

What are the possible causes of bone cancer?

Although bone cancer does not have a clearly defined cause, researchers have identified several factors that increase the likelihood of developing these tumors. Osteosarcoma occurs more frequently in people who have had high-dose external radiation therapy or treatment with certain anticancer drugs; children seem to be particularly susceptible. A small number of bone cancers are due to heredity. For example, children who have had hereditary retinoblastoma (an uncommon cancer of the eye) are at a higher risk of developing osteosarcoma, particularly if they are treated with radiation. Additionally, people who have hereditary defects of bones and people with metal implants, which doctors sometimes use to repair fractures, are more likely to develop osteosarcoma. Ewing sarcoma is not strongly associated with any heredity cancer syndromes, congenital childhood diseases, or previous radiation exposure.

How often does bone cancer occur?

Primary bone cancer is rare. It accounts for much less than 1 percent of all cancers. About 2,300 new cases of primary bone cancer are diagnosed in the United States each year. Different types of bone cancer are more likely to occur in certain populations as with the following:

- Osteosarcoma occurs most commonly between ages 10 and 19. However, people over age 40 who have other conditions, such as Paget disease (a benign condition characterized by abnormal development of new bone cells), are at increased risk of developing this cancer.

- Chondrosarcoma occurs mainly in older adults (over age 40). The risk increases with advancing age. This disease rarely occurs in children and adolescents. ESFTs occur most often in children and adolescents under 19 years of age. Boys are affected more often than girls. These tumors are extremely rare in African-American children.

What are the symptoms of bone cancer?

Pain is the most common symptom of bone cancer, but not all bone cancers cause pain.

Persistent or unusual pain or swelling in or near a bone can be caused by cancer or by other conditions. It is important to see a doctor to determine the cause.

How is bone cancer diagnosed?

To help diagnose bone cancer, the doctor asks about the patient's personal and family medical history. The doctor also performs a physical examination and may order laboratory and other diagnostic tests. These tests may include the following:

- **X-rays:** These can show the location, size, and shape of a bone tumor. If x-rays suggest that an abnormal area may be cancer, the doctor is likely to recommend special imaging tests. Even if x-rays suggest that an abnormal area is benign, the doctor may want to do further tests, especially if the patient is experiencing unusual or persistent pain.

  - **Bone Scan:** This is a test in which a small amount of radioactive material is injected into a blood vessel and travels through the bloodstream; it then collects in the bones and is detected by a scanner.

  - **Computed Tomography (CT or CAT) Scan:** This is a series of detailed pictures of areas inside the body, taken from different angles, that are created by a computer linked to an x-ray machine.

  - **Magnetic Resonance Imaging (MRI):** This procedure uses a powerful magnet linked to a computer to create detailed pictures of areas inside the body without using x-rays.

  - **Positron Emission Tomography (PET) Scan:** With this, a small amount of radioactive glucose (sugar) is injected into a vein, and a scanner is used to make detailed, computerized pictures of areas inside the body where the glucose is used. Because cancer cells often use more glucose than normal cells, the pictures can be used to find cancer cells in the body.

  - **Angiogram:** This is an x-ray of blood vessels.

- **Biopsy:** This is removal of a tissue sample from the bone tumor to determine whether cancer is present. The surgeon may perform a needle biopsy or an incisional biopsy. During a needle biopsy, the surgeon makes a small hole in the bone and removes a sample of tissue from the tumor with a needle-like instrument. In an incisional biopsy, the surgeon cuts into the tumor and removes a sample of tissue. Biopsies are best done by an orthopedic oncologist (a doctor experienced in the treatment of bone cancer. A pathologist (a doctor who identifies disease by studying cells and tissues under a microscope) examines the tissue to determine whether it is cancerous.

- **Blood Tests:** These are used to determine the level of an enzyme called alkaline phosphatase. A large amount of this enzyme is present in the blood when the cells that form bone tissue are very active—when children are growing, when a broken bone is mending, or when a disease or tumor causes production of abnormal bone tissue. Because high levels of alkaline phosphatase are normal in growing children and adolescents, this test is not a completely reliable indicator of bone cancer.

Prosthetics

(Plural form of prosthesis)

A prosthesis is an artificial body part that replaces a natural one. If you have been diagnosed with a type of bone cancer (osteosarcoma, Ewing's sarcoma), you may need a prosthesis.

Treatment of your disease may require one of two types of surgery:

- You may have a limb salvage procedure, in which the bone containing the tumor and some of the surrounding tissues are removed. It will be replaced with either a bone graft or a metal (usually titanium) rod, a type of prosthesis.

- If your tumor has spread beyond the bone to the nerves and blood vessels, amputation of some or your entire limb might be necessary. You will be fitted with an artificial limb or prosthesis.

Such great improvements have been made to prostheses that many teens are able to return to their normal activities, including most sports.

Source: Reprinted with permission from Teens Living with Cancer, a program of Melissa's Living Legacy Teen Cancer Foundation, © 2013. All rights reserved. The Melissa's Living Legacy Teen Cancer Foundation is a non-profit organization providing resources to help teens with cancer have meaningful, life-affirming experiences throughout all stages of their disease. For additional information, visit www.teenslivingwithcancer.org.

What are the treatment options for bone cancer?

Treatment options depend on the type, size, location, and stage of the cancer, as well as the person's age and general health. Treatment options for bone cancer include surgery, chemotherapy, radiation therapy, and cryosurgery.

- **Surgery:** Surgery is the usual treatment for bone cancer. The surgeon removes the entire tumor with negative margins (no cancer cells are found at the edge or border of the tissue removed during surgery). The surgeon may also use special surgical techniques to minimize the amount of healthy tissue removed with the tumor.

  Dramatic improvements in surgical techniques and preoperative tumor treatment have made it possible for most patients with bone cancer in an arm or leg to avoid radical surgical procedures (removal of the entire limb). However, most patients who undergo limb-sparing surgery need reconstructive surgery to maximize limb function.

- **Chemotherapy:** Chemotherapy is the use of anticancer drugs to kill cancer cells. Patients who have bone cancer usually receive a combination of anticancer drugs. However, chemotherapy is not currently used to treat chondrosarcoma.

- **Radiation Therapy:** Also called radiotherapy, this involves the use of high-energy x-rays to kill cancer cells. This treatment may be used in combination with surgery. It is often used to treat, which cannot be treated with chemotherapy, as well as ESFTs. It may also be used for patients who refuse surgery.

- **Cryosurgery:** Cryosurgery is the use of liquid nitrogen to freeze and kill cancer cells. This technique can sometimes be used instead of conventional surgery to destroy the tumor.

Is follow-up treatment necessary? What does it involve?

Yes. Bone cancer sometimes metastasizes, particularly to the lungs, or can recur (come back), either at the same location or in other bones in the body. People who have had bone cancer should see their doctor regularly and should report any unusual symptoms right away. Follow-up varies for different types and stages of bone cancer. Generally, patients are checked frequently by their doctor and have regular blood tests and x-rays. People who have had bone cancer, particularly children and adolescents, have an increased likelihood of developing another type of cancer, such as leukemia, later in life. Regular follow-up care ensures that changes in health are discussed and that problems are treated as soon as possible.

Are clinical trials (research studies) available for people with bone cancer?

Yes. Participation in clinical trials is an important treatment option for many people with bone cancer. To develop new treatments and better ways to use current treatments, the National Cancer Institute (NCI), a part of the National Institutes of Health, is sponsoring clinical trials in many hospitals and cancer centers around the country. Clinical trials are a critical step in the development of new methods of treatment. Before any new treatment can be recommended for general use, doctors conduct clinical trials to find out whether the treatment is safe for patients and effective against the disease.

People interested in taking part in a clinical trial should talk with their doctor. Information about clinical trials is available from NCI's Cancer Information Service (CIS) at 800-4-CANCER (800-422-6237).

More information about clinical trials is available on NCI's Clinical Trials page at http://www.cancer.gov/clinicaltrials.

Chapter 16

Brain Tumors

Brain tumors are the most common solid tumors of childhood, as common as leukemia.

There are tremendous differences among brain tumors in children; some have a very poor outlook while others can be cured with surgery alone. These differences can make understanding pediatric brain tumors, and finding the right treatment for each one, confusing.

What Is A Brain Tumor?

A tumor is any mass caused by abnormal or uncontrolled growth of cells. Tumors in the brain are categorized according to several factors, including where they're located, the type of cells involved, and how quickly they're growing.

Medical terms doctors may use to describe brain tumors include:

- **Low-Grade Vs. High-Grade:** Usually, low-grade tumors are slow growing, while high-grade tumors are fast growing and aggressive. High-grade tumors can invade nearby tissue or spread elsewhere in the body, and are more likely to recur after treatment. They are generally associated with a worse outlook.

- **Localized Vs. Invasive:** A localized tumor is confined to one area and is generally easier to remove, as long as it's in an accessible part of the brain. An invasive tumor has spread to surrounding areas and is more difficult or impossible to remove completely.

About This Chapter: "Brain Tumors," September 2010, reprinted with permission from www.kidshealth.org. This information was provided by KidsHealth®, one of the largest resources online for medically reviewed health information written for parents, kids, and teens. For more articles like this, visit www.KidsHealth.org, or www .TeensHealth.org. Copyright © 1995-2013 The Nemours Foundation. All rights reserved.

- **Primary Vs. Secondary:** Primary brain tumors originate in the brain. Secondary brain tumors are made up of cells that have spread (metastasized) to the brain from somewhere else in the body. In children, most brain tumors are primary.

What Causes A Brain Tumor?

Like all tumors, brain tumors originate when a normal cell begins to grow abnormally and multiply too quickly. Eventually these cells develop into a mass called a tumor. The exact cause of this abnormal growth is unknown, though research continues on possible genetic and environmental causes.

Brain And Spinal Cord: Central Nervous System

A childhood brain or spinal cord tumor is a disease in which abnormal cells form in the tissues of the brain or spinal cord.

Together, the brain and spinal cord make up the central nervous system (CNS).

The brain has three major parts:

- The cerebrum is the largest part of the brain. It is at the top of the head. The cerebrum controls thinking, learning, problem solving, emotions, speech, reading, writing, and voluntary movement.
- The cerebellum is in the lower back of the brain (near the middle of the back of the head). It controls movement, balance, and posture.
- The brain stem connects the brain to the spinal cord. It is in the lowest part of the brain (just above the back of the neck). The brain stem controls breathing, heart rate, and the nerves and muscles used in seeing, hearing, walking, talking, and eating.

The spinal cord connects the brain with nerves in most parts of the body.

The spinal cord is a column of nerve tissue that runs from the brain stem down the center of the back. It is covered by three thin layers of tissue called membranes. These membranes are surrounded by the vertebrae (back bones). Spinal cord nerves carry messages between the brain and the rest of the body. For example, a signal from the brain causes muscles to move or the skin sends a signal to the brain when touched.

Tumors of many different cell types may form in the spinal cord. Low-grade spinal cord tumors usually do not spread. High-grade spinal cord tumors may spread to other places in the spinal cord or to the brain.

Source: Excerpted from PDQ® Cancer Information Summary. National Cancer Institute; Bethesda, MD. Childhood Brain and Spinal Cord Tumors Treatment Overview (PDQ): Patient version. Updated 02/2013. Available at: www.cancer.gov. Accessed May 19, 2013.

Some kids who have certain genetic conditions have a greater chance of developing brain tumors. Diseases such as neurofibromatosis, von Hippel-Lindau disease, and Li-Fraumeni syndrome are all associated with a higher risk of brain tumors.

Signs And Symptoms

A brain tumor can cause symptoms by directly pressing on the surrounding brain, or by causing a buildup of spinal fluid and pressure throughout the brain (a condition known as hydrocephalus). A range of symptoms can develop as a result.

Signs or symptoms vary depending on a child's age and the location of the tumor, but may include:

- Vomiting

- Seizures

- Weakness of the face, trunk, arms, or legs

- Slurred speech

- Difficulty standing or walking

- Poor coordination

- Headache

- In babies, a rapidly enlarging head

Because symptoms might develop gradually and can be like those of other common childhood conditions, brain tumors can be difficult to diagnose. So it's always wise to discuss any symptoms that concern you with your doctor.

Diagnosis

A doctor who suspects that a child has a brain tumor will order imaging studies of the brain: a CT scan, MRI, or possibly both. These procedures let doctors see inside the brain and identify any areas that look abnormal. Although both are painless, they do require children to be very still. Some kids, especially those who are young, may need to be sedated for these scans.

If imaging studies reveal a brain tumor, then surgery is likely to be the next step. A pediatric neurosurgeon will try to remove the tumor; if complete removal is not possible, then partial removal—or at least a biopsy (removal of a sample for microscopic examination)—may be done to confirm the diagnosis.

A pediatric pathologist (a doctor who helps diagnose diseases in children by looking at body tissues and cells under a microscope) will then review the tissue to classify and grade the tumor.

Special tests might be used to analyze the genetic makeup of the tumor cells. Using these tests to get specific information about cancer cells can help doctors identify the tumor and develop the best treatment plan for someone with a brain tumor.

Treatment

Treatment for a brain tumor requires a team of medical specialists. Most pediatric brain tumor patients require some combination of surgery, radiation therapy, and chemotherapy. Advancements in all three treatment areas in the last few decades have contributed to better outcomes.

Surgery

Pediatric neurosurgeons are having more success than ever in helping to cure children with brain tumors, partly because of new technologies in the operating room and partly because it has been learned that an aggressive surgical approach at diagnosis can significantly increase the chance for cure.

Medical Team

The care of a child with a brain tumor is very complicated and requires close coordination between members of the medical team, which typically will include:

- A pediatric neuro-oncologist (a doctor who specializes in treating cancers of the brain or spine)
- A pediatric neurologist (a doctor who specializes in disorders of the nervous system)
- A pediatric neurosurgeon (a surgeon who operates on the brain or spine)
- A pediatric radiation therapist (a specialist who administers radiation therapy)
- Pediatric rehabilitation medicine specialists, including speech, physical, and occupational therapists
- Pediatric psychologists and social workers

These experts will choose a child's therapy very carefully. Finding a treatment that will be effective and cure the child but not cause unacceptable side effects is probably one of the most difficult aspects of treating brain tumors.

Source: "Brain Tumors," Nemours Foundation, September, 2010.

Neurosurgeons may use stereotactic devices, which help target tumors by providing 3D images of the brain during surgery. Staged surgeries are also being used more frequently. This means that instead of trying to remove a large tumor all at once, surgeons will take out only part of the tumor at diagnosis. The patient will then get chemotherapy and/or radiation therapy to shrink the tumor and then return to the operating room a second or even a third time to try to remove the rest of the tumor.

After surgery, some patients may not require any more treatment beyond observation (periodic checkups and imaging scans to watch for problems). Many, however, will require radiation therapy, chemotherapy, or a combination of both.

Radiation Therapy

Radiation therapy—the use of high-energy light to kill rapidly multiplying cells—is very effective in the treatment of many pediatric brain tumors. However, because the developing brain in children younger than 10 years old (and especially those younger than 5) is highly sensitive to its effects, radiation therapy can have serious long-term consequences. These may include seizures, stroke, developmental delays, learning problems, growth problems, and hormone problems.

The decision to use radiation therapy is, therefore, an especially challenging one regarding young children.

The methods for giving radiation therapy have changed significantly over the last several decades. New computer-assisted technologies allow doctors to construct 3-D radiation fields that accurately target tumor tissue while avoiding injury to important brain structures like the hearing centers.

Chemotherapy

Chemotherapy (chemo) is the use of drugs to kill cancer cells. It is often given through a special long-lasting intravenous (IV) catheter called a central line, and may require frequent hospital stays.

Although chemotherapy has many short-term side effects (such as fatigue, nausea, vomiting, and hair loss), it has fewer long-term side effects than radiation therapy. Many children with brain tumors are treated with chemo in order to delay or avoid radiation treatment.

Unlike brain tumors in adults, many pediatric brain tumors are highly sensitive to the effects of chemo, so it is routinely used for many kids with brain tumors.

Common Types Of Brain Tumors

There are many different types of pediatric brain tumors, ranging from those that can be cured with minimal therapy to those that cannot be cured even with aggressive therapy.

Some of the most common types are:

Astrocytomas

Astrocytomas come in four major subtypes: juvenile pilocytic astrocytoma, fibrillary astrocytoma, anaplastic astrocytoma, and glioblastoma multiforme.

An important feature in determining the outlook for patients with astrocytomas is location, because this directly affects the chance for a cure. Tumors that can be completely removed surgically are much more likely to be cured, while those that can't be completely removed are, in general, less curable.

Ependymomas

Ependymomas are treated primarily with surgery and radiation therapy. If the tumor can be completely removed, patients with ependymomas may need no additional treatments. However, some completely removed ependymomas and most incompletely removed ependymomas will require further treatment—usually radiation therapy and sometimes also chemotherapy.

Brainstem Gliomas

Brainstem gliomas refer to a group of tumors of the brainstem that differ primarily by location. Most are curable with surgery and/or radiation therapy except the most common and serious type, the diffuse pontine glioma. These tumors, which originate in a part of the brainstem called the pons, are rarely curable even with aggressive therapy. Treatment for diffuse pontine gliomas usually includes radiation therapy, which lengthens survival and improves quality of life, but is rarely curative.

Medulloblastomas And Primitive Neuroectodermal Tumors (PNETs)

Medulloblastomas and primitive neuroectodermal tumors are very similar brain cancers and appear almost identical under the microscope. Medulloblastomas, by definition, can only occur in the posterior fossa or cerebellum (back part of the brain), while primitive neuroectodermal tumors can occur anywhere in the brain or spinal cord. These cancers are highly sensitive to chemotherapy and radiation therapy, so modern treatment regimens are usually curative. Although treatment regimens are effective, late side effects of therapy can be a significant problem.

Craniopharyngiomas

Craniopharyngiomas are low-grade tumors that arise in the middle of the brain near the pituitary gland. As a result of their location, many patients have endocrinologic (hormone) problems when the tumor is diagnosed and after it is treated.

While craniopharyngiomas can be cured with surgery alone, most pediatric centers do not attempt total removal of the tumor at diagnosis unless it can be accomplished without injury to the sensitive surrounding structures. Total removal of the tumor without consideration of these surrounding structures can cause permanent hormone deficiencies that can be difficult to manage.

Therefore, for most patients, only partial removal of the tumor is done at diagnosis, followed by radiation therapy for any remaining tumor. This approach usually results in effective treatment of the tumor without causing lifelong hormone deficiencies.

Germ Cell Tumors

These brain tumors usually arise from two special areas in the middle of the brain—the areas around the pituitary and pineal glands. Germ cell tumors include two main types, germinomas and nongerminomatous germ cell tumors.

Germinomas are sensitive to chemo and radiation therapy and both are usually used to help achieve an excellent cure rate. Nongerminomatous germ cell tumors include several different types of tumors which, in general, are not as curable as germinomas. Nongerminomatous germ cell tumors are treated with surgery, chemotherapy, and radiation therapy.

Late Effects

Late effects are problems that patients can develop after cancer treatments have ended. For survivors of pediatric brain tumors, late effects may include cognitive delay (problems with learning and thinking), seizures, growth abnormalities, hormone deficiencies, vision and hearing problems, and the possibility of developing a second cancer, including a second brain tumor.

Because these problems sometimes don't become apparent until years after treatment, careful observation and medical follow-up are needed to watch for these.

In some cases, short-term effects might improve with the help of physical, occupational, or speech therapy and may continue to improve as the brain heals.

In other cases, kids may experience side effects that are longer term, including learning disabilities; medical problems such as diabetes, growth delay, or delayed or early puberty; physical disabilities related to movement, speech, or swallowing; and emotional problems linked to the stresses of diagnosis and treatment. Some of these problems may become more severe with the passage of time.

Be aware of the potential for physical and psychological late effects, especially when the time comes to return to school, activities, and friendships. You or your parents can talk to teachers about the impact treatment has had and discuss any necessary accommodations, including a limited schedule, additional rest time or bathroom visits, modifications in homework, testing or recess activities, and medication scheduling. Your doctor can offer advice on how to make the transition easier.

Chapter 17

Breast Cancer

Inside a woman's breast are 15 to 20 sections (lobes). Each lobe is made of many smaller sections (lobules). Lobules have groups of tiny glands that can make milk.

After a baby is born, breast milk flows from the lobules through thin tubes (ducts) to the nipple.

Cancer Cells

Cancer begins in cells, the building blocks that make up all tissues and organs of the body, including the breast.

Normal cells in the breast and other parts of the body grow and divide to form new cells as they are needed. When normal cells grow old or get damaged, they die, and new cells take their place.

Sometimes, this process goes wrong. New cells form when the body doesn't need them, and old or damaged cells don't die as they should. The buildup of extra cells often forms a mass of tissue called a lump, growth, or tumor.

Tumors in the breast can be benign (not cancer) or malignant (cancer).

Benign Tumors: These tumors noncancerous are usually not harmful. They rarely invade the tissues around them and don't spread to other parts of the body. Benign tumors can be removed and usually don't grow back.

About This Chapter: Excerpted from "What You Need To Know About Breast Cancer," National Cancer Institute, September 26, 2012.

Malignant Tumors: These cancerous tumors may be a threat to life. They can invade nearby organs and tissues (such as the chest wall). Malignant tumors can spread to other parts of the body. Often they can be removed but sometimes grow back.

Breast cancer cells can spread by breaking away from a breast tumor. They can travel through blood vessels or lymph vessels to reach other parts of the body. After spreading, cancer cells may attach to other tissues and grow to form new tumors that may damage those tissues.

Types Of Breast Cancer

Breast cancer is the most common type of cancer among women in the United States (other than skin cancer). In 2013, more than 232,000 American women will be diagnosed with breast cancer.

The most common type of breast cancer is ductal carcinoma. This cancer begins in cells that line breast duct. About 7 of every 10 women with breast cancer have ductal carcinoma.

The second most common type of breast cancer is lobular carcinoma. This cancer begins in a lobule of the breast. See the picture of lobules. About 1 of every 10 women with breast cancer has lobular carcinoma.

Other women have a mixture of ductal and lobular type or they have a less common type of breast cancer.

It's A Fact!

Breast cancer also develops in men. In 2013, more than 2,200 American men will learn they have breast cancer.

Source: NCI, September 26, 2012.

Tests

After someone finds out that they have breast cancer, they may need other tests to help choose the best treatment for them.

Lab Tests With Breast Tissue

The breast tissue that was removed during the biopsy can be used in the following special lab tests:

- **Hormone Receptor Tests:** Some breast cancers need hormones to grow. These cancers have hormone receptors for the hormones estrogen, progesterone, or both. If the hormone receptor tests show that the breast cancer has these receptors, then hormone therapy is often recommended as part of the treatment plan.

- **HER2 Test:** Some breast cancers have large amounts of a protein called HER2, which helps them to grow. The HER2 test shows whether a woman's breast cancer has a large amount of HER2. If so, then targeted therapy against HER2 may be a treatment option.

Triple-Negative Breast Cancer

About 15 of every 100 American women with breast cancer have triple-negative breast cancer. These women have breast cancer cells with these characteristics:

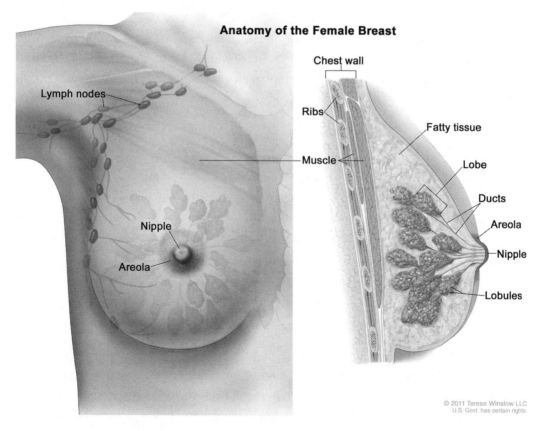

Anatomy of the Female Breast

Figure 17.1. Anatomy of the female breast. (Source: © 2011 Terese Winslow LLC, U.S. Govt. has certain rights.)

- Do not have estrogen receptors (estrogen negative)

- Do not have progesterone receptors (progesterone negative)

- Do not have a large amount of HER2 (HER2 negative)

Staging Tests

Staging tests can show whether cancer cells have spread to other parts of the body.

When breast cancer spreads, cancer cells are often found in the underarm lymph nodes (axillary lymph nodes). Breast cancer cells can spread from the breast to almost any other part of the body, such as the lungs, liver, bones, or brain.

Your doctor needs to learn the stage (extent) of the breast cancer to help patients choose the best treatment. Staging tests may include the following:

- **Lymph Node Biopsy:** If cancer cells are found in a lymph node, then cancer may have spread to other lymph nodes and other places in the body. Surgeons use a method called sentinel lymph node biopsy to remove the lymph node most likely to have breast cancer cells.

  If cancer cells are not found in the sentinel node, the woman may be able to avoid having more lymph nodes removed. The method of removing more lymph nodes to check for cancer cells is called axillary dissection.

- **CT Scan:** An x-ray machine linked to a computer takes a series of detailed pictures of a patient's chest or abdomen. Patients may receive contrast material by mouth and by injection into a blood vessel in their arm or hand. The contrast material makes abnormal areas easier to see. The pictures from a CT scan can show cancer that has spread to the lungs or liver.

- **MRI:** A strong magnet linked to a computer is used to make detailed pictures of a patient's chest, abdomen, or brain. An MRI can show whether cancer has spread to these areas. Sometimes contrast material makes abnormal areas show up more clearly on the picture.

- **Bone Scan:** The doctor injects a small amount of a radioactive substance into a blood vessel. It travels through the bloodstream and collects in the bones. A machine called a scanner detects and measures the radiation. The scanner makes pictures of the bones. Because higher amounts of the substance collect in areas where there is cancer, the pictures can show cancer that has spread to the bones.

- **PET Scan:** You'll receive an injection of a small amount of radioactive sugar. The radioactive sugar gives off signals that the PET scanner picks up. The PET scanner makes a picture of the places in your body where the sugar is being taken up. Cancer cells show up brighter in the picture because they take up sugar faster than normal cells do. A PET scan can show cancer that has spread to other parts of the body.

Stages

The stage of breast cancer depends on the size of the breast tumor and whether it has spread to lymph nodes or other parts of the body.

Doctors describe the stages of breast cancer using the Roman numerals 0, I, II, III, and IV and the letters A, B, and C.

A cancer that is Stage I is early-stage breast cancer, and a cancer that is Stage IV is advanced cancer that has spread to other parts of the body, such as the liver.

The stage often is not known until after surgery to remove the tumor in the breast and one or more underarm lymph nodes.

Stage 0: Stage 0 is carcinoma in situ. In ductal carcinoma in situ (DCIS), abnormal cells are in the lining of a breast duct, but the abnormal cells have not invaded nearby breast tissue or spread outside the duct.

Stage IA: In Stage IA, the breast tumor is no more than two centimeters (three-quarters of an inch) across. Cancer has not spread to the lymph nodes.

Stage IB: In Stage IB, the tumor is no more than two centimeters across. Cancer cells are found in lymph nodes.

Stage IIA: In Stage IIA, the tumor is no more than two centimeters across, and the cancer has spread to underarm lymph nodes. Or, the tumor is between two and five centimeters (three-quarters of an inch to two inches) across, but the cancer hasn't spread to underarm lymph nodes.

Stage IIB: In Stage IIB, the tumor is between two and five centimeters across, and the cancer has spread to underarm lymph nodes. Or, the tumor is larger than five centimeters across, but the cancer hasn't spread to underarm lymph nodes.

Stage IIIA: In Stage IIA, the breast tumor is no more than five centimeters across, and the cancer has spread to underarm lymph nodes that are attached to each other or nearby tissue. Or, the cancer may have spread to lymph nodes behind the breastbone.

Or, the tumor is more than five centimeters across. The cancer has spread to underarm lymph nodes that may be attached to each other or nearby tissue. Or, the cancer may have spread to lymph nodes behind the breastbone but not spread to underarm lymph nodes.

Stage IIIB: In Stage IIIB, the breast tumor can be any size, and it has grown into the chest wall or the skin of the breast. The breast may be swollen or the breast skin may have lumps.

The cancer may have spread to underarm lymph nodes, and these lymph nodes may be attached to each other or nearby tissue. Or, the cancer may have spread to lymph nodes behind the breastbone.

Stage IIIC: In Stage IIIC, the breast cancer can be any size, and it has spread to lymph nodes behind the breastbone and under the arm. Or, the cancer has spread to lymph nodes above or below the collarbone.

Stage IV: In Stage IV, the tumor can be any size, and cancer cells have spread to other parts of the body, such as the lungs, liver, bones, or brain.

Inflammatory breast cancer is a rare type of breast cancer. The breast looks red and swollen because cancer cells block the lymph vessels in the skin of the breast. When a doctor diagnoses inflammatory breast cancer, it's at least Stage IIIB, but it could be more advanced.

Treatment

Women with breast cancer have many treatment options. These include surgery, radiation therapy, hormone therapy, chemotherapy, and targeted therapy. Many women need more than one type of treatment.

The treatment depends mainly on the stage of breast cancer, whether the tumor has hormone receptors, whether the tumor has too much HER2, the patient's general health, and the size of the tumor.

Quick Tip

Before starting treatment, you might want a second opinion about your treatment plan. It may take some time and effort to gather your medical records and see another doctor. In most cases, it's not a problem to take several weeks to get a second opinion. The delay in starting treatment usually will not make treatment less effective. To make sure, you should discuss this delay with your doctor.

Surgery: Surgery is the most common treatment for breast cancer. There are several kinds of surgery. Breast-sparing surgery is an operation to remove the cancer and a small amount of the normal tissue that surrounds it. This is also called breast-conserving surgery. It can be a lumpectomy or a segmental mastectomy (also called a partial mastectomy). Some women will have more tissue removed but not the whole breast. For these women, the surgeon will remove lymph nodes under the arm and some of the lining over the chest muscles below the tumor. Surgery to remove the whole breast (or as much of the breast tissue as possible) is a mastectomy. In some cases, a skin-sparing mastectomy may be an option.

Radiation Therapy: Radiation therapy uses high-energy rays to kill cancer cells. It affects cells only in the part of the body that is treated. Radiation therapy may be used after surgery to destroy breast cancer cells that remain in the chest area. Women usually have radiation therapy after breast-sparing surgery, but it's sometimes used after mastectomy too.

Hormone Therapy: If lab tests show that a patient's breast cancer cells have hormone receptors, then hormone therapy may be an option. Hormone therapy keeps the cancer cells from getting or using the natural hormones (estrogen and progesterone) they need to grow.

Chemotherapy: Chemotherapy uses drugs to kill cancer cells. The drugs for breast cancer are usually given directly into a vein (intravenously) through a thin needle or as a pill. Chemotherapy is often a combination of drugs.

Targeted Therapy: Patients whose breast cancer cells have too much HER2 protein may receive targeted therapy. The targeted therapies used to treat breast cancer block cancer cell growth by blocking the action of the extra HER2 protein. These drugs may be given intravenously or as a pill.

Chapter 18

Cervical Cancer

General Information About Cervical Cancer

Cervical cancer is a disease in which malignant (cancer) cells form in the tissues of the cervix.

The cervix is the lower, narrow end of the uterus (the hollow, pear-shaped organ where a fetus grows). The cervix leads from the uterus to the vagina (birth canal).

Cervical cancer usually develops slowly over time. Before cancer appears in the cervix, the cells of the cervix go through changes known as dysplasia, in which cells that are not normal begin to appear in the cervical tissue. Later, cancer cells start to grow and spread more deeply into the cervix and to surrounding areas.

Cervical cancer in children is rare.

Human papillomavirus (HPV) infection is the major risk factor for development of cervical cancer.

Anything that increases your risk of getting a disease is called a risk factor. Having a risk factor does not mean that you will get cancer; not having risk factors doesn't mean that you will not get cancer. Talk with your doctor if you think you may be at risk.

Infection of the cervix with human papillomavirus (HPV) is the most common cause of cervical cancer. Not all women with HPV infection, however, will develop cervical cancer.

About This Chapter: PDQ® Cancer Information Summary. National Cancer Institute; Bethesda, MD. Cervical Cancer Treatment (PDQ): Patient version. Updated 09/2012. Available at: www.cancer.gov. Accessed May 7, 2013.

Women who do not regularly have a Pap smear to detect HPV or abnormal cells in the cervix are at increased risk of cervical cancer.

Other possible risk factors include the following:

- Giving birth to many children

- Having many sexual partners

- Having first sexual intercourse at a young age

- Smoking cigarettes

- Using oral contraceptives ("the Pill")

- Having a weakened immune system

Remember!

Having a human papillomavirus (HPV) infection is a risk factor for cervical cancer. However, many women with HPV infection or other risk factors will never develop cervical cancer.

There are usually no noticeable signs of early cervical cancer but it can be detected early with regular check-ups.

Early cervical cancer may not cause noticeable signs or symptoms. Women should have regular check-ups, including a Pap smear to check for abnormal cells in the cervix. The prognosis (chance of recovery) is better when the cancer is found early.

Tests that examine the cervix are used to detect (find) and diagnose cervical cancer.

The following procedures may be used:

- **Physical Exam And History:** An exam of the body to check general signs of health, including checking for signs of disease, such as lumps or anything else that seems unusual. A history of the patient's health habits and past illnesses and treatments will also be taken.

- **Pelvic Exam:** An exam of the vagina, cervix, uterus, fallopian tubes, ovaries, and rectum. The doctor or nurse inserts one or two lubricated, gloved fingers of one hand into the vagina and places the other hand over the lower abdomen to feel the size, shape, and position of the uterus and ovaries. A speculum is also inserted into the vagina and the doctor or nurse looks at the vagina and cervix for signs of disease. A Pap test of the cervix is usually done. The doctor or nurse also inserts a lubricated, gloved finger into the rectum to feel for lumps or abnormal areas.

- **Pap Smear:** A procedure to collect cells from the surface of the cervix and vagina. A piece of cotton, a brush, or a small wooden stick is used to gently scrape cells from the cervix and vagina. The cells are viewed under a microscope to find out if they are abnormal. This procedure is also called a Pap test.

- **Human Papillomavirus (HPV) Test:** A laboratory test used to check DNA (genetic material) for certain types of HPV infection. Cells are collected from the cervix and checked to find out if an infection is caused by a type of human papillomavirus that is linked to cervical cancer. This test may be done if the results of a Pap smear show certain abnormal cervical cells. This test is also called the HPV DNA test.

- **Endocervical Curettage:** A procedure to collect cells or tissue from the cervical canal using a curette (spoon-shaped instrument). Tissue samples may be taken and checked under a microscope for signs of cancer. This procedure is sometimes done at the same time as a colposcopy.

- **Colposcopy:** A procedure in which a colposcope (a lighted, magnifying instrument) is used to check the vagina and cervix for abnormal areas. Tissue samples may be taken using a curette (spoon-shaped instrument) and checked under a microscope for signs of disease.

- **Biopsy:** If abnormal cells are found in a Pap smear, the doctor may do a biopsy. A sample of tissue is cut from the cervix and viewed under a microscope by a pathologist to check for signs of cancer. A biopsy that removes only a small amount of tissue is usually

It's A Fact!

Possible signs of cervical cancer include vaginal bleeding and pelvic pain. These and other symptoms may be caused by cervical cancer. Other conditions may cause the same symptoms. Check with your doctor if you have any of the following problems:

- Vaginal bleeding
- Unusual vaginal discharge
- Pelvic pain
- Pain during sexual intercourse

done in the doctor's office. A woman may need to go to a hospital for a cervical cone biopsy (removal of a larger, cone-shaped sample of cervical tissue).

Certain factors affect prognosis (chance of recovery) and treatment options.

The prognosis (chance of recovery) depends on the following factors:

- The patient's age and general health
- Whether or not the patient has a certain type of human papillomavirus
- The stage of the cancer (whether it affects part of the cervix, involves the whole cervix, or has spread to the lymph nodes or other places in the body)
- The type of cervical cancer
- The size of the tumor

Treatment options depend on the following factors:

- The stage of the cancer
- The size of the tumor
- The patient's desire to have children
- The patient's age

Treatment of cervical cancer during pregnancy depends on the stage of the cancer and the stage of the pregnancy. For cervical cancer found early or for cancer found during the last trimester of pregnancy, treatment may be delayed until after the baby is born.

Stages Of Cervical Cancer

After cervical cancer has been diagnosed, tests are done to find out if cancer cells have spread within the cervix or to other parts of the body.

The process used to find out if cancer has spread within the cervix or to other parts of the body is called staging. The information gathered from the staging process determines the stage of the disease. It is important to know the stage in order to plan treatment. The following tests and procedures may be used in the staging process:

- **CT Scan (CAT Scan):** A procedure that makes a series of detailed pictures of areas inside the body, taken from different angles. The pictures are made by a computer linked to an x-ray machine. A dye may be injected into a vein or swallowed to help the organs or tissues show up more clearly. This procedure is also called computed tomography, computerized tomography, or computerized axial tomography.

- **PET Scan (Positron Emission Tomography Scan):** A procedure to find malignant tumor cells in the body. A small amount of radioactive glucose (sugar) is injected into a vein. The PET scanner rotates around the body and makes a picture of where glucose is being used in the body. Malignant tumor cells show up brighter in the picture because they are more active and take up more glucose than normal cells do.

- **Ultrasound Exam:** A procedure in which high-energy sound waves (ultrasound) are bounced off internal tissues or organs and make echoes. The echoes form a picture of body tissues called a sonogram.

- **Chest X-Ray:** An x-ray of the organs and bones inside the chest. An x-ray is a type of energy beam that can go through the body and onto film, making a picture of areas inside the body.

- **Cystoscopy:** A procedure to look inside the bladder and urethra to check for abnormal areas. A cystoscope is inserted through the urethra into the bladder. A cystoscope is a thin, tube-like instrument with a light and a lens for viewing. It may also have a tool to remove tissue samples, which are checked under a microscope for signs of cancer.

- **Laparoscopy:** A surgical procedure to look at the organs inside the abdomen to check for signs of disease. Small incisions (cuts) are made in the wall of the abdomen and a laparoscope (a thin, lighted tube) is inserted into one of the incisions. Other instruments may be inserted through the same or other incisions to perform procedures such as removing organs or taking tissue samples to be checked under a microscope for signs of disease.

- **Pretreatment Surgical Staging:** Surgery (an operation) is done to find out if the cancer has spread within the cervix or to other parts of the body. In some cases, the cervical cancer can be removed at the same time. Pretreatment surgical staging is usually done only as part of a clinical trial.

The results of these tests are viewed together with the results of the original tumor biopsy to determine the cervical cancer stage.

There are three ways that cancer spreads in the body.

The three ways that cancer spreads in the body are through the following:

- **Tissue:** Cancer invades the surrounding normal tissue.

- **Lymph System:** Cancer invades the lymph system and travels through the lymph vessels to other places in the body.

- **Blood:** Cancer invades the veins and capillaries and travels through the blood to other places in the body.

When cancer cells break away from the primary (original) tumor and travel through the lymph or blood to other places in the body, another (secondary) tumor may form. This process is called metastasis. The secondary (metastatic) tumor is the same type of cancer as the primary tumor. For example, if breast cancer spreads to the bones, the cancer cells in the bones are actually breast cancer cells. The disease is metastatic breast cancer, not bone cancer.

The following stages are used for cervical cancer:

Carcinoma in Situ (Stage 0)

In carcinoma in situ (stage 0), abnormal cells are found in the innermost lining of the cervix. These abnormal cells may become cancer and spread into nearby normal tissue.

Stage I

In stage I, cancer is found in the cervix only. Stage I is divided into stages IA and IB, based on the amount of cancer that is found.

- *Stage IA:* A very small amount of cancer that can only be seen with a microscope is found in the tissues of the cervix. Stage IA is divided into stages IA1 and IA2, based on the size of the tumor.

  - In stage IA1, the cancer is not more than 3 millimeters deep and not more than 7 millimeters wide.

  - In stage IA2, the cancer is more than 3 but not more than 5 millimeters deep, and not more than 7 millimeters wide.

- *Stage IB* is divided into stages IB1 and IB2.

  - In stage IB1 the cancer can only be seen with a microscope and is more than 5 millimeters deep and more than 7 millimeters wide; or the cancer can be seen without a microscope and is 4 centimeters or smaller.

- In stage IB2, the cancer can be seen without a microscope and is larger than 4 centimeters.

Stage II

In stage II, cancer has spread beyond the cervix but not to the pelvic wall (the tissues that line the part of the body between the hips) or to the lower third of the vagina. Stage II is divided into stages IIA and IIB, based on how far the cancer has spread.

- *Stage IIA:* Cancer has spread beyond the cervix to the upper two thirds of the vagina but not to tissues around the uterus. Stage IIA is divided into stages IIA1 and IIA2, based on the size of the tumor.

  - In stage IIA1, the tumor can be seen without a microscope and is 4 centimeters or smaller.

  - In stage IIA2, the tumor can be seen without a microscope and is larger than 4 centimeters.

- *Stage IIB:* Cancer has spread beyond the cervix to the tissues around the uterus.

Stage III

In stage III, cancer has spread to the lower third of the vagina, and/or to the pelvic wall, and/or has caused kidney problems. Stage III is divided into stages IIIA and IIIB, based on how far the cancer has spread.

- *Stage IIIA:* Cancer has spread to the lower third of the vagina but not to the pelvic wall.

- *Stage IIIB:* Cancer has spread to the pelvic wall; and/o the tumor has become large enough to block the ureters (the tubes that connect the kidneys to the bladder). This blockage can cause the kidneys to enlarge or stop working.

Stage IV

In stage IV, cancer has spread to the bladder, rectum, or other parts of the body. Stage IV is divided into stages IVA and IVB, based on where the cancer is found.

- *Stage IVA:* Cancer has spread to nearby organs, such as the bladder or rectum.

- *Stage IVB:* Cancer has spread to other parts of the body, such as the liver, lungs, bones, or distant lymph nodes.

Recurrent Cervical Cancer

Recurrent cervical cancer is cancer that has recurred (come back) after it has been treated. The cancer may come back in the cervix or in other parts of the body.

There are different types of treatment for patients with cervical cancer.

Different types of treatment are available for patients with cervical cancer. Some treatments are standard (the currently used treatment), and some are being tested in clinical trials. A treatment clinical trial is a research study meant to help improve current treatments or obtain information on new treatments for patients with cancer. When clinical trials show that a new treatment is better than the standard treatment, the new treatment may become the standard treatment. Patients may want to think about taking part in a clinical trial. Some clinical trials are open only to patients who have not started treatment.

Treatment

Three types of standard treatment are used.

Surgery: Surgery (removing the cancer in an operation) is sometimes used to treat cervical cancer. The following surgical procedures may be used:

- *Conization:* A procedure to remove a cone-shaped piece of tissue from the cervix and cervical canal. A pathologist views the tissue under a microscope to look for cancer cells. Conization may be used to diagnose or treat a cervical condition. This procedure is also called a cone biopsy.

- *Total Hysterectomy:* Surgery to remove the uterus, including the cervix. If the uterus and cervix are taken out through the vagina, the operation is called a vaginal hysterectomy. If the uterus and cervix are taken out through a large incision (cut) in the abdomen, the operation is called a total abdominal hysterectomy. If the uterus and cervix are taken out through a small incision in the abdomen using a laparoscope, the operation is called a total laparoscopic hysterectomy.

- *Radical Hysterectomy:* Surgery to remove the uterus, cervix, part of the vagina, and a wide area of ligaments and tissues around these organs. The ovaries, fallopian tubes, or nearby lymph nodes may also be removed.

- *Modified Radical Hysterectomy:* Surgery to remove the uterus, cervix, upper part of the vagina, and ligaments and tissues that closely surround these organs. Nearby lymph nodes may also be removed. In this type of surgery, not as many tissues and/or organs are removed as in a radical hysterectomy.

- *Bilateral Salpingo-Oophorectomy:* Surgery to remove both ovaries and both fallopian tubes.

- *Pelvic Exenteration:* Surgery to remove the lower colon, rectum, and bladder. In women, the cervix, vagina, ovaries, and nearby lymph nodes are also removed. Artificial openings (stoma) are made for urine and stool to flow from the body to a collection bag. Plastic surgery may be needed to make an artificial vagina after this operation.

- *Cryosurgery:* A treatment that uses an instrument to freeze and destroy abnormal tissue, such as carcinoma in situ. This type of treatment is also called cryotherapy.

- *Laser Surgery:* A surgical procedure that uses a laser beam (a narrow beam of intense light) as a knife to make bloodless cuts in tissue or to remove a surface lesion such as a tumor.

- *Loop Electrosurgical Excision Procedure (LEEP)*: A treatment that uses electrical current passed through a thin wire loop as a knife to remove abnormal tissue or cancer.

Radiation Therapy: Radiation therapy is a cancer treatment that uses high-energy x-rays or other types of radiation to kill cancer cells or keep them from growing. There are two types of radiation therapy. External radiation therapy uses a machine outside the body to send radiation toward the cancer. Internal radiation therapy uses a radioactive substance sealed in needles, seeds, wires, or catheters that are placed directly into or near the cancer. The way the radiation therapy is given depends on the type and stage of the cancer being treated.

Chemotherapy: Chemotherapy is a cancer treatment that uses drugs to stop the growth of cancer cells, either by killing the cells or by stopping them from dividing. When chemotherapy is taken by mouth or injected into a vein or muscle, the drugs enter the bloodstream and can reach cancer cells throughout the body (systemic chemotherapy). When chemotherapy is placed directly into the cerebrospinal fluid, an organ, or a body cavity such as the abdomen, the drugs mainly affect cancer cells in those areas (regional chemotherapy). The way the chemotherapy is given depends on the type and stage of the cancer being treated.

Follow-Up Care

Some of the tests that were done to diagnose the cancer or to find out the stage of the cancer may be repeated. Some tests will be repeated in order to see how well the treatment is working. Decisions about whether to continue, change, or stop treatment may be based on the results of these tests. This is sometimes called re-staging.

Some of the tests will continue to be done from time to time after treatment has ended. The results of these tests can show if your condition has changed or if the cancer has recurred (come back). These tests are sometimes called follow-up tests or check-ups.

Chapter 19

Colorectal Cancer

Colorectal cancer is a disease in which malignant (cancer) cells form in the tissues of the colon or the rectum. The colon is part of the body's digestive system. The digestive system removes and processes nutrients (vitamins, minerals, carbohydrates, fats, proteins, and water) from foods and helps pass waste material out of the body.

The digestive system is made up of the esophagus, stomach, and the small and large intestines. The first six feet of the large intestine are called the large bowel or colon. The last six inches are the rectum and the anal canal. The anal canal ends at the anus (the opening of the large intestine to the outside of the body).

Cancers that develop within the main part of the large intestine are usually referred to as colon cancer. Cancers that develop in the last six inches are called rectal cancer. Because colon cancers and rectal cancers have similar causes, risk factors, and patterns of spread, they are often grouped together and referred to as colorectal cancer.

Most colorectal cancer occurs in people over the age of 40. However, it can occur in children or teens on rare occasions. Genetics play a large role in colorectal cancer risk, so if you have a family history of colorectal cancer, you may need to be tested at a much earlier age than most people.

About This Chapter: Text in this chapter is excerpted from PDQ® Cancer Information Summary. National Cancer Institute; Bethesda, MD. Unusual Cancers of Childhood (PDQ): Patient version. Updated 05/2013. Available at: www.cancer.gov. Accessed June 1, 2013; and it includes excerpts from "What You Need To Know About™ Cancer of the Colon and Rectum," National Cancer Institute, 5/26/2006; revised by David A. Cooke, MD, FACP, June 2013.

How Does Colorectal Cancer Happen?

The lining of the colon (large intestine) absorbs water from undigested waste products, and protects the organ from injury and harmful microorganisms. The cells in the lining are shed rapidly and new ones take their place. In effect, the colon grows a new lining every few days.

Because the cells lining the colon are constantly dividing, there is always a risk that errors (mutations) may occur during the copying of genetic material. While some of these genetic errors are harmless, others can interfere with the normal controls that prevent cells from dividing abnormally and invading other tissues. Cells that accumulate a series of mutations may transform into cancer cells that can spread throughout the body.

Exposure to toxins and age increase the risk of mutations. Some people inherit already damaged genes from their parent, which may place them farther down the road to colorectal cancer, or increase their odds of developing additional mutations.

Most colorectal cancer develops from colon polyps, which are mushroom-like growths of the colon's lining. There is more than one kind of polyp, and some are harmless. However, other types known as colon adenomas consist of mutated cells that are growing unusually quickly. Given enough time, many colon adenomas will eventually transform into colorectal cancer. Prevention of colorectal cancer depends heavily on detecting pre-cancerous polyps and removing them before they have the opportunity to become cancer.

Testing For Colorectal Cancer

Colorectal cancer develops deep inside the body where it cannot be easily seen. There are usually no symptoms of colorectal cancer until is quite advanced, and treatment options are poor. However, if colorectal cancer can be found at an early stage, before there are any symptoms, treatment is often quite successful. Colorectal cancer testing is performed to identify polyps before they have the chance to become cancer, and to find curable, early stage cancers that have not yet caused any symptoms

Testing for colorectal cancer may involve testing stool samples for blood. Colon polyps or cancers may bleed in small amounts, which may be detected by chemical testing. Alternatively, lower endoscopy (sigmoidoscopy or colonoscopy) may be performed. Both involve placing a thin, flexible tube with a fiber-optic light or camera into the large intestine to inspect it from the inside. Sigmoidoscopy inspects the lower third of the large intestine, while colonoscopy checks the entire large intestine.

Colorectal testing is recommended for everyone starting at age 50. However, some people may need to be checked sooner. People with a family history of colorectal cancers generally should be tested when they are 10 years younger than their family member's age of diagnosis.

Certain conditions, or family history of conditions, may require testing for colon cancer in childhood or the teen years. While this is unusual, testing is extremely important in the cases because the risk of colorectal cancer may be very high even at young ages.

Childhood Colon Cancer

Childhood colon cancer is most often part of an inherited syndrome that causes the disease. Some colorectal cancers in young people are linked to a gene mutation that causes polyps (growths in the mucous membrane that lines the colon) to form that may turn into cancer later.

The risk of colorectal cancer is increased by having inherited certain conditions, such as the following:

- Attenuated familial adenomatous polyposis
- Familial adenomatous polyposis
- Lynch syndrome
- Li-Fraumeni syndrome
- MYH-associated polyposis
- Turcot syndrome
- Cowden syndrome
- Juvenile polyposis syndrome
- Peutz-Jeghers syndrome

Colon polyps that form in children who do not have an inherited syndrome are not linked to an increased risk of cancer.

Colon Cancer Symptoms

As noted above, colorectal cancer usually has no symptoms until it is quite advanced. If symptoms do occur, they usually depend on where the tumor forms. Colorectal cancer may cause any of the following signs and symptoms. Check with your doctor if you see any of the following problems:

- Tumors of the rectum or lower colon may cause pain in the abdomen, constipation, or diarrhea.

- Tumors in the part of the colon on the right side of the body may cause:
  - A lump in the abdomen
  - Weight loss for no known reason
  - Loss of appetite
  - Blood in the stool

Other conditions that are not colorectal cancer may cause these same symptoms.

Familial Adenomatous Polyposis (FAP)

Familial adenomatous polyposis (FAP) is an inherited [or genetic] colon condition. It occurs anywhere from one in 7,000 to one in 22,000 live births, and is more common in Western countries. Each child of a patient with FAP has a 50 percent chance of inheriting the disease gene. Males and females are equally likely to be affected.

Classical FAP includes multiple (more than 100) adenomatous (non-cancerous) polyps in the colon and rectum developing after the first 10 years of life. People with FAP also may develop polyps in the upper gastrointestinal tract. In addition, they may have other symptoms such as congenital eye conditions, non-cancerous bone tumors, extra teeth and skin cysts.

People with FAP may have cancerous changes such as thyroid tumors, small bowel cancer, hepatoblastoma [a type of liver cancer], and brain tumors, particularly medulloblastoma.

By age 10 years, only 15 percent of FAP gene carriers have colon polyps. By age 20 years, the probability rises to 75 percent, and by age 30 years, 90 percent will show signs of FAP. Without any treatment, most individuals with FAP will develop colon cancers by the fourth decade of life, and cancers can appear much earlier.

People who carry the gene responsible for FAP or who are at risk for FAP traditionally undergo an annual lower endoscopy starting around puberty to detect polyps, so they can be removed. Because the risk of colorectal cancer is so high in FAP, some patients with the disease choose to undergo colectomy (removal of the large intestine) to remove the cancer-prone tissues.

Some people believe that children at risk should undergo genetic testing for FAP, in part so that those who do not have the FAP-related gene can be spared the yearly sigmoidoscopy. The psychological effects of genetic testing on children and at what age to do so are being researched.

Source: Excerpted and adapted from PDQ® Cancer Information Summary. National Cancer Institute; Bethesda, MD. Genetics of Colorectal Cancer (PDQ): Health professional version. Updated 05/2013. Available at: www.cancer.gov. Accessed June 1, 2013. Revised by David A. Cooke, MD, FACP, June 2013.

Diagnosis

Colorectal cancer is usually diagnosed through biopsies performed during lower endoscopy, which allows for a definite diagnosis. Once cancer has been identified, the next step is determining the extent of the cancer, known as staging.

Tests to stage colorectal cancer may include the following:

- Physical exam and history
- X-ray of the chest
- CT scan
- PET scan
- MRI
- Bone scan
- Biopsy

Other tests used to stage colorectal cancer include the following:

- **Complete Blood Count (CBC):** A procedure in which a sample of blood is drawn and checked for the following:
    - The number of red blood cells, white blood cells, and platelets
    - The amount of hemoglobin (the protein that carries oxygen) in the red blood cells.
    - The portion of the blood sample made up of red blood cells.

- **Kidney Function Test:** A test in which blood or urine samples are checked for the amounts of certain substances released by the kidneys. A higher or lower than normal amount of a substance can be a sign that the kidneys are not working the way they should. This is also called a renal function test.

- **Liver Function Test:** A blood test to measure the blood levels of certain substances released by the liver. A high or low level of certain substances can be a sign of liver disease.

- **Carcinoembryonic Antigen (CEA) Assay:** A test that measures the level of CEA in the blood. CEA is released into the bloodstream from both cancer cells and normal cells. When found in higher than normal amounts, it can be a sign of colon cancer or other conditions.

Prognosis

The prognosis (chance of recovery) depends on the following:

- Whether the entire tumor was removed by surgery

- Whether the cancer has spread to other parts of the body, such as the lymph nodes, liver, pelvis, or ovaries

Treatment

Treatment for colorectal cancer in children may include the following:

- Surgery to remove the tumor when it has not spread

- Radiation therapy and chemotherapy for tumors in the rectum or lower colon

- Combination chemotherapy

Colon Cancer Staging

If tests show an abnormal area (such as a polyp), a biopsy to check for cancer cells may be necessary. Often, the abnormal tissue can be removed during colonoscopy or sigmoidoscopy. A pathologist checks the tissue for cancer cells using a microscope.

If the biopsy shows that cancer is present, your doctor needs to know the extent (stage) of the disease to plan the best treatment. The stage is based on whether the tumor has invaded nearby tissues, whether the cancer has spread and, if so, to what parts of the body.

Doctors describe colorectal cancer by the following stages:

- **Stage 0:** The cancer is found only in the innermost lining of the colon or rectum. Carcinoma in situ is another name for Stage 0 colorectal cancer.

- **Stage I:** The tumor has grown into the inner wall of the colon or rectum. The tumor has not grown through the wall.

- **Stage II:** The tumor extends more deeply into or through the wall of the colon or rectum. It may have invaded nearby tissue, but cancer cells have not spread to the lymph nodes.

- **Stage III:** The cancer has spread to nearby lymph nodes, but not to other parts of the body.

- **Stage IV:** The cancer has spread to other parts of the body, such as the liver or lungs.

- **Recurrence:** This is cancer that has been treated and has returned after a period of time when the cancer could not be detected. The disease may return in the colon or rectum, or in another part of the body.

Source: from "What You Need To Know About™ Cancer of the Colon and Rectum," NCI, 5/26/2006 Reviewed by David A. Cooke, MD, FACP, June 2013.

Children with certain familial colon cancer syndromes may be treated with:

- Surgery to remove the colon before cancer forms
- Medicine to decrease the number of polyps in the colon

Treatment Methods

The choice of treatment depends mainly on the location of the tumor in the colon or rectum and the stage of the disease. Treatment for colorectal cancer may involve *surgery, chemotherapy, biological therapy,* or *radiation therapy.* Some people have a combination of treatments. These treatments are described below.

Colon cancer sometimes is treated differently from rectal cancer. Treatments for colon and rectal cancer are described separately below. Your doctor can describe your treatment choices and the expected results. You and your doctor can work together to develop a treatment plan that meets your needs.

Cancer treatment is either local therapy or systemic therapy:

- *Local Therapy:* Surgery and radiation therapy are local therapies. They remove or destroy cancer in or near the colon or rectum. When colorectal cancer has spread to other parts of the body, local therapy may be used to control the disease in those specific areas.
- *Systemic Therapy:* Chemotherapy and biological therapy are systemic therapies. The drugs enter the bloodstream and destroy or control cancer throughout the body.

Because cancer treatments often damage healthy cells and tissues, *side effects* are common. Side effects depend mainly on the type and extent of the treatment. Side effects may not be the same for each person, and they may change from one treatment session to the next. Before treatment starts, your health care team will explain possible side effects and suggest ways to help you manage them.

You may want to talk to your doctor about taking part in a clinical trial, a research study of new treatment methods.

Surgery: Surgery is the most common treatment for colorectal cancer:

- *Colonoscopy:* A small malignant polyp may be removed from your colon or upper rectum with a colonoscope. Some small tumors in the lower rectum can be removed through your anus without a colonoscope.
- *Laparoscopy:* Early colon cancer may be removed with the aid of a thin, lighted tube (laparoscope). Three or four tiny cuts are made into your abdomen. The surgeon sees

inside your abdomen with the laparoscope. The tumor and part of the healthy colon are removed. Nearby lymph nodes also may be removed. The surgeon checks the rest of your intestine and your liver to see if the cancer has spread.

- *Open Surgery:* The surgeon makes a large cut into your abdomen to remove the tumor and part of the healthy colon or rectum. Some nearby lymph nodes are also removed. The surgeon checks the rest of your intestine and your liver to see if the cancer has spread.

When a section of your colon or rectum is removed, the surgeon can usually reconnect the healthy parts. However, sometimes reconnection is not possible. In this case, the surgeon creates a new path for waste to leave your body. The surgeon makes an opening (stoma) in the wall of the abdomen, connects the upper end of the intestine to the stoma, and closes the other end. The operation to create the stoma is called a colostomy. A flat bag fits over the stoma to collect waste, and a special adhesive holds it in place.

For most people, the stoma is temporary. It is needed only until the colon or rectum heals from surgery. After healing takes place, the surgeon reconnects the parts of the intestine and closes the stoma. Some people, especially those with a tumor in the lower rectum, need a permanent stoma.

People who have a colostomy may have irritation of the skin around the stoma. Your doctor, your nurse, or an enterostomal therapist can teach you how to clean the area and prevent irritation and infection.

The time it takes to heal after surgery is different for each person. You may be uncomfortable for the first few days. Medicine can help control your pain. Before surgery, you should discuss the plan for pain relief with your doctor or nurse. After surgery, your doctor can adjust the plan if you need more pain relief.

It is common to feel tired or weak for a while. Also, surgery sometimes causes constipation or diarrhea. Your health care team monitors you for signs of bleeding, infection, or other problems requiring immediate treatment.

Chemotherapy: Chemotherapy uses anticancer drugs to kill cancer cells. The drugs enter the bloodstream and can affect cancer cells all over the body.

Anticancer drugs are usually given through a vein, but some may be given by mouth. You may be treated in an outpatient part of the hospital, at the doctor's office, or at home. Rarely, a hospital stay may be needed.

The side effects of chemotherapy depend mainly on the specific drugs and the dose. The drugs can harm normal cells that divide rapidly:

- *Blood Cells:* These cells fight infection, help blood to clot, and carry oxygen to all parts of your body. When drugs affect your blood cells, you are more likely to get infections, bruise or bleed easily, and feel very weak and tired.

- *Cells In Hair Roots:* Chemotherapy can cause hair loss. Your hair will grow back, but it may be somewhat different in color and texture.

- *Cells That Line The Digestive Tract:* Chemotherapy can cause poor appetite, nausea and vomiting, diarrhea, or mouth and lip sores.

Chemotherapy for colorectal cancer can cause the skin on the palms of the hands and bottoms of the feet to become red and painful. The skin may peel off.

Your health care team can suggest ways to control many of these side effects. Most side effects usually go away after treatment ends.

Biological Therapy: Some people with colorectal cancer that has spread receive a monoclonal *antibody*, a type of biological therapy. The monoclonal antibodies bind to colorectal cancer cells. They interfere with cancer cell growth and the spread of cancer. People receive monoclonal antibodies through a vein at the doctor's office, hospital, or clinic. Some people receive chemotherapy at the same time.

During treatment, your health care team will watch for signs of problems. Some people get medicine to prevent a possible allergic reaction. The side effects depend mainly on the monoclonal antibody used. Side effects may include rash, fever, abdominal pain, vomiting, diarrhea, blood pressure changes, bleeding, or breathing problems. Side effects usually become milder after the first treatment.

Radiation Therapy: Radiation therapy (also called radiotherapy) uses high-energy rays to kill cancer cells. It affects cancer cells only in the treated area.

Doctors use different types of radiation therapy to treat cancer. Sometimes people receive two types:

- *External Radiation:* The radiation comes from a machine. The most common type of machine used for radiation therapy is called a linear accelerator. Most patients go to the hospital or clinic for their treatment, generally 5 days a week for several weeks.

- *Internal Radiation (Implant Radiation Or Brachytherapy)*: The radiation comes from radioactive material placed in thin tubes put directly into or near the tumor. The patient stays in the hospital, and the implants generally remain in place for several days. Usually they are removed before the patient goes home.

- *Intraoperative Radiation Therapy (IORT):* In some cases, radiation is given during surgery.

Side effects depend mainly on the amount of radiation given and the part of your body that is treated. Radiation therapy to your abdomen and pelvis may cause nausea, vomiting, diarrhea, bloody stools, or urgent bowel movements. It also may cause urinary problems, such as being unable to stop the flow of urine from the bladder. In addition, your skin in the treated area may become red, dry, and tender. The skin near the anus is especially sensitive.

You are likely to become very tired during radiation therapy, especially in the later weeks of treatment. Resting is important, but doctors usually advise patients to try to stay as active as they can.

Although the side effects of radiation therapy can be distressing, your doctor can usually treat or control them. Also, side effects usually go away after treatment ends.

Treatment For Colon Cancer

Most patients with colon cancer are treated with surgery. Some people have both surgery and chemotherapy. Some with advanced disease get biological therapy.

A colostomy is seldom needed for people with colon cancer.

Although radiation therapy is rarely used to treat colon cancer, sometimes it is used to relieve pain and other symptoms.

Treatment For Rectal Cancer

For all stages of rectal cancer, surgery is the most common treatment. Some patients receive surgery, radiation therapy, and chemotherapy. Some with advanced disease get biological therapy.

About one out of eight people with rectal cancer needs a permanent colostomy.

Radiation therapy may be used before and after surgery. Some people have radiation therapy before surgery to shrink the tumor, and some have it after surgery to kill cancer cells that may remain in the area. At some hospitals, patients may have radiation therapy during surgery. People also may have radiation therapy to relieve pain and other problems caused by the cancer.

Rehabilitation

Rehabilitation is an important part of cancer care. Your health care team makes every effort to help you return to normal activities as soon as possible.

If you have a stoma, you need to learn to care for it. Doctors, nurses, and enterostomal therapists can help. Often, enterostomal therapists visit you before surgery to discuss what to expect. They teach you how to care for the stoma after surgery. They talk about lifestyle issues, including emotional, physical, and sexual concerns. Often they can provide information about resources and support groups.

Follow-Up Care

Follow-up care after treatment for colorectal cancer is important. Even when the cancer seems to have been completely removed or destroyed, the disease sometimes returns because undetected cancer cells remained somewhere in the body after treatment. Your doctor monitors your recovery and checks for recurrence of the cancer. Checkups help ensure that any changes in health are noted and treated if needed.

Checkups may include a physical exam (including a digital rectal exam), lab tests (including fecal occult blood test and CEA test), colonoscopy, x-rays, CT scans, or other tests.

Chapter 20

Germ Cell Tumors

Childhood Extracranial Germ Cell Tumors

There are three types of extracranial germ cell tumors.

As a fetus develops, certain cells form sperm in the testicles or eggs in the ovaries. These are called germ cells.

A germ cell can travel to other parts of the body and may turn into a rare kind of cancer called a germ cell tumor. This chapter covers germ cell tumors that occur *extracranially* (everywhere except for the brain). Extracranial germ cell tumors may be benign (not cancerous) or malignant (cancerous).

Extracranial germ cell tumors are grouped into mature teratomas, immature teratomas, or malignant germ cell tumors:

Mature Teratomas: Mature teratomas are the most common type of extracranial germ cell tumor. The cells of mature teratomas look very much like normal cells. Mature teratomas are benign and not likely to become cancer.

Immature Teratomas: Immature teratomas have cells that look very different from normal cells. Immature teratomas are not cancer. They often contain several different types of tissue such as hair, muscle, and bone.

About This Chapter: PDQ® Cancer Information Summary. National Cancer Institute; Bethesda, MD. Child Extracranial Germ Cell Tumors Treatment (PDQ): Patient version. Updated 12/2012. Available at: www.cancer.gov. Accessed May 7, 2013.

Malignant Germ Cell Tumors: Malignant germ cell tumors are cancer. The following are the three types of malignant germ cell tumors:

- **Yolk Sac Tumors:** Tumors that make a hormone called alpha-fetoprotein

- **Germinomas:** Tumors that make a hormone called beta-human chorionic gonadotropin

- **Choriocarcinomas:** Tumors that make a hormone called beta-human chorionic gonadotropin

Gonadal germ cell tumors form in the testicles or ovaries.

- **Testicular Germ Cell Tumors:** Testicular germ cell tumors usually occur before the age of four years or in teenagers and young adults.

- **Testicular Germ Cell Tumors In Teens And Young Adults:** These are different from those that form in early childhood. They are more like testicular cancer in adults. Testicular germ cell tumors are divided into two main types, seminoma and nonseminoma. Boys older than 14 years with testicular germ cell tumors are treated in pediatric cancer centers, but the treatment is similar to that used in adults.

- **Ovarian Germ Cell Tumors:** Ovarian germ cell tumors form in egg-making cells in an ovary. These tumors are more common in teen girls and young women. Most ovarian germ cell tumors are benign teratomas.

> Extracranial germ cell tumors are rare and may be benign or malignant. They are most common in teenagers 15 to 19 years old.

Extragonadal germ cell tumors form in areas other than the testicles or ovaries.

- **Extragonadal, Extracranial Germ Cell Tumors In Young Children:** Most germ cell tumors that are not in the testicles, ovaries, or brain, form along the midline of the body. Locations of these germ cell tumors include the sacrum (the triangle-shaped bone in the lower spine that forms part of the pelvis) and the coccyx (the small bone at the bottom of the spine, also called the tailbone). In younger children, extragonadal extracranial germ cell tumors usually occur at birth or in early childhood.

- **Extragonadal, Extracranial Germ Cell Tumors In Older Children, Teens, And Young Adults:** These germ cell tumors are often in the mediastinum (within the chest).

It's A Fact!

The cause of most childhood extracranial germ cell tumors is unknown.

Having certain inherited disorders can increase the risk of developing an extracranial germ cell tumor. Having a risk factor does not mean that you will get cancer; not having risk factors doesn't mean that you will not get cancer.

Possible risk factors for extracranial germ cell tumors include the following:

- Having the following genetic syndromes may increase the risk of developing childhood germ cell tumors:
  - Klinefelter syndrome may increase the risk of developing germ cell tumors in the mediastinum (within the chest).
  - Swyer syndrome may increase the risk of developing germ cell tumors in the testes or ovaries.
- Having an undescended testicle may increase the risk of developing a testicular germ cell tumor.

Signs of childhood extracranial germ cell tumors depend on the type of tumor and where it is in the body.

Different tumors may cause the following signs and symptoms. Other conditions may cause these same symptoms. Check with a doctor for any of the following problems:

- Most tumors of the sacrum and coccyx can be seen as a lump.
- A testicular tumor may cause a painless lump in the testicles.
- An ovarian germ cell tumor may cause the following symptoms:
  - Pain or a lump in the abdomen
  - Fever
  - Constipation

- No menstruation

- Unusual vaginal bleeding

Imaging studies and blood tests are used to detect (find) and diagnose childhood extracranial germ cell tumors.

Certain factors affect prognosis (chance of recovery) and treatment options.

The prognosis (chance of recovery) and treatment options depend on the following:

- The type of germ cell tumor

- Where the tumor first began to grow

- The stage of the cancer (whether it has spread to nearby areas or to other places in the body)

- Whether the tumor can be completely removed by surgery

- The patient's age and general health

- Whether the cancer has just been diagnosed or has recurred (come back)

The prognosis for childhood extracranial germ cell tumors, especially ovarian germ cell tumors, is good.

Stages Of Childhood Extracranial Germ Cell Tumors

After a childhood extracranial germ cell tumor has been diagnosed, tests are done to find out if cancer cells have spread from where the tumor started to nearby areas or to other parts of the body.

The process used to find out if cancer has spread from where the tumor started to other parts of the body is called staging. The information gathered from the staging process determines the stage of the disease. It is important to know the stage in order to plan treatment.

The following stages are commonly used for childhood nonseminoma testicular germ cell tumors:

- **Stage I:** Cancer is found only in the testicle and is completely removed by surgery. Tumor marker levels return to normal after surgery.

- **Stage II:** Cancer is removed by surgery and some cancer cells remain in the scrotum or cancer that can only be seen with a microscope has spread to the scrotum or spermatic cord. Tumor marker levels do not return to normal after surgery and may increase.

- **Stage III:** Cancer has spread to one or more lymph nodes in the abdomen and is not completely removed by surgery. The cancer that remains after surgery can be seen without a microscope.

- **Stage IV:** Cancer has spread to distant parts of the body such as the liver.

The following stages may be used for childhood ovarian germ cell tumors:

- **Stage I:** Cancer is in the ovary and can be completely removed by surgery.

- **Stage II:** In stage II, one of the following is true:

  - Cancer is not completely removed by surgery. The remaining cancer can be seen with a microscope only.

  - Cancer has spread to the lymph nodes and can be seen with a microscope only.

  - Cancer has spread to the capsule (outer covering) of the ovary.

- **Stage III:** In stage III, one of the following is true:

  - Cancer is not completely removed by surgery. The remaining cancer can be seen without a microscope.

  - Cancer has spread to lymph nodes and the lymph nodes are 2 centimeters or larger.

  - Cancer is found in fluid in the abdomen.

- **Stage IV:** Cancer has spread to the lung, liver, brain, or bone.

The following stages are commonly used for extragonadal extracranial germ cell tumors:

- **Stage I:** Cancer is in one place and can be completely removed by surgery. For tumors at the base of the tailbone, the cancer and tailbone are completed removed by surgery. Tumor marker levels return to normal after surgery.

- **Stage II:** Cancer has spread to nearby tissues and/or lymph nodes and is not completely removed by surgery. The cancer remaining after surgery can be seen with a microscope only. Tumor marker levels do not return to normal after surgery and may increase.

- **Stage III:** In stage III, one of the following is true:

  - Cancer is not completely removed by surgery. The cancer remaining after surgery can be seen without a microscope.

  - Cancer has spread to lymph nodes and is larger than 2 centimeters in diameter.

- **Stage IV:** Cancer has spread to distant parts of the body, including the liver.

- **Recurrent:** Recurrent childhood extracranial germ cell tumor is cancer that has recurred (come back) after it has been treated. The cancer may come back in the same place or in other parts of the body.

Treatment

Different types of treatments are available for children with extracranial germ cell tumors. Some treatments are standard (the currently used treatment), and some are being tested in clinical trials. A treatment clinical trial is a research study meant to help improve current treatments or obtain information on new treatments for patients with cancer. When clinical trials show that a new treatment is better than the standard treatment, the new treatment may become the standard treatment.

Because cancer in children is rare, taking part in a clinical trial should be considered. Some clinical trials are open only to patients who have not started treatment.

Treatment will be overseen by a pediatric oncologist, a doctor who specializes in treating children with cancer. The pediatric oncologist works with other health care providers who are experts in treating children with extracranial germ cell tumors and who specialize in certain areas of medicine. These may include the following specialists: pediatric surgeon pediatric hematologist, radiation oncologist, pediatric nurse specialist, and others.

Three types of standard treatment listed below are used:

- **Surgery:** Surgery to completely remove the tumor is done whenever possible. If the tumor is very large, chemotherapy may be given first, to make the tumor smaller and decrease the amount of tissue that needs to be removed during surgery.

- **Watchful Waiting:** Watchful waiting is closely monitoring a patient's condition without giving any treatment until symptoms appear or change. For childhood extracranial germ cell tumors, this includes physical exams, imaging tests, and tumor marker tests.

- **Chemotherapy:** Chemotherapy is a cancer treatment that uses drugs to stop the growth of cancer cells, either by killing the cells or by stopping them from dividing.

Children with extracranial germ cell tumors should have their treatment planned by a team of health care providers who are experts in treating cancer in children.

Taking Part In A Clinical Trial

For some patients, taking part in a clinical trial may be the best treatment choice. Clinical trials are part of the cancer research process. Clinical trials are done to find out if new cancer treatments are safe and effective or better than the standard treatment.

Many of today's standard treatments for cancer are based on earlier clinical trials. Patients who take part in a clinical trial may receive the standard treatment or be among the first to receive a new treatment.

Patients who take part in clinical trials also help improve the way cancer will be treated in the future. Even when clinical trials do not lead to effective new treatments, they often answer important questions and help move research forward.

Patients can enter clinical trials before, during, or after starting their cancer treatment.

Some clinical trials only include patients who have not yet received treatment. Other trials test treatments for patients whose cancer has not gotten better. There are also clinical trials that test new ways to stop cancer from recurring (coming back) or reduce the side effects of cancer treatment.

Chapter 21

Leukemia

What You Need To Know About Leukemia

What is leukemia?

Leukemia is cancer that starts in the tissue that forms blood. To understand cancer, it helps to know how normal blood cells form.

Most blood cells develop from cells in the bone marrow called stem cells. Bone marrow is the soft material in the center of most bones. Stem cells mature into different kinds of blood cells. Each kind has a special job:

- White blood cells help fight infection. There are several types of white blood cells.

- Red blood cells carry oxygen to tissues throughout the body.

- Platelets help form blood clots that control bleeding.

Stem cells can mature into different types of white blood cells. First, a stem cell matures into either a myeloid stem cell or a lymphoid stem cell:

- A myeloid stem cell matures into a myeloid blast. The blast can form a red blood cell, platelets, or one of several types of white blood cells.

About This Chapter: Text in this chapter is excerpted from the following documents "What You Need to Know About Leukemia," National Cancer Institute, November 25, 2008; PDQ® Cancer Information Summary. National Cancer Institute; Bethesda, MD. Childhood Acute Lymphoblastic Leukemia Treatment (PDQ): Patient version. Updated 03/2013. Available at: www.cancer.gov. Accessed May 9, 2013; and PDQ® Cancer Information Summary. National Cancer Institute; Bethesda, MD. Childhood Acute Myeloid Leukemia/Other Myeloid Malignancies Treatment (PDQ): Patient version. Updated 04/2013. Available at: www.cancer.gov. Accessed May 9, 2013. Revised by David A. Cooke, MD, FACP, June 2013.

- A lymphoid stem cell matures into a lymphoid blast. The blast can form one of several types of white blood cells, such as B cells or T cells. The white blood cells that form from myeloid blasts are different from the white blood cells that form from lymphoid blasts.

In a person with leukemia, genetically abnormal strains of bone marrow stem cells produce abnormal white blood cells. The abnormal cells are leukemia cells. Unlike normal blood cells, leukemia cells don't die when they should. They may crowd out normal white blood cells, red blood cells, and platelets. This makes it hard for normal blood cells to do their work.

What are different types of leukemia?

The types of leukemia can be grouped based on how quickly the disease develops and gets worse.

Leukemia is either chronic (which usually gets worse slowly) or acute (which usually gets worse quickly):

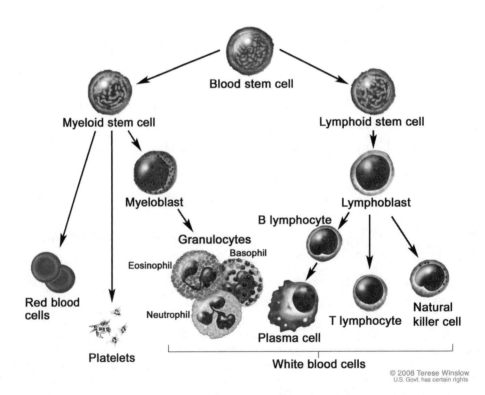

© 2008 Terese Winslow
U.S. Govt. has certain rights

Figure 21.1. Blood cells maturing from stem cells. (Source: © 2008 Terese Winslow, U.S. Govt. has certain rights.)

- **Chronic Leukemia:** Early in the disease, the leukemic bone marrow cells are only a small proportion of the marrow, so most of the white cells in the blood come from normal marrow. People may not have any symptoms at first. Doctors often find chronic leukemia during a routine checkup—before there are any symptoms. Slowly, chronic leukemia gets worse. As the number of leukemia cells in the marrow increases, the normal marrow is crowded out. People may begin to get symptoms, such as swollen lymph nodes or infections related to excessive leukemic cells or inadequate numbers of normal white cells. When symptoms do appear, they are usually mild at first and get worse gradually.

- **Acute Leukemia:** The leukemic marrow cells have different genetic mutations than in the chronic forms that result in very aggressive cancers. Abnormal marrow cells divide rapidly and take over the bone marrow. The number of leukemia cells in the blood increases rapidly. Acute leukemia usually worsens quickly.

The types of leukemia also can be grouped based on the type of white blood cell that is affected. Leukemia can start in lymphoid cells or myeloid cells. Leukemia that affects lymphoid cells is called lymphoid, lymphocytic, or lymphoblastic leukemia. Leukemia that affects myeloid cells is called myeloid, myelogenous, or myeloblastic leukemia.

There are four common types of leukemia:

- **Chronic Lymphocytic Leukemia (CLL):** CLL affects lymphoid cells and usually grows slowly. It accounts for more than 15,000 new cases of leukemia each year. Most often, people diagnosed with the disease are over age 55. It almost never affects children.

- **Chronic Myeloid Leukemia (CML):** CML affects myeloid cells and usually grows slowly at first. It accounts for nearly 5,000 new cases of leukemia each year. It mainly affects adults.

- **Acute Lymphocytic (Lymphoblastic) Leukemia (ALL):** ALL affects lymphoid cells and grows quickly. It accounts for more than 5,000 new cases of leukemia each year. ALL is the most common type of leukemia in young children. It also affects adults.

- **Acute Myeloid Leukemia (AML):** AML affects myeloid cells and grows quickly. It accounts for more than 13,000 new cases of leukemia each year. It occurs in both adults and children.

Hairy cell leukemia is a rare type of chronic leukemia. Hairy cell leukemia and other rare types of leukemia account for fewer than 6,000 new cases of leukemia each year.

What are the risk factors for leukemia?

No one knows the exact causes of leukemia. Doctors seldom know why one person gets leukemia and another doesn't. However, research shows that certain risk factors increase the chance that a person will get this disease. The risk factors may be different for the different types of leukemia:

- **Radiation:** People exposed to very high levels of radiation are much more likely than others to get acute myeloid leukemia, chronic myeloid leukemia, or acute lymphocytic leukemia. Very high levels of radiation have been caused by atomic bomb explosions (such as those in Japan during World War II). People, especially children, who survive atomic bomb explosions are at increased risk of leukemia. Another source of exposure to high levels of radiation is medical treatment for cancer and other conditions. Radiation therapy for cancer can increase the risk of later developing leukemia. Dental x-rays and other diagnostic x-rays (such as CT scans) expose people to much lower levels of radiation. It's not known yet whether this low level of radiation to children or adults is linked to leukemia. Researchers are studying whether having many x-rays may increase the risk of leukemia. They are also studying whether CT scans during childhood are linked with increased risk of developing leukemia.

- **Smoking:** Smoking cigarettes increases the risk of acute myeloid leukemia.

- **Benzene:** Exposure to benzene in the workplace can cause acute myeloid leukemia. It may also cause chronic myeloid leukemia or acute lymphocytic leukemia. Benzene is used widely in the chemical industry. It's also found in cigarette smoke and gasoline.

- **Chemotherapy:** Cancer patients treated with certain types of cancer-fighting drugs sometimes later get acute myeloid leukemia or acute lymphocytic leukemia. For example, being treated with drugs known as alkylating agents or topoisomerase inhibitors is linked with a small chance of later developing acute leukemia.

- **Inherited Diseases:** Down syndrome and certain other inherited diseases increase the risk of developing acute leukemia.

- **Blood Disorders:** People with certain blood disorders are at increased risk of acute myeloid leukemia.

- **HTLV-1 Infection:** People with human T-cell leukemia virus type 1 (HTLV-1) infection are at increased risk of a rare type of leukemia known as adult T-cell leukemia. Although the HTLV-1 virus may cause this rare disease, adult T-cell leukemia and other types of leukemia are not contagious.

- **Family History of Leukemia:** It's rare for more than one person in a family to have leukemia. When it does happen, it's most likely to involve chronic lymphocytic leukemia. However, only a few people with chronic lymphocytic leukemia have a father, mother, brother, sister, or child who also has the disease.

Having one or more risk factors does not mean that a person will get leukemia. Most people who have risk factors never develop the disease.

Childhood Acute Lymphoblastic Leukemia

Childhood acute lymphoblastic leukemia (ALL) is a type of cancer in which the bone marrow makes too many immature lymphocytes (a type of white blood cell). This type of cancer usually gets worse quickly if it is not treated.

ALL is the most common type of cancer in children.

ALL is due to genetic mutations lymphoid stem cells or precursor cells. Ordinarily, a lymphoid stem cell becomes a lymphoblast cell, and then transforms into one of three types of lymphocytes (white blood cells):

- B lymphocytes that make antibodies to help fight infection
- T lymphocytes that help B lymphocytes make the antibodies that help fight infection
- Natural killer cells that attack cancer cells and viruses

In ALL, the lymphoid precursor cells do not transform normally into lymphocytes, or result in lymphocytes that do not function as they should.

What are possible signs of childhood ALL?

Possible signs of childhood ALL include fever and bruising, due to low levels of normally functioning cells in the blood. These and other symptoms may be caused by childhood ALL. Other conditions may cause the same symptoms. Check with your doctor for any of the following problems:

- Fever
- Easy bruising or bleeding
- Petechiae (flat, pinpoint, dark-red spots under the skin caused by bleeding)
- Bone or joint pain
- Painless lumps in the neck, underarm, stomach, or groin

- Pain or feeling of fullness below the ribs

- Weakness, feeling tired, or looking pale

- Loss of appetite

What tests are used to detect and diagnose childhood ALL?

Tests that examine the blood and bone marrow are used to detect (find) and diagnose childhood ALL. The following tests and procedures may be used:

- **Physical Exam And History:** This is exam of the body to check general signs of health, including checking for signs of disease, such as lumps or anything else that seems unusual. A history of the patient's health habits and past illnesses and treatments will also be taken.

- **Complete Blood Count (CBC) With Differential:** CBC with differential is a procedure in which a sample of blood is drawn and checked for the following:

  - Number of red blood cells and platelets

  - Number and type of white blood cells

  - Amount of hemoglobin (the protein that carries oxygen) in the red blood cells

  - Portion of the sample made up of red blood cells

- **Bone Marrow Aspiration And Biopsy:** This procedure is the removal of bone marrow, blood, and a small piece of bone by inserting a hollow needle into the hipbone or breastbone. A pathologist views the bone marrow, blood, and bone under a microscope to look for signs of cancer.

- **Cytogenetic Analysis:** In this laboratory test, cells in a sample of blood or bone marrow are viewed under a microscope to look for certain changes in the chromosomes in the lymphocytes. For example, in Philadelphia chromosome-positive ALL, part of one chromosome is moved to another chromosome. This is called the "Philadelphia chromosome." Other tests, such as fluorescence in situ hybridization (FISH), may also be done to look for certain changes in the chromosomes.

- **Immunophenotyping:** In this test, cells in a sample of blood or bone marrow are looked at under a microscope to find out if malignant lymphocytes (cancer) began from the B lymphocytes or the T lymphocytes.

- **Blood Chemistry Studies:** In this procedure, a blood sample is checked to measure the amounts of certain substances released into the blood by organs and tissues in the body.

An unusual (higher or lower than normal) amount of a substance can be a sign of disease in the organ or tissue that makes it.

- **Chest X-Ray:** An x-ray is taken of the organs and bones inside the chest.

Which factors affect chance of recovery and treatment options?

The prognosis (chance of recovery) depends on these factors:

- Age at diagnosis, gender, and race
- The number of white blood cells at diagnosis
- Whether the leukemia cells began from B lymphocytes or T lymphocytes
- Whether there are certain changes in the chromosomes of lymphocytes.
- Whether the child has Down syndrome
- Whether the leukemia has spread to the brain, spinal cord, or testicles
- How quickly and how low the leukemia cell count drops after initial treatment

The treatment options depend on the following:

- Whether the leukemia cells began from B lymphocytes or T lymphocytes
- Whether the child has standard-risk or high-risk ALL
- The age of the child at diagnosis
- Whether there are certain changes in the chromosomes of lymphocytes, such as the Philadelphia chromosome

Once childhood ALL has been diagnosed, tests are done to find out if the cancer has spread to the brain, spinal cord, testicles, or to other parts of the body.

What are the three phases of childhood ALL treatment?

- **Induction Therapy:** This is the first phase of treatment. The goal is to kill the leukemia cells in the blood and bone marrow. This puts the leukemia into remission. This is also called the remission induction phase.

- **Consolidation/Intensification Therapy:** This is the second phase of therapy. It begins once the leukemia is in remission. The goal of consolidation/intensification therapy is to kill any remaining leukemia cells that may not be active but could begin to regrow and cause a relapse.

- **Maintenance Therapy:** This is the third phase of treatment. The goal is to kill any remaining leukemia cells that may regrow and cause a relapse. Often the cancer treatments are given in lower doses than those used for induction and consolidation/intensification therapy. This is also called the continuation therapy phase.

What standard treatments are used for ALL?

Four types of standard treatment are used: chemotherapy, radiation therapy, chemotherapy with stem cell transplant, and targeted therapy.

Chemotherapy: Chemotherapy is a cancer treatment that uses drugs to stop the growth of cancer cells, either by killing the cells or by stopping them from dividing. When chemotherapy is taken by mouth or injected into a vein or muscle, the drugs enter the bloodstream and can reach cancer cells throughout the body (systemic chemotherapy). When chemotherapy is placed directly into the cerebrospinal fluid (intrathecal), an organ, or a body cavity such as the abdomen, the drugs mainly affect cancer cells in those areas (regional chemotherapy). Combination chemotherapy is treatment using more than one anticancer drug.

The way the chemotherapy is given depends on the child's risk group. Children with high-risk ALL receive more anticancer drugs, higher doses of anticancer drugs, and receive treatment for a longer time than children with standard-risk ALL.

Radiation Therapy: Radiation therapy is a cancer treatment that uses high-energy x-rays or other types of radiation to kill cancer cells or keep them from growing. There are two types of radiation therapy. External radiation therapy uses a machine outside the body to send radiation toward the cancer. Internal radiation therapy uses a radioactive substance sealed in needles, seeds, wires, or catheters that are placed directly into or near the cancer. External radiation therapy may be used to treat childhood ALL that has spread, or may spread, to the brain and spinal cord.

Chemotherapy With Stem Cell Transplant: Stem cell transplant is a method of giving high doses of chemotherapy and sometimes radiation therapy, and then replacing the blood-forming cells destroyed by the cancer treatment. Stem cells (immature blood cells) are removed from the blood or bone marrow of a donor. After the patient receives treatment, the donor's stem cells are given to the patient through an infusion. These re-infused stem cells grow into (and restore) the patient's blood cells. The stem cell donor doesn't have to be related to the patient.

Leukemia Treatment Team

Children with leukemia should have their treatment planned by a team of doctors with expertise in treating childhood leukemia. Treatment will be overseen by a pediatric oncologist, a doctor who specializes in treating children with cancer. The pediatric oncologist works with other pediatric health professionals who are experts in treating children with leukemia and who specialize in certain areas of medicine. These may include the following specialists:

- Hematologist
- Medical oncologist
- Pediatric surgeon
- Radiation oncologist
- Neurologist
- Pathologist
- Radiologist
- Pediatric nurse specialist
- Social worker
- Rehabilitation specialist
- Psychologist

Regular follow-up exams are very important. Treatment can cause side effects long after it has ended. These are called late effects. Radiation therapy to the brain may cause changes in mood, feelings, thinking, learning, or memory.

Source: Excerpted from "Childhood Acute Lymphoblastic Leukemia Treatment (PDQ®)," National Cancer Institute. Updated March 6, 2013.

Stem cell transplant is rarely used as initial treatment for children and teenagers with ALL. It is used more often as part of treatment for ALL that relapses (comes back after treatment).

Targeted Therapy: Targeted therapy is a treatment that uses drugs or other substances to identify and attack specific cancer cells without harming normal cells.

Tyrosine kinase inhibitors (TKIs) are targeted therapy drugs that block the enzyme, tyrosine kinase, which causes stem cells to become more white blood cells or blasts than the body needs. For example, imatinib mesylate (Gleevec) is a TKI used in the treatment of children with Philadelphia chromosome-positive ALL.

New kinds of targeted therapies are also being studied in the treatment of childhood ALL.

Childhood Acute Myeloid Leukemia And Other Myeloid Malignancies

What is childhood acute myeloid leukemia?

Childhood acute myeloid leukemia (AML) is a type of cancer in which the bone marrow makes a large number of abnormal blood cells. Cancers that are acute usually get worse quickly if they are not treated. Cancers that are chronic usually get worse slowly. Acute myeloid leukemia (AML) is also called acute myelogenous leukemia, acute myeloblastic leukemia, acute granulocytic leukemia, or acute nonlymphocytic leukemia.

In AML, the myeloid stem cells usually become a type of immature white blood cell called myeloblasts (or myeloid blasts). The myeloblasts, or leukemia cells, in AML are abnormal and do not become healthy white blood cells. The leukemia cells can build up in the blood and bone marrow so there is less room for healthy white blood cells, red blood cells, and platelets. When this happens, infection, anemia, or easy bleeding may occur. The leukemia cells can spread outside the blood to other parts of the body, including the central nervous system (brain and spinal cord), skin, and gums. Sometimes leukemia cells form a solid tumor called a granulocytic sarcoma or chloroma.

There are subtypes of AML based on the type of blood cell that is affected. The treatment of AML is different when it is a subtype called acute promyelocytic leukemia (APL) or when the child has Down syndrome.

What are risk factors for developing myeloid malignancies?

Risk factors for developing childhood AML, childhood CML, JMML, TMD, and MDS are similar. Possible risk factors include the following:

- Having a brother or sister, especially a twin, with leukemia

- Being Hispanic

- Being exposed to cigarette smoke or alcohol before birth

- Having a history of MDS or aplastic anemia

- Past treatment with chemotherapy or radiation therapy

- Being exposed to ionizing radiation or chemicals such as benzene

- Having certain genetic disorders, such as Down syndrome, Fanconi anemia, neurofibromatosis type 1, Noonan syndrome, and Shwachman-Diamond syndrome

What are symptoms of AML and other myeloid malignancies?

Possible signs of childhood AML, childhood CML, JMML, or MDS include fever, feeling tired, and easy bleeding or bruising.

These and other symptoms may be caused by childhood AML, childhood CML, JMML, or MDS. Other conditions may cause the same symptoms. Check with a doctor for the following problems:

- Fever with or without an infection
- Night sweats
- Shortness of breath

It's A Fact!

Myeloid diseases can affect the blood and bone marrow.

Chronic Myelogenous Leukemia: In chronic myelogenous leukemia (CML), too many bone marrow stem cells become a type of white blood cell called granulocytes. Some of these bone marrow stem cells never become mature white blood cells. These are called blasts. Over time, the granulocytes and blasts crowd out the red blood cells and platelets in the bone marrow. CML is rare in children.

Juvenile Myelomonocytic Leukemia: Juvenile myelomonocytic leukemia (JMML) is a rare childhood cancer that occurs more often in children around the age of two years. In JMML, too many bone marrow stem cells become two types of white blood cells called myelocytes and monocytes. Some of these bone marrow stem cells never become mature white blood cells. These immature cells, called blasts, are unable to do their usual work. Over time, the myelocytes, monocytes, and blasts crowd out the red blood cells and platelets in the bone marrow. When this happens, infection, anemia, or easy bleeding may occur.

Transient Myeloproliferative Disorder: Transient myeloproliferative disorder (TMD) is a disorder of the bone marrow that can develop in newborns who have Down syndrome. This disorder usually goes away on its own within the first three weeks of life. Infants who have Down syndrome and TMD have an increased chance of developing AML before the age of three years.

Myelodysplastic Syndromes: In myelodysplastic syndromes (MDS), the bone marrow makes too few red blood cells, white blood cells, and platelets. These blood cells may not mature and enter the blood. The treatment for MDS depends on how much lower than normal the number of red blood cells, white blood cells, or platelets is. MDS may progress to AML.

Source: Excerpted from "Childhood Acute Myeloid Leukemia/Other Myeloid Malignancies Treatment (PDQ®)," National Cancer Institute. Updated April 4, 2013.

- Weakness or feeling tired

- Easy bruising or bleeding

- Petechiae

- Pain in the bones or joints

- Pain or feeling of fullness below the ribs

- Painless lumps in the neck, underarm, stomach, groin, or other parts of the body. When seen in childhood AML, these lumps, called leukemia cutis, may be blue or purple.

- Painless lumps that are sometimes around the eyes. These lumps, called chloromas, are sometimes seen in childhood AML and may be blue-green.

- An eczema-like skin rash

Which factors affect chance of recovery and treatment options for childhood AML?

The prognosis (chance of recovery) and treatment options for childhood AML depend on the following:

- Age of the child at diagnosis

- Race or ethnic group of the child

- Whether the child is greatly overweight

- Number of white blood cells in the blood at diagnosis

- Whether the AML was caused by previous anticancer treatment

- The subtype of AML

- Whether there are certain chromosome or gene changes in the leukemia cells

- Whether the child has Down syndrome. Most children with AML and Down syndrome can be cured of their leukemia.

- Whether the child has leukemia in the central nervous system (brain and spinal cord)

- How quickly the leukemia responds to initial treatment

- Whether the AML is newly diagnosed or has recurred (come back) after being treated

- The length of time since treatment ended, for AML that has recurred

What about recovery and treatment for CML?

The prognosis and treatment options for childhood CML depend on how long it has been since the patient was diagnosed and how many blast cells are in the blood.

How is treatment planned for childhood acute myeloid leukemia?

In childhood acute myeloid leukemia (AML), the subtype of AML and whether the leukemia has spread outside the blood and bone marrow are used, instead of the stage, to plan treatment. The following tests and procedures may be used to determine if the leukemia has spread:

- **Lumbar Puncture:** This procedure is used to collect cerebrospinal fluid (CSF) from the spinal column. This is done by placing a needle into the spinal column. This procedure is also called an LP or spinal tap.

- **Biopsy:** Biopsy is the removal of cells or tissues from the testicles, ovaries, or skin so they can be viewed under a microscope to check for signs of cancer. This is done only if something unusual about the testicles, ovaries, or skin is found during the physical exam.

What standard treatments are used for childhood AML and other myeloid malignancies?

Seven types of standard treatment are used for childhood AML, childhood CML, JMML, TMD, or MDS. The way the chemotherapy is given depends on the type of cancer being treated.

Chemotherapy: In AML, the leukemia cells may spread to the brain and/or spinal cord. Anticancer drugs given by mouth or vein to treat AML cannot cross the blood-brain barrier and enter the fluid that surrounds the brain and spinal cord. Instead, an anticancer drug is injected into the fluid-filled space to kill leukemia cells that may have spread there (intrathecal chemotherapy).

Radiation: As with other types of leukemia, internal or external radiation may be used. External radiation therapy may be used to treat childhood AML that has spread, or may spread, to the brain and spinal cord. When used this way, it is called central nervous system (CNS) sanctuary therapy or CNS prophylaxis.

Stem Cell Transplant: Stem cell transplant is sometimes used with myeloid malignancies.

Targeted Therapy With A Tyrosine Kinase Inhibitor: Imatinib (Gleevec) is one of the TKIs used to treat childhood CML. TKIs may be used in combination with other anticancer drugs as adjuvant therapy (treatment given after the initial treatment, to lower the risk that the cancer will come back).

Other Drug Therapy: Lenalidomide may be used to lessen the need for transfusions in patients who have myelodysplastic syndromes caused by a specific chromosome change.

Arsenic trioxide and all-trans retinoic acid (ATRA) are anticancer drugs that kill leukemia cells, stop the leukemia cells from dividing, or help the leukemia cells mature into white blood cells. These drugs are used in the treatment of a subtype of AML called acute promyelocytic leukemia (APL).

Watchful Waiting: Watchful waiting is closely monitoring a patient's condition without giving any treatment until symptoms appear or change. It is sometimes used to treat MDS or TMD.

Are new treatments being tested?

Patients may want to think about taking part in a clinical trial.

For some patients, taking part in a clinical trial may be the best treatment choice. Clinical trials are part of the cancer research process. Clinical trials are done to find out if new cancer treatments are safe and effective or better than the standard treatment.

Information on new clinical trials is available at the National Cancer Institute website at http://cancer.gov/clinicaltrials.

It's A Fact!

Supportive care is given to lessen the problems caused by the disease or its treatment. Supportive care may include the following:

- Transfusion therapy: Transfusion is a way of giving red blood cells, white blood cells, or platelets to replace blood cells destroyed by disease or cancer treatment. The blood may be donated from another person or it may have been taken from the person earlier and stored until needed.

- Drug therapy, such as antibiotics.

- Leukapheresis: Leukapheresis is a procedure in which a special machine is used to remove white blood cells from the blood. Blood is taken from the patient and put through a blood cell separator where the white blood cells are removed. The rest of the blood is then returned to the patient's bloodstream.

Source: Excerpted from "Childhood Acute Myeloid Leukemia/Other Myeloid Malignancies Treatment (PDQ®)," National Cancer Institute. Updated April 4, 2013.

Chapter 22

Lymphoma

Childhood Hodgkin Lymphoma

What is childhood Hodgkin lymphoma?

Childhood Hodgkin lymphoma is a type of cancer that develops in the lymph system, which is part of the body's immune system. The lymph system includes the following:

- **Lymph:** Colorless, watery fluid that travels through the lymph system and carries white blood cells called lymphocytes. Lymphocytes protect the body against infections and the growth of tumors.

- **Lymph Vessels:** A network of thin tubes that collect lymph from different parts of the body and return it to the bloodstream.

- **Lymph Nodes:** Small, bean-shaped structures that filter lymph and store white blood cells that help fight infection and disease. Lymph nodes are located along the network of lymph vessels found throughout the body. Clusters of lymph nodes are found in the underarm, pelvis, neck, abdomen, and groin.

- **Thymus:** An organ in which lymphocytes grow and multiply. The thymus is in the chest behind the breastbone.

About This Chapter: This chapter includes information from the following documents: PDQ® Cancer Information Summary. National Cancer Institute; Bethesda, MD. Childhood Hodgkin Lymphoma Treatment (PDQ): Patient version. Updated 01/2013; and, PDQ® Cancer Information Summary. National Cancer Institute; Bethesda, MD. Childhood Non-Hodgkin Lymphoma Treatment (PDQ): Patient version. Updated 3/2013. Both available at: www.cancer.gov. Accessed May 11, 2013.

Other parts of the lymph system include the spleen, tonsils, and bone marrow.

Because lymph tissue is found throughout the body, Hodgkin lymphoma can start in almost any part of the body and spread to almost any tissue or organ in the body.

Lymphomas are divided into two general types: Hodgkin lymphoma and non-Hodgkin lymphoma. Hodgkin lymphoma often occurs in teens (age 15 to 19). The treatment for children and teens may be different than treatment for adults.

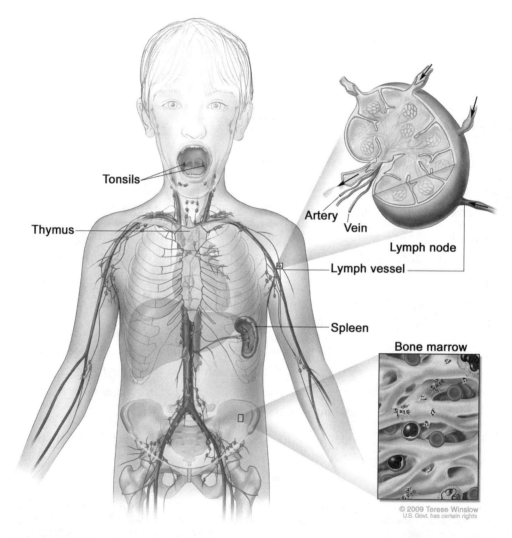

Figure 22.1. Anatomy of the lymph system. (Source: © 2008 Terese Winslow, U.S. Govt. has certain rights.)

Why do people develop childhood Hodgkin lymphoma?

Anything that increases your risk of getting a disease is called a risk factor. Having a risk factor does not mean that you will get cancer; not having risk factors doesn't mean that you will not get cancer. Risk factors for childhood Hodgkin lymphoma include the following:

- Being infected with the Epstein-Barr virus

- Being infected with the human immunodeficiency virus (HIV)

- Having certain inherited diseases of the immune system

- Having a personal history of mononucleosis ("mono")

Being exposed to common infections before the age of five may decrease the risk of Hodgkin lymphoma in children because of the effect it has on the immune system.

What are the symptoms of childhood Hodgkin lymphoma?

These and other symptoms may be caused by childhood Hodgkin lymphoma or by other conditions. Check with a doctor for any of the following problems:

- Painless, swollen lymph nodes in the neck, chest, underarm, or groin

- Fever for no known reason

- Weight loss for no known reason

- Night sweats

- Fatigue

- Anorexia

- Itchy skin

It's A Fact!

There are two types of childhood Hodgkin lymphoma.

- **Classical Hodgkin Lymphoma:** The most common type of Hodgkin lymphoma is the classical type.
- **Nodular Lymphocyte-Predominant Hodgkin Lymphoma:** This is a rare type of Hodgkin lymphoma. It is marked by the presence of an abnormal cell called a popcorn cell.

Source: NCI, January 30, 2013.

- Pain in the lymph nodes after drinking alcohol

Fever, weight loss, and night sweats are called B symptoms.

How is childhood Hodgkin lymphoma diagnosed?

If you have symptoms such as swollen lymph nodes or other signs that suggest Hodgkin lymphoma, your doctor may perform a physical exam, ask about your medical and family history, order blood tests, or have chest x-rays or other imaging procedures done.

However, a biopsy is the definitive way to diagnose childhood Hodgkin lymphoma. This is the removal of all or part of a lymph node. It is removed during one of the following procedures:

- **Thoracoscopy**: This is an exam of the inside of the chest, using a thoracoscope. A thoracoscope is a thin, tube-like instrument with a light and a lens for viewing.

- **Mediastinoscopy:** In this procedure, a scope is used to examine the organs in the area between the lungs and nearby lymph nodes.

- **Laparoscopy:** This procedure uses a laparoscope, inserted through the abdominal wall, to examine the inside of the abdomen.

Excisional biopsy is removal of an entire lymph node. Incisional biopsy is the removal of part of a lymph node. Core biopsy is the removal of tissue from a lymph node using a wide needle. Fine-needle aspiration biopsy is the removal tissue from a lymph node using a fine needle.

A pathologist views the tissue under a microscope to look for cancer cells, especially Reed-Sternberg cells. Reed-Sternberg cells are large, abnormal lymphocytes that may contain more than one nucleus. These cells are found in Hodgkin lymphoma.

Immunophenotyping may be done on tissue that was removed: This is a test in which the cells in a sample of blood or bone marrow are looked at under a microscope to find out what type of malignant (cancerous) lymphocytes are causing the lymphoma.

What affects chances of recovery and treatment options?

The prognosis (chance of recovery) and treatment options depend on the stage of the cancer, the size of the tumor, the type of the Hodgkin's lymphoma, and whether there are B symptoms at diagnosis. Other factors include certain features of the cancer cells, whether there are too many white blood cells or too few red blood cells at diagnosis, how well the tumor responds to initial treatment with chemotherapy, and whether the cancer is newly diagnosis or has recurred (come back).

> ## Remember!
>
> Most children and teenagers with newly diagnosed Hodgkin lymphoma can be cured.
>
> Source: NCI, January 30, 2013.

What is staging?

After childhood Hodgkin lymphoma has been diagnosed, tests are done to find out if cancer cells have spread within the lymph system or to other parts of the body.

The process used to find out if cancer has spread within the lymph system or to other parts of the body is called staging. The information gathered from the staging process determines the stage of the disease. Treatment is based on the stage and other factors that affect prognosis. The following tests and procedures may be used in the staging process:

- **CT Scan:** A computer linked to an x-ray machine makes a series of detailed pictures of areas inside the body, such as the neck, chest, abdomen, and pelvis. A dye may be injected into a vein or swallowed to help the organs or tissues show up more clearly.

- **Positron Emission Tomography (PET) Scan:** A small amount of radioactive glucose (sugar) is injected into a vein. The PET scanner rotates around the body and makes a picture of where glucose is being used in the body. Malignant tumor cells show up brighter in the picture because they are more active and take up more glucose than normal cells do.

- **Magnetic Resonance Imaging (MRI):** A magnet, radio waves, and a computer are used to make a series of detailed pictures of areas inside the body.

- **Bone Marrow Aspiration And Biopsy:** The doctor inserts a hollow needle into the hipbone or breastbone to remove bone marrow, blood, and a small piece of bone by. A pathologist views the bone marrow, blood, and bone under a microscope to look for abnormal cells.

The following stages are used for childhood Hodgkin lymphoma:

- **Stage I:** Cancer is found in one of the following places in the lymph system:

  - One or more lymph nodes in one lymph node group

  - Waldeyer's ring

- Thymus

- Spleen

- **Stage IE:** Cancer is found outside the lymph system in one organ or area.

- **Stage II:** Cancer is found in two or more lymph node groups either above or below the diaphragm (the thin muscle below the lungs that helps breathing and separates the chest from the abdomen).

- **Stage IIE:** Cancer is found in one or more lymph node groups either above or below the diaphragm and outside the lymph nodes in a nearby organ or area.

- **Stage III:** Cancer is found in lymph node groups above and below the diaphragm (the thin muscle below the lungs that helps breathing and separates the chest from the abdomen).

- **Stage IIIE:** Cancer is found in lymph node groups above and below the diaphragm and outside the lymph nodes in a nearby organ or area.

- **Stage IIIS:** Cancer is found in lymph node groups above and below the diaphragm, and in the spleen.

- **Stage IIIE,S:** Cancer is found in lymph node groups above and below the diaphragm, outside the lymph nodes in a nearby organ or area, and in the spleen.

- **Stage IV:** The cancer is found in one of the following combinations:

  - Outside the lymph nodes throughout one or more organs, and may be in lymph nodes near those organs.

It's A Fact!

Stages of childhood Hodgkin lymphoma may include A, B, E, and S:

- **A:** The patient does not have fever, weight loss, or night sweats.
- **B:** The patient has B symptoms (fever, weight loss, and night sweats).
- **E:** Cancer is found in an organ or tissue that is not part of the lymph system but which may be next to an involved area of the lymph system.
- **S:** Cancer is found in the spleen.

Source: NCI, January 30, 2013.

- Outside the lymph nodes in one organ and has spread to areas far away from that organ.

- In the lung, liver, bone marrow, or cerebrospinal fluid (CSF). The cancer has not spread to the lung, liver, bone marrow, or CSF from nearby areas.

- **Recurrent:** Disease has recurred (come back) after it has been treated.

What treatments are used for childhood Hodgkin lymphoma?

The treatment of Hodgkin lymphoma in teens and young adults may be different than the treatment for children. Some teens and young adults are treated with an adult regimen.

Five types of standard treatment are used:

Chemotherapy: Chemotherapy uses drugs to stop the growth of cancer cells, either by killing the cells or by stopping them from dividing. When chemotherapy is taken by mouth or injected into a vein or muscle, the drugs enter the bloodstream and can reach cancer cells throughout the body (systemic chemotherapy). When chemotherapy is placed directly into the cerebrospinal fluid, an organ, or a body cavity such as the abdomen, the drugs mainly affect cancer cells in those areas (regional chemotherapy). Combination chemotherapy is treatment using more than one anticancer drug.

The way the chemotherapy is given depends on the risk group. For example, children with low-risk Hodgkin lymphoma receive fewer cycles of treatment, fewer anticancer drugs, and lower doses of anticancer drugs than children with high-risk lymphoma.

Radiation Therapy: Radiation therapy uses high-energy x-rays or other types of radiation to kill cancer cells or keep them from growing. There are two types of radiation therapy. External radiation therapy uses a machine outside the body to send radiation toward the cancer. Internal radiation therapy uses a radioactive substance sealed in needles, seeds, wires, or catheters that are placed directly into or near the cancer.

Radiation therapy may be given, based on the child's risk group and chemotherapy regimen. External radiation therapy is used for childhood Hodgkin lymphoma. The radiation is given only to the lymph nodes or other areas with cancer.

Targeted Therapy: Targeted therapy is a type of treatment that uses drugs or other substances to identify and attack specific cancer cells without harming normal cells. One type of targeted therapy being used in the treatment of childhood Hodgkin lymphoma is monoclonal antibody therapy.

Monoclonal antibody therapy is a cancer treatment that uses antibodies made in the laboratory from a single type of immune system cell. These antibodies can identify substances on cancer cells or normal substances that may help cancer cells grow. The antibodies attach to the substances and kill the cancer cells, block their growth, or keep them from spreading. Monoclonal antibodies are given by infusion. They may be used alone or to carry drugs, toxins, or radioactive material directly to cancer cells.

Surgery: Surgery may be done to remove as much of the tumor as possible in some cases of childhood Hodgkin lymphoma.

High-Dose Chemotherapy With Stem Cell Transplant: This treatment is a way of giving high doses of chemotherapy and replacing blood-forming cells destroyed by the cancer treatment. Stem cells (immature blood cells) are removed from the blood or bone marrow of the patient or a donor and are frozen and stored. After the chemotherapy is completed, the stored stem cells are thawed and given back to the patient through an infusion. These re-infused stem cells grow into (and restore) the body's blood cells.

New types of treatment are being tested in clinical trials. For some patients, taking part in a clinical trial may be the best treatment choice. Clinical trials are part of the cancer research process. Clinical trials are done to find out if new cancer treatments are safe and effective or better than the standard treatment.

Childhood Non-Hodgkin Lymphoma

What is childhood non-Hodgkin lymphoma?

Childhood non-Hodgkin lymphoma is a disease in which malignant (cancer) cells form in the lymph system.

Because lymph tissue is found throughout the body, childhood non-Hodgkin lymphoma can begin in almost any part of the body. Cancer can spread to the liver and many other organs and tissues.

The specific type of lymphoma is determined by how the cells look under a microscope. The four major types of childhood non-Hodgkin lymphoma are:

- B-cell non-Hodgkin lymphoma (Burkitt and Burkitt-like lymphoma) and Burkitt leukemia
- Diffuse large B-cell lymphoma
- Lymphoblastic lymphoma
- Anaplastic large cell lymphoma

There are other types of lymphoma that occur in children. These include the following:

- Lymphoproliferative disease associated with a weakened immune system
- Rare non-Hodgkin lymphomas that are more common in adults than in children

What are the symptoms of childhood non-Hodgkin lymphoma?

Possible signs of childhood non-Hodgkin lymphoma include breathing problems and swollen lymph nodes. Other conditions may cause the same symptoms. Check with a doctor for trouble breathing, wheezing, coughing, or high-pitched breathing sounds. Swelling of the head, neck, upper body, or arms are also possible signs, as is trouble swallowing. Other signs include painless swelling of the lymph nodes in the neck, underarm, stomach, or groin, and in boys, painless lump or swelling in a testicle. Fever or weight loss for no known reason and night sweats are also possible signs.

What are the stages of childhood non-Hodgkin lymphoma?

The following stages are used for childhood non-Hodgkin lymphoma:

- **Stage I:** Cancer is found in one group of lymph nodes or one area outside the lymph nodes, but no cancer is found in the abdomen or mediastinum (area between the lungs).

- **Stage II:** Cancer is found in one area outside the lymph nodes and in nearby lymph node; or in two or more areas above or below the diaphragm; or cancer started in the stomach, appendix, or intestines and can be removed by surgery.

- **Stage III:** Cancer is found in at least one area above and below the diaphragm; or cancer started in the chest; or cancer started in the abdomen and spread throughout the abdomen; or in the area around the spine.

- **Stage IV:** Cancer is found in the bone marrow, brain, or cerebrospinal fluid (CSF). Cancer may also be found in other parts of the body.

- **Recurrent:** Disease has recurred (come back) after it has been treated. Childhood non-Hodgkin lymphoma may come back in the lymph system or in other parts of the body.

What affects chances of recovery and treatment options?

The prognosis (chance of recovery) and treatment options for childhood non-Hodgkin lymphoma depend on the following:

- Age of patient
- Type of lymphoma

- Stage of the cancer
- Number of places outside of the lymph nodes to which the cancer has spread
- Whether the lymphoma has spread to the bone marrow or central nervous system (brain and spinal cord)
- Whether there are certain changes in the chromosomes
- The type of initial treatment
- Whether the lymphoma responds to initial treatment
- Patient's general health

What types of treatment are used for non-Hodgkin lymphoma?

Four types of standard treatment are used for childhood non-Hodgkin lymphoma: chemotherapy, radiation therapy (in certain patients), high-dose chemotherapy with stem cell transplant, and targeted therapy. These treatments are described earlier in this chapter.

New types of treatment are being tested in clinical trials. Patients may want to think about taking part in a clinical trial.

Some cancer treatments cause side effects months or years after treatment has ended.

Side effects from cancer treatment that begin during or after treatment and continue for months or years are called late effects. Late effects of cancer treatment may include the following:

- Physical problems
- Changes in mood, feelings, thinking, learning, or memory
- Second cancers (new types of cancer)

Some late effects may be treated or controlled. It is important to talk with your doctors about the effects cancer treatment can have.

It's A Fact

Childhood non-Hodgkin lymphoma is also described as low-stage or high-stage. Treatment is based on whether the cancer is low-stage or high-stage. Low-stage lymphoma has not spread beyond the area in which it began. High-stage lymphoma has spread beyond the area in which it began. Stage I and stage II are usually considered low-stage. Stage III and stage IV are usually considered high-stage.

Source: NCI, March 6, 2013.

Chapter 23

Melanoma And Other Skin Cancers

The Skin

Your skin protects your body from heat, injury, and infection. It also protects your body from damage caused by ultraviolet (UV) radiation (such as from the sun or sunlamps). Your skin stores water and fat. It helps control body heat. Also, your skin makes vitamin D. The skin has two main layers:

- **Epidermis:** The epidermis is the top layer of your skin. It's mostly made of flat cells called squamous cells. Below the squamous cells deeper in the epidermis are round cells called basal cells. Cells called melanocytes are scattered among the basal cells. They are in the deepest part of the epidermis. Melanocytes make the pigment (color) found in skin. When skin is exposed to UV radiation, melanocytes make more pigment, causing the skin to darken, or tan.

- **Dermis:** The dermis is the layer under the epidermis. The dermis contains many types of cells and structures, such as blood vessels, lymph vessels, and glands. Some of these glands make sweat, which helps cool your body. Other glands make sebum. Sebum is an oily substance that helps keep your skin from drying out. Sweat and sebum reach the surface of your skin through tiny openings called pores.

About This Chapter: Text in this chapter is excerpted from "What You Need To Know About™ Melanoma and Other Skin Cancers," National Cancer Institute (NCI), January 11, 2011. Available at: www.cancer.gov. Accessed May 12, 2013.

Cancer Cells

Cancer begins in cells, the building blocks that make up tissues. Tissues make up the skin and other organs of the body.

Normal cells grow and divide to form new cells as the body needs them. When normal cells grow old or get damaged, they usually die, and new cells take their place.

But sometimes this process goes wrong. New cells form when the body doesn't need them, and old or damaged cells don't die as they should. The buildup of extra cells often forms a mass of tissue called a growth or tumor.

Growths on the skin can be benign (not cancer) or malignant (cancer). Benign growths are not as harmful as malignant growths.

- **Benign Growths** (such as *moles*):
    - Are rarely a threat to life
    - Generally can be removed and usually don't grow back
    - Don't invade the tissues around them
    - Don't spread to other parts of the body

- **Malignant Growths** (such as melanoma, basal cell cancer, or squamous cell cancer):
    - May be a threat to life
    - Often can be removed but sometimes grow back
    - May invade and damage nearby organs and tissues
    - May spread to other parts of the body

Types Of Skin Cancer

Skin cancers are named for the type of cells that become malignant (cancer). The following are the three most common types:

- **Melanoma:** Melanoma begins in melanocytes (pigment cells). Most melanocytes are in the skin. Melanoma can occur on any skin surface. In men, it's often found on the skin on the head, on the neck, or between the shoulders and the hips. In women, it's often found on the skin on the lower legs or between the shoulders and the hips. Melanoma is rare in people with dark skin. When it does develop in people with dark skin, it's usually found under the fingernails, under the toenails, on the palms of the hands, or on the soles of the feet.

- **Basal Cell Skin Cancer:** Basal cell skin cancer begins in the basal cell layer of the skin. It usually occurs in places that have been in the sun. For example, the face is the most common place to find basal cell skin cancer. In people with fair skin, basal cell skin cancer is the most common type of skin cancer.

- **Squamous Cell Skin Cancer:** Squamous cell skin cancer begins in squamous cells. In people with dark skin, squamous cell skin cancer is the most common type of skin cancer, and it's usually found in places that are not in the sun, such as the legs or feet. However, in people with fair skin, squamous cell skin cancer usually occurs on parts of the skin that have been in the sun, such as the head, face, ears, and neck.

Unlike moles, skin cancer can invade the normal tissue nearby. Also, skin cancer can spread throughout the body. Melanoma is more likely than other skin cancers to spread to other parts of the body. Squamous cell skin cancer sometimes spreads to other parts of the body, but basal cell skin cancer rarely does.

When skin cancer cells do spread, they break away from the original growth and enter blood vessels or lymph vessels. The cancer cells may be found in nearby *lymph nodes*. The cancer cells can also spread to other tissues and attach there to form new tumors that may damage those tissues.

The spread of cancer is called *metastasis*.

Skin Cancer Risk Factors

When you're told that you have skin cancer, it's natural to wonder what may have caused the disease. The main risk factor for skin cancer is exposure to sunlight (UV radiation), but there are also other risk factors. A risk factor is something that may increase the chance of getting a disease. People with certain risk factors are more likely than others to develop skin cancer. Some risk factors vary for the different types of skin cancer. Studies have shown that the following are risk factors for the three most common types of skin cancer:

- **Sunlight:** Sunlight is a source of UV radiation. It's the most important risk factor for any type of skin cancer. The sun's rays cause skin damage that can lead to cancer.

- **Severe, Blistering Sunburns:** People who have had at least one severe, blistering sunburn are at increased risk of skin cancer. Although people who burn easily are more likely to have had sunburns as a child, sunburns during adulthood also increase the risk of skin cancer.

- **Lifetime Sun Exposure:** The total amount of sun exposure over a lifetime is a risk factor for skin cancer.

> ## It's A Fact!
> Skin cancer is the most common type of cancer in the United States. Each year, more than 68,000 Americans are diagnosed with melanoma, and another 48,000 are diagnosed with an early form of the disease that involves only the top layer of skin.
>
> Source: NCI, January 11, 2011.

- **Tanning:** Although a tan slightly lowers the risk of sunburn, even people who tan well without sunburning have a higher risk of skin cancer because of more lifetime sun exposure.

- **Sunlamps And Tanning Booths:** Artificial sources of UV radiation, such as sunlamps and tanning booths, can cause skin damage and skin cancer. Health care providers strongly encourage people, especially young people, to avoid using sunlamps and tanning booths. The risk of skin cancer is greatly increased by using sunlamps and tanning booths before age 30.

- **Personal History:** People who have had melanoma have an increased risk of developing other melanomas. Also, people who have had basal cell or squamous cell skin cancer have an increased risk of developing another skin cancer of any type.

- **Family History:** Melanoma sometimes runs in families. Having two or more close relatives (mother, father, sister, brother, or child) who have had this disease is a risk factor for developing melanoma. Other types of skin cancer also sometimes run in families. Rarely, members of a family will have an inherited disorder, such as xeroderma pigmentosum or nevoid basal cell carcinoma syndrome, that makes the skin more sensitive to the sun and increases the risk of skin cancer.

- **Skin That Burns Easily:** Having fair (pale) skin that burns in the sun easily, blue or gray eyes, red or blond hair, or many freckles increases the risk of skin cancer.

- **Certain Medical Conditions Or Medicines:** Medical conditions or medicines (such as some antibiotics, hormones, or antidepressants) that make your skin more sensitive to the sun increase the risk of skin cancer. Also, medical conditions or medicines that suppress the immune system increase the risk of skin cancer.

Sunlight can be reflected by sand, water, snow, ice, and pavement. The sun's rays can get through clouds, windshields, windows, and light clothing.

In the United States, skin cancer is more common where the sun is strong. For example, more people in Texas than Minnesota get skin cancer. Also, the sun is stronger at higher elevations, such as in the mountains. Doctors encourage people to limit their exposure to sunlight.

Basal Cell And Squamous Cell Skin Cancer: Other Risk Factors

The following risk factors increase the risk of basal cell and squamous cell skin cancers:

- Old scars, burns, ulcers, or areas of inflammation on the skin

- Exposure to arsenic at work

- Radiation therapy

The risk of squamous cell skin cancer is increased by the following:

- **Actinic Keratosis:** Actinic keratosis is a type of flat, scaly growth on the skin. It is most often found on areas exposed to the sun, especially the face and the backs of the hands. The growth may appear as a rough red or brown patch on the skin. It may also appear as cracking or peeling of the lower lip that does not heal. Without treatment, this scaly growth may turn into squamous cell skin cancer.

Melanoma Risk And Moles

The following risk factors increase the risk of melanoma:

Dysplastic Nevus: A dysplastic nevus is a type of mole that looks different from a common mole. A dysplastic nevus may be bigger than a common mole, and its color, surface, and border may be different. It's usually wider than a pea and may be longer than a peanut. A dysplastic nevus can have a mixture of several colors, from pink to dark brown. Usually, it's flat with a smooth, slightly scaly or pebbly surface, and it has an irregular edge that may fade into the surrounding skin.

A dysplastic nevus is more likely than a common mole to turn into cancer. However, most do not change into melanoma. A doctor will remove a dysplastic nevus if it looks like it might have changed into melanoma.

More Than 50 Common Moles: Usually, a common mole is smaller than a pea, has an even color (pink, tan, or brown), and is round or oval with a smooth surface. Having many common moles increases the risk of developing melanoma.

Source: NCI, January 11, 2011.

- **HPV (Human Papillomavirus):** Certain types of HPV can infect the skin and may increase the risk of squamous cell skin cancer. These HPVs are different from the HPV types that cause cervical cancer and other cancers in the female and male genital areas.

Symptoms of Melanoma

Often the first sign of melanoma is a change in the shape, color, size, or feel of an existing mole. Melanoma may also appear as a new mole. (See the "Checking For Melanoma" box to learn what to look for.)

Melanomas can vary greatly in how they look. Many show all of the ABCDE features. However, some may show changes or abnormal areas in only one or two of the ABCDE features.

In more advanced melanoma, the texture of the mole may change. The skin on the surface may break down and look scraped. It may become hard or lumpy. The surface may ooze or bleed. Sometimes the melanoma is itchy, tender, or painful.

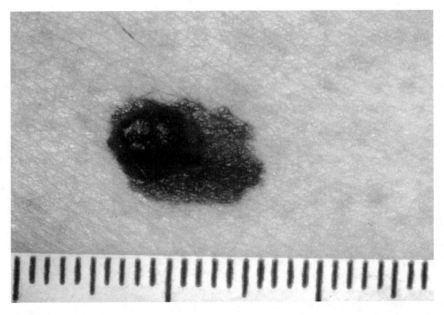

Figure 23.1. Asymmetrical melanoma. (Source: NCI Visuals Online, AV-8809-4035).

Symptoms Of Basal Cell And Squamous Cell Skin Cancers

A change on the skin is the most common sign of skin cancer. This may be a new growth, a sore that doesn't heal, or a change in an old growth. Not all skin cancers look the same. Usually, skin cancer is not painful.

Common symptoms of basal cell or squamous cell skin cancer include:

- A lump that is small, smooth, shiny, pale, or waxy

- A lump that is firm and red

- A sore or lump that bleeds or develops a crust or a scab

- A flat red spot that is rough, dry, or scaly and may become itchy or tender

- A red or brown patch that is rough and scaly

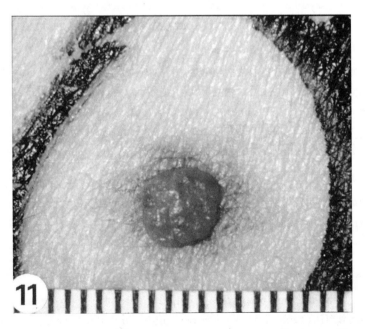

Figure 23.2. Dysplastic nevi. (Source: NCI Visuals Online, AV-8500-3698).

Checking For Melanoma

Thinking of **"ABCDE"** can help you remember what to look for when checking a mole:

- **Asymmetry:** The shape of one half does not match the other half.

- **Border That Is Irregular:** The edges are often ragged, notched, or blurred in outline. The pigment may spread into the surrounding skin.

- **Color That Is Uneven:** Shades of black, brown, and tan may be present. Areas of white, gray, red, pink, or blue may also be seen.

- **Diameter:** There is a change in size, usually an increase. Melanomas can be tiny, but most are larger than the size of a pea (larger than six millimeters or about one-quarter of an inch).

- **Evolving:** The mole has changed over the past few weeks or months.

Diagnosis

If you have a change on your skin, your doctor must find out whether or not the problem is from cancer. You may need to see a dermatologist, a doctor who has special training in the diagnosis and treatment of skin problems. Your doctor will check the skin all over your body to see if other unusual growths are present.

If your doctor suspects that a spot on the skin is cancer, you may need a biopsy. For a biopsy, your doctor may remove all or part of the skin that does not look normal. The sample goes to a lab. A pathologist checks the sample under a microscope. Sometimes it's helpful for more than one pathologist to check the tissue for cancer cells. You may have the biopsy in a doctor's office or as an outpatient in a clinic or hospital. You'll probably have local anesthesia.

There are four common types of skin biopsies:

- **Shave Biopsy:** The doctor uses a thin, sharp blade to shave off the abnormal growth.

- **Punch Biopsy:** The doctor uses a sharp, hollow tool to remove a circle of tissue from the abnormal area.

- **Incisional Biopsy:** The doctor uses a scalpel to remove part of the growth.

- **Excisional Biopsy:** The doctor uses a scalpel to remove the entire growth and some tissue around it. This type of biopsy is most commonly used for growths that appear to be melanoma.

Staging

If the biopsy shows that you have skin cancer, your doctor needs to learn the stage (extent) of the disease to help you choose the best treatment. The stage is based on these factors:

- The size (width) of the growth

- How deeply it has grown beneath the top layer of skin

- Whether cancer cells have spread to nearby lymph nodes or to other parts of the body

When skin cancer spreads from its original place to another part of the body, the new tumor has the same kind of abnormal cells and the same name as the primary (original) tumor. For example, if skin cancer spreads to the lung, the cancer cells in the lung are actually skin cancer cells. The disease is metastatic skin cancer, not lung cancer. For that reason, it's treated as skin cancer, not as lung cancer. Doctors sometimes call the new tumor "distant" disease.

Blood tests and an imaging test such as a chest x-ray, a CT scan, an MRI, or a PET scan may be used to check for the spread of skin cancer. For example, if a melanoma growth is thick, your doctor may order blood tests and an imaging test.

For squamous cell skin cancer or melanoma, the doctor will also check the lymph nodes near the cancer on the skin. If one or more lymph nodes near the skin cancer are enlarged (or if the lymph node looks enlarged on an imaging test), your doctor may use a thin needle to remove a sample of cells from the lymph node (fine-needle aspiration biopsy). A pathologist will check the sample for cancer cells.

Even if the nearby lymph nodes are not enlarged, the nodes may contain cancer cells. The stage is sometimes not known until after surgery to remove the growth and one or more nearby lymph nodes. For thick melanoma, surgeons may use a method called sentinel lymph node biopsy to remove the lymph node most likely to have cancer cells. Cancer cells may appear first in the sentinel node before spreading to other lymph nodes and other places in the body.

Stages Of Melanoma

The following are the stages of melanoma:

- **Stage 0:** The melanoma involves only the top layer of skin. It is called melanoma in situ.

- **Stage I:** The tumor is no more than one millimeter thick (about the width of the tip of a sharpened pencil.) The surface may appear broken down. Or, the tumor is between one and two millimeters thick, and the surface is not broken down.

How To Check Your Skin

Your doctor or nurse may suggest that you do a regular skin self-exam to check for the development of a new skin cancer.

The best time to do this exam is after a shower or bath. Check your skin in a room with plenty of light. Use a full-length mirror and a hand-held mirror.

It's best to begin by learning where your birthmarks, moles, and other marks are and their usual look and feel.

Check for anything new, including the following:

- A new mole (that looks different from your other moles)
- A new red or darker color flaky patch that may be a little raised
- A new flesh-colored firm bump
- A change in the size, shape, color, or feel of a mole
- A sore that doesn't heal

Check yourself from head to toe in the following way:

- Look at your face, neck, ears, and scalp. You may want to use a comb or a blow dryer to move your hair so that you can see better. You also may want to have a relative or friend check through your hair. It may be hard to check your scalp by yourself.
- Look at the front and back of your body in the mirror. Then, raise your arms and look at your left and right sides.
- Bend your elbows. Look carefully at your fingernails, palms, forearms (including the undersides), and upper arms.
- Examine the back, front, and sides of your legs. Also look around your genital area and between your buttocks.
- Sit and closely examine your feet, including your toenails, your soles, and the spaces between your toes.

By checking your skin regularly, you'll learn what is normal for you. It may be helpful to record the dates of your skin exams and to write notes about the way your skin looks. If your doctor has taken photos of your skin, you can compare your skin to the photos to help check for changes. If you find anything unusual, see your doctor.

Source: NCI, January 11, 2011.

- **Stage II:** The tumor is between one and two millimeters thick, and the surface appears broken down. Or, the thickness of the tumor is more than two millimeters, and the surface may appear broken down.

- **Stage III:** The melanoma cells have spread to at least one nearby lymph node. Or, the melanoma cells have spread from the original tumor to tissues nearby.

- **Stage IV:** Cancer cells have spread to the lung or other organs, skin areas, or lymph nodes far away from the original growth. Melanoma commonly spreads to other parts of the skin, tissue under the skin, lymph nodes, and lungs. It can also spread to the liver, brain, bones, and other organs.

Stages Of Other Skin Cancers

The following are the stages of basal cell and squamous cell skin cancers:

- **Stage 0:** The cancer involves only the top layer of skin. It is called carcinoma in situ. Bowen disease is an early form of squamous cell skin cancer. It usually looks like a reddish, scaly or thickened patch on the skin. If not treated, the cancer may grow deeper into the skin.

- **Stage I:** The growth is as large as two centimeters wide (more than three-quarters of an inch or about the size of a peanut).

- **Stage II:** The growth is larger than two centimeters wide.

- **Stage III:** The cancer has invaded below the skin to cartilage, muscle, or bone. Or, cancer cells have spread to nearby lymph nodes. Cancer cells have not spread to other places in the body.

- **Stage IV:** The cancer has spread to other places in the body. Basal cell cancer rarely spreads to other parts of the body, but squamous cell cancer sometimes spreads to lymph nodes and other organs.

Treatment Methods

Treatment for skin cancer depends on the type and stage of the disease, the size and place of the tumor, and your general health and medical history. In most cases, the goal of treatment is to remove or destroy the cancer completely. Most skin cancers can be cured if found and treated early.

Sometimes all of the skin cancer is removed during the biopsy. In such cases, no more treatment is needed.

If you do need more treatment, your doctor can describe your treatment choices and what to expect. You and your doctor can work together to develop a treatment plan that meets your needs.

Surgery is the usual treatment for people with skin cancer. In some cases, the doctor may suggest chemotherapy, photodynamic therapy, or radiation therapy. People with melanoma may also have biological therapy.

You may have a team of specialists to help plan your treatment. Your doctor may refer you to a specialist, or you may ask for a referral. Specialists who treat skin cancer include dermatologists and surgeons. Some people may also need a reconstructive or plastic surgeon.

People with advanced skin cancer may be referred to a medical oncologist or radiation oncologist. Your health care team may also include an oncology nurse, a social worker, and a registered dietitian.

Because skin cancer treatment may damage healthy cells and tissues, unwanted side effects sometimes occur. Side effects depend mainly on the type and extent of the treatment. Side effects may not be the same for each person. Before treatment starts, your health care team will tell you about possible side effects and suggest ways to help you manage them.

Many skin cancers can be removed quickly and easily. But some people may need supportive care to control pain and other symptoms, to relieve the side effects of treatment, and to help them cope with the feelings that a diagnosis of cancer can bring.

You may want to talk with your doctor about taking part in a clinical trial, a research study of new treatment methods.

Surgery

In general, the surgeon will remove the cancerous growth and some normal tissue around it. This reduces the chance that cancer cells will be left in the area.

There are several methods of surgery for skin cancer. The method your doctor uses depends mainly on the type of skin cancer, the size of the cancer, and where it was found on your body. Your doctor can further describe these methods of surgery:

- **Excisional Skin Surgery:** This is a common treatment to remove any type of skin cancer. After numbing the area of skin, the surgeon removes the growth (tumor) with a scalpel. The surgeon also removes a border (a margin) of normal skin around the growth. The margin of skin is examined under a microscope to be certain that all the cancer cells have been removed. The thickness of the margin depends on the size of the tumor.

- **Mohs Surgery (Also Called Mohs Micrographic Surgery):** This method is often used for basal cell and squamous cell skin cancers. After numbing the area of skin, a specially trained surgeon shaves away thin layers of the tumor. Each layer is examined under a microscope. The surgeon continues to shave away tissue until no cancer cells can be seen under the microscope. In this way, the surgeon can remove all the cancer and only a small bit of healthy tissue.

  Some people will have radiation therapy after Mohs surgery to make sure all of the cancer cells are destroyed.

- **Electrodesiccation And Curettage:** This method is often used to remove a small basal cell or squamous cell skin cancer. After the doctor numbs the area to be treated, the cancer is removed with a sharp tool shaped like a spoon (called a curette). The doctor then uses a needle-shaped electrode to send an electric current into the treated area to control bleeding and kill any cancer cells that may be left. This method is usually fast and simple. It may be performed up to three times to remove all of the cancer.

- **Cryosurgery:** This method is an option for an early-stage or a very thin basal cell or squamous cell skin cancer. Cryosurgery is often used for people who are not able to have other types of surgery. The doctor applies liquid nitrogen (which is extremely cold) directly to the skin growth to freeze and kill the cancer cells. This treatment may cause swelling. It also may damage nerves, which can cause a loss of feeling in the damaged area.

For people with cancer that has spread to the lymph nodes, the surgeon may remove some or all of the nearby lymph nodes. Additional treatment may be needed after surgery.

If a large area of tissue is removed, the surgeon may do a skin graft. The doctor uses skin from another part of the body to replace the skin that was removed. After numbing the area, the surgeon removes a patch of healthy skin from another part of the body, such as the upper thigh. The patch is then used to cover the area where skin cancer was removed. If you have a skin graft, you may have to take special care of the area until it heals.

The time it takes to heal after surgery is different for each person. You may have pain for the first few days. Medicine can help control your pain. Before surgery, you should discuss the plan for pain relief with your doctor or nurse. After surgery, your doctor can adjust the plan if you need more pain relief.

Surgery nearly always leaves some type of scar. The size and color of the scar depend on the size of the cancer, the type of surgery, the color of your skin, and how your skin heals.

For any type of surgery, including skin grafts or reconstructive surgery, follow your doctor's advice on bathing, shaving, exercise, or other activities.

Chemotherapy

Chemotherapy uses drugs to kill cancer cells. Drugs for skin cancer can be given in many ways.

Put Directly On The Skin

A cream or lotion form of chemotherapy may be used to treat very thin, early-stage basal cell or squamous cell skin cancer (Bowen disease). It may also be used if there are several small skin cancers. The doctor will show you how to apply the cream or lotion to the skin one or two times a day for several weeks.

The cream or lotion contains a drug that kills cancer cells only in the top layer of the skin:

- *Fluorouracil (Another Name Is 5-FU):* This drug is used to treat early-stage basal cell and squamous cell cancers.

- *Imiquimod:* This drug is used to treat early-stage basal cell cancer.

These drugs may cause your skin to turn red or swell. Your skin also may itch, ooze, or develop a rash. Your skin may be sore or sensitive to the sun after treatment. These skin changes usually go away after treatment is over.

A cream or lotion form of chemotherapy usually does not leave a scar. If healthy skin becomes too red or raw when the skin cancer is treated, your doctor may stop treatment.

Swallowed Or Injected

People with melanoma may receive chemotherapy by mouth or through a vein (intravenous). You may receive one or more drugs. The drugs enter the bloodstream and travel throughout the body.

If you have melanoma on an arm or leg, you may receive drugs directly into the bloodstream of that limb. The flow of blood to and from the limb is stopped for a while. This allows a high dose of drugs in the area with the melanoma. Most of the chemotherapy remains in that limb.

You may receive chemotherapy in an outpatient part of the hospital, at the doctor's office, or at home. Some people need to stay in the hospital during treatment.

The side effects depend mainly on which drugs are given and how much. Chemotherapy kills fast-growing cancer cells, but the drugs can also harm normal cells that divide rapidly:

- *Blood Cells:* When drugs lower the levels of healthy blood cells, you're more likely to get infections, bruise or bleed easily, and feel very weak and tired. Your health care team will check for low levels of blood cells. If your levels are low, your health care team may stop the chemotherapy for a while or reduce the dose of the drug. There are also medicines that can help your body make new blood cells.

- *Cells In Hair Roots:* Chemotherapy may cause hair loss. If you lose your hair, it will grow back after treatment, but the color and texture may be changed.

- *Cells That Line The Digestive Tract:* Chemotherapy can cause a poor appetite, nausea and vomiting, diarrhea, or mouth and lip sores. Your health care team can give you medicines and suggest other ways to help with these problems. They usually go away when treatment ends.

Photodynamic Therapy

Photodynamic therapy (PDT) uses a drug along with a special light source, such as a laser light, to kill cancer cells. PDT may be used to treat very thin, early-stage basal cell or squamous cell skin cancer (Bowen disease).

The drug is either rubbed into the skin or injected intravenously. The drug is absorbed by cancer cells. It stays in cancer cells longer than in normal cells. Several hours or days later, a special light is focused on the cancer. The drug becomes active and destroys the cancer cells.

The side effects of PDT are usually not serious. PDT may cause burning or stinging pain. It also may cause burns, swelling, or redness. It may scar healthy tissue near the growth. If you have PDT, you will need to avoid direct sunlight and bright indoor light for at least six weeks after treatment.

Biological Therapy

Some people with advanced melanoma receive a drug called biological therapy. Biological therapy for melanoma is treatment that may improve the body's natural defense (immune system response) against cancer.

One drug for melanoma is interferon. It's injected intravenously (usually at a hospital or clinic) or injected under the skin (at home or in a doctor's office). Interferon can slow the growth of melanoma cells.

Another drug used for melanoma is interleukin-2. It's given intravenously. It can help the body destroy cancer cells. Interleukin-2 is usually given at the hospital.

Other drugs may be given at the same time to prevent side effects. The side effects differ with the drug used, and from person to person. Biological therapies commonly cause a rash or swelling. You may feel very tired during treatment. These drugs may also cause a headache, muscle aches, a fever, or weakness.

Follow-Up Care

After treatment for skin cancer, you'll need regular checkups (such as every three to six months for the first year or two). Your doctor will monitor your recovery and check for any new skin cancers. Regular checkups help ensure that any changes in your health are noted and treated if needed.

During a checkup, you'll have a physical exam. People with melanoma may have x-rays, blood tests, and scans of the chest, liver, bones, and brain.

People who have had melanoma have an increased risk of developing a new melanoma, and people with basal or squamous cell skin cancers have a risk of developing another skin cancer of any type. It's a good idea to get in a routine for checking your skin for new growths or other changes. Keep in mind that changes are not a sure sign of skin cancer. Still, you should tell your doctor about any changes right away.

Follow your doctor's advice about how to reduce your risk of developing skin cancer again.

Chapter 24

Neuroblastoma: Cancer Of The Nervous System

Neuroblastoma

Neuroblastoma is a solid cancerous tumor in the nerve tissue of your neck, chest, abdomen, or pelvis. It usually originates in your adrenal glands, which sit on top of your kidneys.

Your neuroblastoma has often spread beyond its primary site when you are first diagnosed, usually to your bone marrow (70 percent) and bones (56 percent). It can also metastasize (spread) to your lymph nodes, liver, brain, and the area around your eyes.

What does staging mean?

Once a neuroblastoma is found, more tests will be done to find out if the cancer has spread from where it started to other parts of your body. Your doctor needs to know the stage or extent of your disease to plan your treatment:

- **Stage I:** Your tumor is able to be completely removed.

- **Stage II:** Your tumor is confined to one side of your body and only the lymph nodes on the same side as the tumor are positive for disease. The tumor can be either totally or partially removed by surgery.

- **Stage III:** Your tumor has crossed over the midline or, if it is one-sided, your lymph nodes on the opposite side have disease.

- **Stage IV:** Your disease has spread or metastasized beyond its original site.

About This Chapter: Reprinted with permission from Teens Living with Cancer, a program of Melissa's Living Legacy Teen Cancer Foundation, © 2013. All rights reserved. The Melissa's Living Legacy Teen Cancer Foundation is a non-profit organization providing resources to help teens with cancer have meaningful, life-affirming experiences throughout all stages of their disease. For additional information, visit www.teenslivingwithcancer.org.

Neuroblastoma In Numbers

- Neuroblastoma accounts for about 7 percent of all childhood cancer diagnoses.
- It is estimated that 800 to 900 children in the United States will be diagnosed with neuroblastoma each year.
- Ninety percent of children who are diagnosed with neuroblastoma are younger than five years of age and only three percent are older than ten years. Guess that puts you in the minority—how lucky can you get?

Source: Teens Living With Cancer, 2013

So, what happens now?

Your treatment options are related to your age at diagnosis, the tumor location and the stage of disease. More than one method of treatment may be used, depending on your needs:

- Surgery is used to remove as much of the cancer as possible. If the cancer cannot be removed, surgery may be limited to a biopsy (when a small piece of tissue is taken and examined under the microscope for signs of cancer).

- Radiation therapy uses high-energy rays to damage or kill cancer cells and shrink tumors.

- Chemotherapy uses drugs to kill cancer cells and shrink tumors. It may be given after the tumor has been surgically removed to kill any remaining cancer cells (adjuvant therapy—after another type of therapy) or before surgery to shrink the cancer (neoadjuvant—therapy—before another type of therapy).

- Bone marrow transplantation, a procedure in which healthy bone marrow replaces marrow destroyed by high dose chemotherapy or radiation, may be considered.

Unfortunately, most cases of neuroblastoma are advanced at diagnosis and may have some biological factors known to make treatment difficult. If this is the case, you may be treated with more intensive and higher dose chemotherapy and radiation. High dose therapy is frequently followed by a bone marrow or stem cell transplantation.

What are my chances?

Your chances for a complete recovery are dependent on your age at the time of diagnosis and the initial stage of your disease. For low stages of disease (I, II), survival rates are around 90 percent. Discovery of new treatments for advanced stages of neuroblastoma are increasingly effective and have improved outcomes. Remember that statistics are only averages—and you are certainly above average.

Chapter 25

Soft Tissue Sarcomas

What is childhood soft tissue sarcoma?

Childhood soft tissue sarcoma is a disease in which malignant (cancer) cells form in soft tissues of the body. Soft tissues of the body connect, support, and surround other body parts and organs. The soft tissues include the following:

- Muscles
- Tendons (bands of tissue that connect muscles to bones)
- Synovial tissues (tissues around joints)
- Fat
- Blood vessels
- Lymph vessels
- Nerves

Soft tissue sarcoma may be found anywhere in the body. In children, the tumors form most often in the arms, legs, or trunk (chest and abdomen).

There are many different types of soft tissue sarcomas. The cells of each type of sarcoma look different under a microscope.

About This Chapter: This chapter includes text from two documents: PDQ® Cancer Information Summary. National Cancer Institute; Bethesda, MD. Childhood Soft Tissue Sarcoma Treatment (PDQ): Patient version. Updated 03/2013; and, PDQ® Cancer Information Summary. National Cancer Institute; Bethesda, MD. Childhood Rhabdomyosarcoma Treatment (PDQ): Patient version. Updated 04/2013. Both available at: www.cancer.gov. Both accessed May 16, 2013.

Rhabdomyosarcoma—which often begins in skeletal muscles—is the most common soft tissue sarcoma in children. Other common types occur in joint tissue, connective tissue, and nerve tissue.

Soft tissue sarcoma occurs in children and adults. Soft tissue sarcoma in children may respond differently to treatment, and may have a better outcome than soft tissue sarcoma in adults.

Soft Tissue Sarcoma Types

Soft tissue tumors are grouped based on the type of soft tissue cell where they first formed. Examples include the following:

- **Fibrous (Connective) Tissue Tumors:** Desmoid tumor, dermatofibrosarcoma, fibrosarcoma, and low-grade fibromyxoid sarcoma.

- **Fibrohistiocytic Tumors:** Malignant fibrous histiocytoma (MFH), which is also called undifferentiated pleomorphic sarcoma or spindle cell sarcoma. Plexiform histiocytic tumor is another type.

- **Fat Tissue Tumors:** Liposarcoma.

- **Smooth Muscle Tumors:** Leiomyosarcoma.

- **Peripheral Nervous System Tumors:** Malignant schwannoma: (malignant peripheral nerve sheath tumor).

- **Bone And Cartilage Tumors:** Extraosseous osteosarcoma, extraosseous myxoid chondrosarcoma, mesenchymal chondrosarcoma.

- **PEComas (Perivascular Epithelioid Cell Tumors):** Angiomyolipoma, lymphangioleiomyomatosis, clear cell "sugar" tumor.

- **Tumors With More Than One Type Of Tissue:** Malignant mesenchymoma, malignant triton tumor, malignant ectomesenchymoma.

- **Tumors Of Unknown Origin:** The place where the tumor first formed is not known: alveolar soft part sarcoma, clear cell sarcoma (malignant melanoma of soft parts), desmoplastic small round cell tumor, epithelioid sarcoma, synovial sarcoma, undifferentiated soft tissue sarcoma.

- **Blood And Lymph Vessel Tumors:** Angiosarcoma, hemangioendothelioma, hemangiopericytoma, lymphangiosarcoma.

Source: NCI, March 15, 2013.

What are the possible risk factors for childhood soft tissue sarcoma?

Risk factors for childhood soft tissue sarcoma include having the following inherited disorders:

- Li-Fraumeni Syndrome

- Neurofibromatosis Type 1 (NF1)

- Familial Adenomatous Polyposis (FAP)

Other risk factors include the following:

- Having AIDS (acquired immune deficiency syndrome) and Epstein-Barr virus infection

- Having retinoblastoma in both eyes

- Past treatment with radiation therapy

How is soft tissue sarcoma diagnosed?

The doctor performs a physical exam and may use the following tests and procedures to diagnose soft tissue sarcoma:

- X-rays is a type of energy beam that can go through the body onto film, making pictures of areas inside the body. A series of x-rays may be done to check the lump or painful area.

- Magnetic resonance imaging (MRI) uses a magnet, radio waves, and a computer to make a series of detailed pictures of areas inside the body. This procedure is also called nuclear magnetic resonance imaging (NMRI).

- A biopsy is the removal of tissue or fluid for examination by a pathologist, who views the tissue under a microscope to look for cancer cells.

- In order to plan the best treatment, a large sample of tissue may be removed during the biopsy to find out the type of soft tissue sarcoma and do laboratory tests to look for changes in chromosomes, test the body's immune response, and discover the severity of the tumor.

After childhood soft tissue sarcoma has been diagnosed, tests are done to find out if cancer cells have spread to other parts of the body.

The process used to find out if cancer has spread within the soft tissue or to other parts of the body is called staging. There is no standard staging system for childhood soft tissue sarcoma. Two methods that are commonly used for staging are based on the amount of tumor remaining after surgery to remove the tumor and/or the grade and size of the tumor and whether it has spread to the lymph nodes or other parts of the body. It is important to know the stage in order to plan treatment.

The following tests and procedures may be used in the staging process:

- **Sentinel lymph node biopsy** is the removal of the sentinel lymph node during surgery. The sentinel lymph node is the first lymph node to receive lymphatic drainage from a tumor. It is the first lymph node the cancer is likely to spread to from the tumor. A radioactive substance and/or blue dye is injected near the tumor. The substance or dye flows through the lymph ducts to the lymph nodes. The first lymph node to receive the substance or dye is removed. A pathologist views the tissue under a microscope to look for cancer cells. If cancer cells are not found, it may not be necessary to remove more lymph nodes.

- **Computerized tomography (CT) scan** is a procedure that makes a series of detailed pictures of areas inside the body, taken from different angles. The pictures are made by a computer linked to an x-ray machine. A dye may be injected into a vein or swallowed to help the organs or tissues show up more clearly. The results of the sentinel lymph node biopsy and CT (also called a CAT scan) scan are viewed together with the results of the diagnostic tests and initial surgery to determine the stage of the soft tissue sarcoma.

How is childhood soft tissue sarcoma treated?

Seven types of standard treatment are used to treat soft tissue sarcoma.

Surgery: Surgery to completely remove the soft tissue sarcoma is done whenever possible. If the tumor is very large, radiation therapy or chemotherapy may be given first, to make the tumor smaller and decrease the amount of tissue that needs to be removed during surgery. The following types of surgery may be used:

- **Wide Local Excision:** Removal of the tumor along with some normal tissue around it.

- **Amputation:** Surgery to remove part or all of a limb or appendage, such as the arm or hand.

- **Limb-Sparing Surgery:** Removal of the tumor in an arm or leg without amputation, so the use and appearance of the limb is saved. Radiation therapy or chemotherapy may be given first to shrink the tumor. The tumor is then removed in a wide local excision. Tissue and bone that are removed may be replaced with a graft using tissue and bone taken from another part of the patient's body, or with an implant such as artificial bone.

- **Lymphadenectomy:** Removal of the lymph nodes that contain cancer.

> **The most common sign of childhood soft tissue sarcoma is a pain-less lump or swelling in soft tissues of the body.**
>
> A sarcoma may appear as a painless lump under the skin, often on an arm, a leg, or the trunk. There may be no other symptoms at first. As the sarcoma grows larger and presses on nearby organs, nerves, muscles, or blood vessels, symptoms may occur, including pain or weakness.
>
> Other conditions may cause the same symptoms that soft tissue sarcomas do. A doctor should be consulted if any of these problems occur.
>
> Source: NCI, March 15, 2013.

A second surgery may be needed to remove any remaining cancer cells or check the area around where the tumor was removed for cancer cells and then remove them.

Even if the doctor removes all the cancer that can be seen at the time of the surgery, some patients may be given radiation therapy or chemotherapy after surgery to kill any cancer cells that are left. Treatment given after the surgery, to lower the risk that the cancer will come back, is called adjuvant therapy.

Radiation Therapy: Radiation therapy is a cancer treatment that uses high-energy x-rays or other types of radiation to kill cancer cells or keep them from growing. There are two types of radiation therapy.

External radiation therapy uses a machine outside the body to send radiation toward the cancer.

Stereotactic radiation therapy aims radiation directly to a tumor, causing less damage to normal tissue around the tumor. The total dose of radiation is divided into several smaller doses given over several days.

Internal radiation therapy uses a radioactive substance sealed in needles, seeds, wires, or catheters that are placed directly into or near the cancer.

Chemotherapy: Chemotherapy uses drugs to stop the growth of cancer cells, either by killing the cells or by stopping them from dividing. When chemotherapy is taken by mouth or injected into a vein or muscle, the drugs enter the bloodstream and can reach cancer cells throughout the body (systemic chemotherapy). When chemotherapy is placed directly into the cerebrospinal fluid, an organ, or a body cavity such as the abdomen, the drugs mainly affect cancer cells in those areas (regional chemotherapy). Combination chemotherapy is the use of more than one anticancer drug.

Hormone Therapy: Hormone therapy is a cancer treatment that removes hormones or blocks their action and stops cancer cells from growing. Hormones are substances made by glands in the body and circulated in the bloodstream. Some hormones can cause certain cancers to grow. If tests show that the cancer cells have places where hormones can attach (receptors), drugs, surgery, or radiation therapy is used to reduce the production of hormones or block them from working. Antiestrogens (drugs that block estrogen) may be used to treat childhood soft tissue sarcoma.

Watchful Waiting: Watchful waiting is closely monitoring a patient's condition without giving any treatment until symptoms appear or change. Watchful waiting may be done when complete removal of the tumor is not possible, no other treatments are available, and the tumor does not place any vital organs in danger.

Nonsteroidal Anti-Inflammatory Drugs: Nonsteroidal anti-inflammatory drugs (NSAIDs) are drugs (such as aspirin, ibuprofen, and naproxen) that are commonly used to decrease fever, swelling, pain, and redness. In the treatment of soft tissue sarcomas, an NSAID called sulindac may be used to help block the growth of cancer cells.

Liver Transplant: The liver is removed and replaced with a healthy one from a donor.

Are clinical trials (research studies) available?

Yes. Information about clinical trials for specific types of soft tissue sarcoma is available from the NCI website at http://cancer.gov/clinicaltrials.

Patients may want to think about taking part in a clinical trial. For some patients, taking part in a clinical trial may be the best treatment choice. Clinical trials are part of the cancer research process. Clinical trials are done to find out if new cancer treatments are safe and effective or better than the standard treatment.

Childhood Rhabdomyosarcoma
What is childhood rhabdomyosarcoma?

Rhabdomyosarcoma is a type of sarcoma. Sarcoma is cancer of soft tissue (such as muscle), connective tissue (such as tendon or cartilage), or bone. Rhabdomyosarcoma usually begins in muscles that are attached to bones and that help the body move. Rhabdomyosarcoma is the most common type of soft tissue sarcoma in children. It can begin in many places in the body.

There are three main types of rhabdomyosarcoma:

- **Embryonal:** This type occurs most often in the head and neck area or in the genital or urinary organs. It is the most common type.

- **Alveolar:** This type occurs most often in the arms or legs, chest, abdomen, genital organs, or anal area. It usually occurs during the teen years.

- **Anaplastic:** This type rarely occurs in children.

What causes rhabdomyosarcoma?

Anything that increases the risk of getting a disease is called a risk factor. Having a risk factor does not mean that you will get cancer; not having risk factors doesn't mean that you will not get cancer. Risk factors for rhabdomyosarcoma include having the following inherited diseases: Li-Fraumeni syndrome, pleuropulmonary blastoma, neurofibromatosis type 1 (NF1), Beckwith-Wiedemann syndrome, Costello syndrome, and Noonan syndrome. Children who had a high birth weight or were larger than expected at birth may have an increased risk of embryonal rhabdomyosarcoma. In most cases, the cause of rhabdomyosarcoma is not known.

What are the signs or symptoms of childhood rhabdomyosarcoma?

Lumps and other symptoms may be caused by childhood rhabdomyosarcoma. The symptoms that occur depend on where the cancer forms. Other conditions may cause the same symptoms. Check with a doctor for any of the following problems:

- A lump or swelling that keeps getting bigger or does not go away. It may be painful.

- Bulging of the eye

- Headache

- Trouble urinating or having bowel movements

- Blood in the urine

- Bleeding in the nose, throat, vagina, or rectum

Remember!

A possible sign of childhood rhabdomyosarcoma is a lump or swelling that keeps getting bigger.

Source: NCI, April 2, 2013

What affects the prognosis (chance of recovery) and treatment options for childhood soft tissue sarcoma?

The prognosis and treatment options depend on the type of soft tissue sarcoma, the stage of the cancer (the amount of tumor remaining after surgery to remove it or whether the tumor has spread to other places in the body), the location, grade, and size of the tumor, and how deep under the skin the tumor is. The patient's age, whether the patient also has NF1, whether the cancer has just been diagnosed or has recurred (come back), and how the tumor responds to therapy also affect the prognosis.

Chapter 26

Testicular Cancer

What is testicular cancer?

Testicular cancer is a disease in which malignant (cancer) cells form in the tissues of one or both testicles.

The testicles are two egg-shaped glands located inside the scrotum (a sac of loose skin that lies directly below the penis). The testicles are held within the scrotum by the spermatic cord, which also contains the vas deferens and vessels and nerves of the testicles.

The testicles are the male sex glands and produce testosterone and sperm. Germ cells within the testicles produce immature sperm that travel through a network of tubules (tiny tubes) and larger tubes into the epididymis (a long coiled tube next to the testicles) where the sperm mature and are stored. Almost all testicular cancers start in the germ cells.

What are the risk factors for testicular cancer?

Anything that increases the chance of getting a disease is called a risk factor. Having a risk factor does not mean that you will get cancer; not having risk factors doesn't mean that you will not get cancer. People who think they may be at risk should discuss this with their doctor. Risk factors for testicular cancer include the following:

- Having had an undescended testicle
- Having had abnormal development of the testicles

About This Chapter: Excerpted from PDQ® Cancer Information Summary. National Cancer Institute; Bethesda, MD. Testicular Cancer Treatment (PDQ): Patient version. Updated 05/2012. Available at: www.cancer.gov. Accessed May 20, 2013.

Seminomas And Nonseminomas

The two main types of testicular germ cell tumors are seminomas and nonseminomas. These two types grow and spread differently and are treated differently. Nonseminomas tend to grow and spread more quickly than seminomas. Seminomas are more sensitive to radiation. A testicular tumor that contains both seminoma and nonseminoma cells is treated as a nonseminoma.

Source: National Cancer Institute, May 2012.

- Having a personal history of testicular cancer
- Having a family history of testicular cancer (especially in a father or brother)
- Being white

What are symptoms of testicular cancer?

Possible signs of testicular cancer include swelling or discomfort in the scrotum. These and other symptoms may be caused by testicular cancer. Other conditions may cause the same symptoms. A doctor should be consulted if any of the following problems occur:

- A painless lump or swelling in either testicle
- A change in how the testicle feels
- A dull ache in the lower abdomen or the groin
- A sudden build-up of fluid in the scrotum
- Pain or discomfort in a testicle or in the scrotum

How is testicular cancer diagnosed?

Tests that examine the testicles and blood are used to detect (find) and diagnose testicular cancer. The following tests and procedures may be used:

- **Physical Exam And History:** This is an exam of the body to check general signs of health, including checking for signs of disease, such as lumps or anything else that seems unusual. The testicles will be examined to check for lumps, swelling, or pain. Health care providers will also take a history of the patient's health habits, past illnesses, and treatments.
- **Ultrasound Exam:** In this procedure, high-energy sound waves (ultrasound) are bounced off internal tissues or organs and make echoes. The echoes form a picture of body tissues called a sonogram.

- **Serum Tumor Marker Test:** For this procedure, a sample of blood is examined to measure the amounts of certain substances released into the blood by organs, tissues, or tumor cells in the body. Certain substances are linked to specific types of cancer when found in increased levels in the blood. These are called tumor markers. The following three tumor markers are used to detect testicular cancer: 1. Alpha-fetoprotein (AFP); 2. Beta-human chorionic gonadotropin (B-hCG); and 3. Lactate dehydrogenase (LDH)

Tumor marker levels are measured before radical inguinal orchiectomy and biopsy, to help diagnose testicular cancer.

- **Radical Inguinal Orchiectomy And Biopsy:** This is a procedure to remove the entire testicle through an incision in the groin. A tissue sample from the testicle is then viewed under a microscope to check for cancer cells. (The surgeon does not cut through the scrotum into the testicle to remove a sample of tissue for biopsy, because if cancer is present, this procedure could cause it to spread into the scrotum and lymph nodes. It's important to choose a surgeon who has experience with this kind of surgery.) If cancer is found, the cell type (seminoma or nonseminoma) is determined in order to help plan treatment.

What can affect my prognosis (chance of recovery) and treatment options?

The prognosis and treatment options depend on the following factors:

- Stage of the cancer (whether it is in or near the testicle or has spread to other places in the body, and blood levels of AFP, B-hCG, and LDH)

- Type of cancer

- Size of the tumor

- Number and size of retroperitoneal lymph nodes. These are lymph nodes located deep in the abdomen.

After testicular cancer has been diagnosed, tests are done to find out if cancer cells have spread within the testicles or to other parts of the body.

The process used to find out if cancer has spread within the testicles or to other parts of the body is called staging. The information gathered from the staging process determines the stage of the disease. It is important to know the stage in order to plan treatment.

Testicular cancer can usually be cured.

Questions For Your Doctor: Before The Orchiectomy

This list of questions is intended to be used after you have been diagnosed with testicular cancer, but before you have received any treatment. These questions will help you make the most of your visit to the urologist in preparation for an orchiectomy. It is not an exhaustive list of questions, so be sure to look it over before you see the doctor and add any others that might apply to your specific situation.

These are general questions that most people have when they learn that they have testicular cancer and need to have the cancerous testicle removed.

- Why do you think I have cancer? How sure are you?
- Why do you have to remove the whole testicle?
- What happens if they discover that it is not cancer?
- Can you do anything before actually removing the testicle to make sure that it is necessary to remove it?
- Do I have any other choice of treatment(s)?
- How will this surgery affect my sex life?
- In addition to measuring my tumor markers, are you ordering any other tests before the surgery?
- What are your qualifications to treat testicular cancer?
- Have you treated someone for this kind of cancer before? If so, how many?

Removing the testicle because of testicular cancer usually does not interfere with fertility or testosterone production. However, it does happen and additional treatments are more likely to interfere with these functions. If your "good" testicle is not completely normal in size and function or if fertility is very important to you, you may want to mention this to the doctor and emphasize the next five questions.

- What is my prognosis for fertility following treatment?
- Should I bank sperm before the operation, just in case?
- How can I find out more about the sperm banking service?
- Will losing this testicle stop me from producing testosterone and "being a man?"
- Can you order a baseline measurement of my testosterone and LH levels before the surgery, just in case?

How is testicular cancer treated?

Different types of treatments are available for patients with testicular cancer. Some treatments are standard (the currently used treatment), and some are being tested in clinical trials. A treatment clinical trial is a research study meant to help improve current treatments or obtain information on new treatments for patients with cancer.

The five types of standard treatment are described below.

Surgery: Surgery to remove the testicle (radical inguinal orchiectomy) and some of the lymph nodes may be done at diagnosis and staging. Tumors that have spread to other places in the body may be partly or entirely removed by surgery.

Even if the doctor removes all the cancer that can be seen at the time of the surgery, some patients may be given chemotherapy or radiation therapy after surgery to kill any cancer cells that are left. Treatment given after the surgery, to lower the risk that the cancer will come back, is called adjuvant therapy.

Radiation Therapy: Radiation therapy is a cancer treatment that uses high-energy x-rays or other types of radiation to kill cancer cells. There are two types of radiation therapy. External radiation therapy uses a machine outside the body to send radiation toward the cancer. Internal radiation therapy uses a radioactive substance sealed in needles, seeds, wires, or catheters that are placed directly into or near the cancer.

Chemotherapy: Chemotherapy is a cancer treatment that uses drugs to stop the growth of cancer cells, either by killing the cells or by stopping the cells from dividing. When chemotherapy is taken by mouth or injected into a vein or muscle, the drugs enter the bloodstream and can reach cancer cells throughout the body. This is called systemic chemotherapy. When chemotherapy is placed directly into the cerebrospinal fluid, an organ, or a body cavity such as the abdomen, the drugs mainly affect cancer cells in those areas. This is called regional chemotherapy.

Watchful Waiting: Watchful waiting is closely monitoring a patient's condition without giving any treatment until symptoms appear or change. This is also called observation.

High-Dose Chemotherapy With Stem Cell Transplant: High-dose chemotherapy with stem cell transplant is a method of giving high doses of chemotherapy and replacing blood-forming cells destroyed by the cancer treatment. Immature blood cells called stem cells are removed from the blood or bone marrow of the patient or a donor and are frozen and stored. After the chemotherapy is completed, the stored stem cells are thawed and given back to the patient through an infusion. These re-infused stem cells grow into (and restore) the body's blood cells.

Can men still have children after treatment for testicular cancer?

Certain treatments for testicular cancer can cause infertility that may be permanent. Patients who may wish to have children should consider sperm banking before having treatment. Sperm banking is the process of freezing sperm and storing it for later use.

Are clinical trials (research studies) available for men with testicular cancer?

New types of treatment are being tested in clinical trials (research studies). Patients may want to think about taking part in a clinical trial.

For some patients, taking part in a clinical trial may be the best treatment choice. Clinical trials are part of the cancer research process. Clinical trials are done to find out if new cancer treatments are safe and effective or better than the standard treatment.

Many of today's standard treatments for cancer are based on earlier clinical trials. Patients who take part in a clinical trial may receive the standard treatment or be among the first to receive a new treatment. Patients who take part in clinical trials also help improve the way cancer will be treated in the future. Even when clinical trials do not lead to effective new treatments, they often answer important questions and help move research forward.

Information about clinical trials is available from the National Cancer Institute's website at http://www.cancer.gov/clinicaltrials.

What does follow-up treatment involve?

Some of the tests that were done to diagnose the cancer or to find out the stage of the cancer may be repeated. Some tests will be repeated in order to see how well the treatment is working. Decisions about whether to continue, change, or stop treatment may be based on the results of these tests. This is sometimes called re-staging.

Some of the tests will continue to be done from time to time after treatment has ended. The results of these tests can show if your condition has changed or if the cancer has recurred (come back). These tests are sometimes called follow-up tests or check-ups.

Men who have had testicular cancer have an increased risk of developing cancer in the other testicle. A patient is advised to regularly check the other testicle and report any unusual symptoms to a doctor right away.

Long-term clinical exams are very important. Testicular cancer survivors will probably have check-ups frequently during the first year after surgery and less often after that.

Chapter 27

Thyroid Cancer

Thyroid cancer is rare compared to other cancers. In the United States in 2010 an estimated 45,000 patients were diagnosed with thyroid cancer compared to over 200,000 patients with breast cancer and 140,000 patients with colon cancer. However, fewer than 2000 patients die of thyroid cancer each year. In 2008 when statistics were last collected, over 450,000 patients were alive and living with thyroid cancer. Thyroid cancer is usually very treatable and is often cured with surgery and, if indicated, radioactive iodine. Even when thyroid cancer is more advanced, effective and well-tolerated treatment is available for the most common forms of thyroid cancer.

It is interesting that the number of individuals—both men and women—with newly diagnosed thyroid cancer is increasing at a rate faster than for other types of cancer. The reason for this is unclear. Even though the diagnosis of cancer is terrifying, the outlook for patients with thyroid cancer is usually excellent.

What are the symptoms of thyroid cancer?

Thyroid cancer often arises in a lump or nodule in the thyroid and does not cause any symptoms. Lab tests generally do not help to find thyroid cancer. Thyroid tests such as TSH are usually normal even when a cancer is present. The best way to find a thyroid cancer is to make sure that your thyroid gland does not have nodules and is not enlarged. Neck examination by your doctor is the best way to do that. Often, thyroid nodules are discovered incidentally on imaging tests like CT scans and neck ultrasound done for completely unrelated reasons. Occasionally, patients themselves find thyroid nodules by noticing a lump in their neck while looking in a mirror, buttoning their collar, or fastening a necklace. Rarely, thyroid cancers and nodules do cause symptoms. In these cases, patients may complain of pain in the neck, jaw, or ear. If a nodule is large enough to compress the windpipe or esophagus, it may cause difficulty with breathing, swallowing, or cause a "tickle in the throat." Even less commonly, hoarseness can be caused if a cancer invades the nerve that controls the vocal cords.

The important points to remember are that cancers arising in thyroid nodules generally do not cause symptoms, thyroid tests are typically normal even when cancer is present, and the best way to find a thyroid nodule is to make sure your doctor checks your neck.

What causes thyroid cancer?

Thyroid cancer is more common in people who have a history of exposure to high doses of radiation, have a family history of thyroid cancer, and are older than 40 years of age. However, for most patients, we do not know the specific reason why thyroid cancers develop.

High-dose radiation exposure, especially during childhood, increases the risk of developing thyroid cancer in susceptible patients. Prior to the 1960s, x-ray treatments were often used for conditions such as acne, inflamed tonsils, adenoids, lymph nodes, or to treat enlargement of a gland in the chest called the thymus. All these treatments have been associated with an increased risk of developing thyroid cancer later in life. Even x-ray therapy used to treat serious cancers such as Hodgkin disease (cancer of the lymph nodes) or breast cancer has been associated with an increased risk for developing thyroid cancer if the treatment included exposure to the head, neck or chest. Routine x-ray exposure such as dental x-rays, chest x-rays, mammograms have not been shown to cause thyroid cancer.

Thyroid cancer can also be caused by radioactive iodine released during nuclear disasters such as the 1986 accident at the Chernobyl power plant in Russia or the 2011 nuclear disaster in Fukushima, Japan related to the tsunami. Children are usually the most affected and often develop cancers within a few years of exposure. However, even adults exposed during these accidents develop thyroid cancer with increased frequency, sometimes as many as 40 years later.

You can be protected from developing thyroid cancer in the event of a nuclear disaster by taking potassium iodide. This prevents the absorption of radioactive iodine and has been demonstrated to reduce the risk of thyroid cancer. The American Thyroid Association recommends that anyone living within 200 miles of a nuclear accident be given potassium iodide. If you live in a state containing a nuclear reactor and want more information about potassium iodide, check the recommendations from your state at the following link: http://www.thyroid .org/web-links-for-state-information-about-potassium-iodide.

> ## What is the thyroid gland?
>
> The thyroid gland is a butterfly-shaped endocrine gland that is normally located in the lower front of the neck. The thyroid's job is to make thyroid hormones, which are secreted into the blood and then carried to every tissue in the body. Thyroid hormone helps the body use energy, stay warm and keep the brain, heart, muscles, and other organs working as they should.
>
> Source: American Thyroid Association, 2012

How is thyroid cancer diagnosed?

A diagnosis of thyroid cancer is usually made by a fine needle aspiration biopsy of a thyroid nodule or after the nodule is removed during surgery. Although thyroid nodules are very common, less than one in ten harbors a thyroid cancer.

What are the types of thyroid cancer?

- **Papillary Thyroid Cancer:** Papillary thyroid cancer is the most common type, making up about 70 percent to 80 percent of all thyroid cancers. Papillary thyroid cancer can occur at any age. Papillary cancer tends to grow slowly and often spreads to lymph nodes in the neck. However, unlike many other cancers, papillary cancer has a generally excellent outlook even if there is spread to the lymph nodes.

- **Follicular Thyroid Cancer**: Follicular thyroid cancer, which makes up about 10 percent to 15 percent of all thyroid cancers in the United States, tends to occur in somewhat older patients than does papillary cancer. As with papillary cancer, follicular cancer first can spread to lymph nodes in the neck. Follicular cancer is also more likely than papillary cancer to grow into blood vessels and from there to spread to distant areas, particularly the lungs and bones.

- **Medullary Thyroid Cancer:** Medullary thyroid cancer, which accounts for 5 percent to 10 percent of all thyroid cancers, is more likely to run in families and be associated with other endocrine problems. In family members of an affected person, a test for a genetic mutation in the RET proto-oncogene can lead to an early diagnosis of medullary thyroid cancer and, subsequently, curative surgery to remove it.

- **Anaplastic Thyroid Cancer:** Anaplastic thyroid cancer is the most advanced and aggressive thyroid cancer and is the least likely to respond to treatment. Fortunately, anaplastic thyroid cancer is rare and found in less than 2 percent of patients with thyroid cancer.

What is the treatment for thyroid cancer?

Surgery

The primary therapy for all forms of thyroid cancer is surgery. The generally accepted approach at the present time is to remove the entire thyroid gland in what is called a total thyroidectomy. Some patients will have thyroid cancer present in the lymph nodes of the neck or upper chest. These lymph nodes are removed at the time of thyroid surgery or sometimes, as a later procedure. After surgery, patients need to be on thyroid hormone for the rest of their life. Often, thyroid cancer is cured by surgery alone, especially if the cancer is small. If the cancer is larger, if it has spread to lymph nodes or if your doctor feels that you are at high risk for recurrent cancer, radioactive iodine may be used to destroy any remaining thyroid cancer cells after the thyroid gland is removed.

Radioactive Iodine Therapy

Thyroid cells and most thyroid cancers absorb and concentrate iodine very readily. That is why radioactive iodine can be used so effectively to destroy all remaining normal and cancerous thyroid tissue after. The procedure to destroy or ablate thyroid tissue is called a radioactive iodine ablation. This produces high concentrations of radioactive iodine in thyroid tissues damaging the DNA in the thyroid cells, eventually causing the cells to die. Since other tissues in the body do not efficiently absorb or concentrate iodine, radioactive iodine used during the ablation procedure has little or no effect on tissues outside of the thyroid. Two risks are known to happen. In some patients, the radioactive iodine can affect the glands that produce saliva and lead to a having a dry mouth. In other patients, when high dose of radioactive iodine are necessary, there may be a small risk of developing other cancers later. These risks are small but increase as the doses of radioactive iodine increase. The potential risks of treatment can be minimized by using the smallest dose possible. Balancing potential risks against the benefits of radioactive iodine therapy is an important discussion that you should have with your doctor if radioactive iodine therapy is recommended.

If your doctor recommends radioactive iodine therapy, your TSH will need to be elevated prior to the treatment. This can be done in two ways. The first is by stopping to take thyroid hormone pill (levothyroxine) for four to six weeks. This causes you to become hypothyroid and high levels of TSH will be produced by your body naturally. However, hypothyroidism causes fatigue that can sometimes be significant. To minimize the symptoms of hypothyroidism your doctor may prescribe T3 (Cytomel, liothyronine), which is a short-acting form of thyroid hormone that is usually taken after the levothyroxine is stopped until the final two weeks before treatment. Alternatively, TSH can be increased sufficiently without making you hypothyroid simply by injecting TSH into you! Recombinant human TSH (rhTSH, Thyrogen) can be given as two injections in the several days prior to radioactive iodine treatment. The benefit of this approach is that you can stay on thyroid hormone and do not become hypothyroid. You may also be asked to go on a low iodine diet for one to two weeks prior to treatment. This will leave your body iodine depleted, which improves absorption of radioactive iodine, and helps maximize the treatment effect.

Once the TSH level is high enough, a pretherapy iodine scan is often done by administering a small dose of radioactive iodine. This scan determines how much thyroid tissue needs to be destroyed and allows the doctor to calculate how large a dose of therapeutic radioactive iodine needs to be administered. When used correctly, radioactive iodine therapy has proven to be safe and well tolerated and it has even been able to cure cases of thyroid cancer that have spread to other parts of the body like the lungs.

Treatment Of Advanced Thyroid Cancer

Thyroid cancer that spreads (metastasizes) to distant locations in the body occurs rarely but can be a serious problem. Surgery and radioactive iodine remain the best way to treat such cancers as long as these treatments continue to work. However, for more advanced cancers, or when radioactive iodine therapy is no longer effective, other means of treatment are needed. External beam radiation directs precisely focused x-rays to areas that need to be treated—often metastases to bones or other organs. This can kill or slow the growth of specific tumors. Cancer that has spread more widely requires additional treatment. New chemotherapy agents that have shown promise treating other advanced cancers are increasingly available for treatment of thyroid cancer. These drugs rarely cure advanced cancers that have spread widely throughout the body. However, they can often slow down or partially reverse the growth of the cancer. These treatments are usually given by an oncologist (cancer specialist) and often require care at a regional or university medical center.

What is the follow-up for patients with thyroid cancer?

Periodic follow-up examinations are essential for all patients with thyroid cancer because the thyroid cancer can return—sometimes many years after successful initial treatment. These follow-up visits include a careful history and physical examination, with particular attention to the neck area. Neck ultrasound is also a very important tool to visualize the inside of the neck and look for nodules, lumps or cancerous lymph nodes that might indicate the cancer has recurred. Blood tests are also important for thyroid cancer patients. All patients who have undergone thyroidectomy require thyroid hormone replacement with levothyroxine once the thyroid is removed. The dose of levothyroxine prescribed by your doctor will in part be determined by the extent of your thyroid cancer. More extensive cancers require higher doses of levothyroxine to suppress TSH. In cases of minimal or very low-risk cancers, it's safe to keep TSH in the normal range. The TSH level is the most sensitive indicator of whether the levothyroxine dose is correctly adjusted and should be followed regularly by your doctor.

Another very important blood test is measurement of thyroglobulin. Thyroglobulin is a protein produced by thyroid tissue and most types of thyroid cancer and is usually checked at least once annually. Following thyroidectomy and radioactive iodine ablation, thyroglobulin levels should be undetectable for life. Therefore, a detectable thyroglobulin level should raise a suspicion for possible cancer recurrence. Detectable thyroglobulin levels may require additional tests and possible further treatment with radioactive iodine and surgery. Thyroglobulin is generally measured either when you're on thyroid hormone with a low or normal TSH, or after TSH is elevated either by stopping thyroid hormone for three to six weeks, or after injection of Thyrogen (see section on radioactive iodine therapy above). Measurement of thyroglobulin may not be possible in up to 25 percent of patients who have interfering thyroglobulin antibodies present in their blood. In these patients, other means of follow-up are often used.

In addition to routine blood tests, your doctor may want to periodically repeat a whole-body iodine scan to determine if any thyroid cells remain. Whole body scanning is also done after your TSH level is raised, either by stopping your thyroid hormone or by administering Thyrogen injections. Increasingly, these scans are only done for high-risk patients and have been largely replaced by routine neck ultrasound and thyroglobulin measurements that have a higher diagnostic sensitivity especially when done together.

What is the prognosis of thyroid cancer?

Patients with papillary thyroid cancer who have a primary tumor that is confined to the thyroid gland have an excellent outlook. Ten-year survival for such patients is 100 percent and death from

> **It's A Fact!**
>
> Overall, the prognosis of thyroid cancer is excellent––especially for patients younger than 45 years of age and those with small cancers.
>
> Source: American Thyroid Association, 2012

thyroid cancer anytime thereafter is extremely rare. For patients over 45 years of age, or those with larger or more aggressive tumors, the prognosis remains very good but the risk of cancer recurrence is higher. The prognosis is not quite as good in patients whose cancer cannot be completely removed with surgery or destroyed with radioactive iodine treatment. Nonetheless, these patients often are able to live a long time and continue to feel well despite the fact that they continue to live with cancer. It is important to talk to your doctor about your individual profile of cancer and expected prognosis. It will be necessary to have lifelong monitoring, even after successful treatment.

Part Three
Cancer Awareness, Diagnosis, And Treatment

Chapter 28

Bumps And Lumps: When Do They Require Medical Attention?

At some point, you may develop a bump or a lump in the genital area. These bumps can be nothing, or their appearance could signal a more serious condition. If you are concerned, talk to your doctor. If you're a girl, you can ask your gynecologist. There are several bumps and lumps that should not be ignored in the genital area.

The two types of lumps and bumps that you should not ignore are skin cancer and infections. Both can have serious consequences if you ignore them. There are also bumps in the genital area that are harmless and don't need treatment.

Skin Cancer

Skin cancer is extremely rare in teens in the genital area, but not impossible. If you find a black spot that continues to enlarge, it could be **melanoma.** This type of skin cancer can be deadly if you don't get it treated. It can be completely flat and can develop in non-sun-exposed skin. Non-melanoma skin cancer usually looks like a non-healing skin-colored or reddish bump that often bleeds easily and does not go away.

There are six important signs that can help you figure out if you should ask your doctor about a spot that you think might be a melanoma—-just think A through E:

- **A—Asymmetry:** A spot that is not the same on both sides is asymmetrical.

- **B—Borders:** When the outline of your spot is wavy, rigid, or uneven—you should ask.

About This Chapter: "Bumps and Lumps: When Do They Require Medical Attention?" reprinted with permission from the Palo Alto Medical Foundation Teen Health website, http://www.pamf.org/teen. © 2013 Palo Alto Medical Foundation. All rights reserved. Authors: Renata Mullen, M D., and Marlana Jean Shile.

- **C—Color:** If your spot is a different color or changes color overtime, make a note and have your doctor take a look.

- **D—Diameter:** Melanomas are usually larger than the diameter of the eraser on your pencil (more than one-quarter of an inch or 5 millimeters).

- **E—Elevation or Evolution:** If the spot that you are worried about is raised above your skin (a bump) or if you notice it changing over time (evolving), it might be more than just a dot.

Infections

Infections that can have serious consequences if not treated are genital warts, syphilis, and possibly herpes.

Genital Warts

Genital warts are small skin-colored bumps, usually multiple. They may eventually go away, stay the same, or become more numerous. They are contagious and caused by HPV (genital human papilloma virus); they have been linked to cervical cancer in women. HPV is the most common sexually transmitted infection, but now there is an HPV vaccine available, currently recommended for all girls, and probably for boys in the future. It is a good idea to get the HPV vaccine as early as possible and before you are sexually active, but it is never too late. If you think you have genital warts, you should see an ob-gyn if female and a dermatologist if male.

Syphilis

Syphilis looks like a sore and can appear in the genital area or on the lips and mouth. It is a bacterium, so it can be treated with antibiotics. It presents as a sore and will eventually go away within a few weeks. However, this doesn't mean the infection is cured. It is still there and it needs to be treated. You can develop serious problems if it is left untreated.

Herpes

Herpes presents as painful blisters in the genital area. Although the herpes infection itself is not particularly dangerous, the biggest problem is that it tends to come back in the same area multiple times. Some people have outbreaks as frequently as once a month. It is contagious and can also be a problem in pregnancy. See a doctor for medication to prevent or treat outbreaks.

Harmless Bumps

You can also get bumps in the genital area that are harmless. These include cysts, angiomas, and mollusca.

- **Cysts:** Cysts are yellowish round lumps under the skin, which feel like a small ball or pebble that can easily be moved around. These may enlarge slightly, but in general stay about the same and do not cause any problems. They are caused usually by blocked hair follicles. No treatment is needed.

- **Angiomas:** Angiomas are small collections of blood vessels and are either bright red or slightly purplish. These do not usually enlarge or bleed. No treatment is needed.

- **Mollusca:** Mollusca are viral in origin and in the genital area are usually sexually transmitted. They are usually skin colored, tiny (one to two millimeters in size), and multiple. They will go away with time, but this may take up to three years. Although they don't cause any disease or increase your chance of cancer, they do represent a sexually transmitted disease and are usually a sign of unprotected sexual intercourse. Therefore, if you develop these, you should see your doctor and get tested for the possibility of other sexually transmitted diseases, such as HIV, syphilis, chlamydia, and hepatitis.

  With the exception of syphilis, these other diseases do not cause you to develop any bumps in the genital area. The people who are most likely to develop sexually transmitted diseases are those who have sex at an early age, have a greater number of sexual partners, and do not use a condom.

Chapter 29

Questions To Ask Your Doctor About Cancer

Questions To Ask Your Doctor When You Find Out You Have Cancer

Learning that you have cancer can be a shock, and you may feel overwhelmed at first. When you meet with your doctor, you will hear a lot of information. These questions may help you to find out more about your cancer and what to expect going forward.

Questions About The Cancer

- What type of cancer do I have?

- Can you explain my test results to me? Will I need more tests before treatment begins?

- What is the stage of my cancer? Has my cancer spread to other areas of my body?

- What is my chance of recovery?

- How will cancer and its treatment affect my body?

Questions About Finding A Specialist And Getting A Second Opinion

- How do I decide where to go for treatment?

- Will I need a specialist(s) for my cancer treatment?

About This Chapter: From "Questions To Ask Your Doctor When You Find Out You Have Cancer," "Questions To Ask Your Doctor About Treatment," and "Questions To Ask Your Doctor When You Have Finished Treatment," National Cancer Institute (NCI), February 14, 2012. Available at: www.cancer.gov. Accessed May 4, 2013.

- Will you help me find a doctor to give me another opinion on the best treatment plan for me?

Questions About Clinical Trials

- Would a clinical trial (research study) be right for me?

- How do I find out about studies for my type and stage of cancer?

Questions About Lifestyle, Finances, And Resources

- How will my daily activities, such as work or school, change?

- How can I get help if I feel anxious or upset about having cancer? If I need help coping with family responsibilities?

- What costs will my insurance cover? Who can answer my questions about how to pay for treatment?

- How can I get help with financial and legal issues (for example, getting financial assistance, preparing a will or an advance directive)?

- How can I get help with my spiritual needs?

- Can you suggest a support group that might help me?

Questions To Ask Your Doctor About Treatment

You may want to ask your doctor some of the following questions before you decide on your cancer treatment.

Questions About Cancer Treatment

- What are the ways to treat my type and stage of cancer?

- What are the benefits and risks of each of these treatments?

- What treatment do you recommend? Why do you think it is best for me?

- When will I need to start treatment?

- Will I need to be in the hospital for treatment? If so, for how long?

- What is my chance of recovery with this treatment?

- How will we know if the treatment is working?

Questions About Finding A Specialist And Getting A Second Opinion

- Will I need a specialist(s) for my cancer treatment?

- Will you help me find a doctor to give me another opinion on the best treatment plan for me?

Questions About Clinical Trials

- Would a clinical trial (research study) be right for me?

- How do I find out about studies for my type and stage of cancer?

Questions About Surgery

- Is surgery an option for me? If so, what kind of surgery do you suggest?

- How long will I stay in the hospital?

- If I have pain, how will it be controlled?

Questions About Other Types Of Treatment (Such As Radiation Therapy Or Chemotherapy)

- Where will I go for treatment?

- How is the treatment given?

- How long will each treatment session take?

- How many treatment sessions will I have?

- Should a family member or friend come with me to my treatment sessions?

Questions About Side Effects From Cancer Treatment

- What are the possible side effects of the treatment?

- What side effects may happen during or between my treatment sessions?

- Are there any side effects that I should call you about right away?

- Are there any lasting effects of the treatment?

- Will this treatment affect my ability to have children?

- How can I prevent or treat side effects?

Questions About Medicines And Other Products You Might Be Taking

- Do I need to tell you about the medicines I am taking now?

- Should I tell you about dietary supplements (such as vitamins, minerals, herbs, or fish oil) that I am taking?

- Could any drugs or supplements change the way that cancer treatment works?

Questions To Ask Your Doctor When You Have Finished Treatment

When you have finished your cancer treatment, you will talk with your doctor about next steps and follow-up care. You may want to ask your doctor some of the following questions:

- How long will it take for me to get better and feel more like myself?

- What kind of care should I expect after my treatment?

- What long-term health issues can I expect as a result of my cancer and its treatment?

- What is the chance that my cancer will return?

Seeking A Second Opinion

Feeling comfortable about your care provider is as important to your treatment as the therapy itself. Many physicians recommend second opinions; many insurance companies require it before covering treatment.

Getting a second opinion is more than just another hoop to jump through in the maze of your cancer treatment. It's a valuable tool to verify facts, like the stage, location, even the existence of the disease at all. A second opinion may provide access to potentially new treatments or clinical trials that are available.

Tell your oncologist that you'd like to seek a second opinion. This is common practice and will not offend your doctor in any way. They may even be able to help direct you to other oncologists in the area. You should also contact your insurance carrier to make sure they will cover the second opinion visit.

Be sure to take a copy of your records, scans, and test results with you to the appointment. This will help avoid having to repeat certain tests that can be costly and time-consuming.

Source: "Seeking a Second Opinion," © Seattle Cancer Care Alliance (www.seattlecca.org), 2013. All rights reserved. Reprinted with permission.

- What symptoms should I tell you about?

- What can I do to be as healthy as possible?

- Which doctor(s) should I see for my follow-up care? How often?

- What tests do I need after treatment is over? How often will I have the tests?

- What records do I need to keep about my treatment?

- Can you suggest a support group that might help me?

Chapter 30

Specialized Children's Cancer Centers

What are children's cancer centers?

Children's cancer centers are hospitals or units in hospitals that specialize in the diagnosis and treatment of cancer in children and adolescents. Most children's, or pediatric, cancer centers treat patients up to the age of 20.

Are there standards for children's cancer centers?

The following groups have established standards for children's cancer centers or programs:

- The National Cancer Institute (NCI)-sponsored Children's Oncology Group (COG), formerly two separate groups known as the Children's Cancer Group (CCG) and the Pediatric Oncology Group (POG), is a network of children's cancer centers that meet strict quality assurance standards. The COG Web site can be found at http://www .childrensoncologygroup.org/.

- The American Academy of Pediatrics (AAP) updated its Guidelines for Pediatric Cancer Centers in 2004. This document describes the personnel and facilities needed to provide state-of-the-art care for children and adolescents with cancer. This policy statement is available at http://aappolicy.aappublications.org/cgi/content/full/ pediatrics;113/6/1833.

- The American Society of Pediatric Hematology/Oncology (ASPHO) established standard requirements for programs treating children with cancer and blood disorders. The ASPHO website is available at http://www.aspho.org/.

About This Chapter: Excerpted from "Care For Children And Adolescents With Cancer," National Cancer Institute (NCI), May 19, 2008. Reviewed by David Cooke, MD, FACP, May 2013.

These groups agree that a childhood cancer center should be staffed by a team of trained pediatric oncologists (doctors who specialize in childhood cancer) and other specialists. Other members of the health professional team usually include pediatric surgeons, specialist surgeons (such as neurosurgeons and urologic surgeons), radiation oncologists, pathologists, nurses, consulting pediatric specialists, psychiatrists, oncology social workers, nutritionists, and home health care professionals—all with expertise in treating children and adolescents with cancer. Together, these professionals offer comprehensive care.

Why might a family look for a specialized children's cancer center when a child or adolescent is diagnosed with cancer?

Because childhood cancer is relatively rare, it is important to seek treatment in centers that specialize in the treatment of children with cancer. Specialized cancer programs at comprehensive, multidisciplinary cancer centers follow established protocols (step-by-step guidelines for treatment). These protocols are carried out using a team approach. The team of health professionals is involved in designing the appropriate treatment and support program for the child and the child's family. In addition, these centers participate in specially designed and monitored research studies that help develop more effective treatments and address issues of long-term childhood cancer survival.

When children go to a specialized cancer center, does it mean their treatment will be part of a research study?

Not necessarily. Participation in research studies is always voluntary. Parents and patients may choose to receive treatment as part of a clinical trial (research study); only patients and parents who wish to do so take part. However, a large number of children who go to pediatric cancer centers take part in clinical trials. About 55 percent to 65 percent of children diagnosed with cancer by or before age 14 enter an NCI-sponsored clinical trial. However, this percentage decreases to about 10 percent for children diagnosed between ages 15 and 19.

It's A Fact!

Survival rates for childhood cancer have risen sharply over the past 25 years. In the United States, more than 80 percent of children with cancer are alive five years after diagnosis, compared with about 62 percent in the mid-1970s. Much of this dramatic improvement is due to the development of improved therapies at children's cancer centers, where the majority of children with cancer have their treatment.

What is a clinical trial or research study?

In cancer research, a clinical trial is a study designed to show how a particular strategy—for instance, a promising anticancer drug, a new diagnostic test, or a possible way to prevent cancer—affects the people who receive it.

Treatment clinical studies fall into the following three categories:

- Phase I studies evaluate what dose is safe, how a new drug should be given (for example, by mouth, injected into a vein, or injected into the muscle), and how often. Phase I trials usually include a small number of patients and take place at only one or a few locations.

- Phase II studies investigate the safety and effectiveness of the treatment and how it affects the human body. Phase II clinical trials usually focus on a particular type of cancer and include fewer than 100 patients.

- Phase III studies, which usually involve a larger number of patients at many locations, compare the new treatment (or new use of a standard one) with the current standard therapy.

What are the benefits of taking part in a clinical trial?

One advantage is the possibility that a new treatment (or diagnostic test or preventive measure) will turn out to be better than a more established method. Patients who take part in approaches that prove to be better have the first chance to benefit from them. In phase III clinical trials, in which one treatment is compared with another, patients receive either the most advanced and accepted treatment for the kind of cancer they have—known as the "standard" treatment—or a new treatment that has shown promise of being at least as beneficial as the standard treatment.

People who take part in clinical trials receive specialized care under a very precise set of directions, or protocol. To ensure quality care, highly trained and experienced cancer specialists design, review, and approve each protocol. In addition, all participants in clinical trials are carefully monitored during the study and are followed afterwards.

Participants are often included in a network of clinical trials carried out around the country. In this network, doctors and researchers share their ideas and experience, and patients receive the benefit of the shared knowledge.

What are the risks of taking part in a clinical trial?

Clinical trials can involve risks as well as benefits. All cancer treatments have side effects, but treatments being studied may have side effects that are not yet understood as well as the side effects of standard treatments. The potential risks and benefits of each study are explained during the informed consent process, when patients and families discuss all aspects of the study with their doctors or nurses before deciding whether to participate.

What about costs? Do insurance or managed care plans cover treatment at a children's cancer center?

Some health plans cover part or all of the cost of care at children's cancer centers, but benefits vary from plan to plan. Questions or concerns about health care costs should be discussed with a medical social worker or the hospital or clinic billing office. Financial assistance and resources to cover health care costs may be available.

Can children with cancer be treated at the National Cancer Institute?

Children with cancer can receive treatment in clinical trials at the National Institutes of Health (NIH) Clinical Center in Bethesda, Maryland. Two branches of the NCI that study specific types of cancer have their own contact points:

- **The Pediatric Oncology Branch (POB)** conducts clinical trials for a wide variety of childhood cancers at the NIH Clinical Center. To refer children, teenagers, or young adults, the patient's health care provider should contact the POB office at 877-624-4878 between 8:30 a.m. and 5:00 p.m., Eastern time. The attending physician will discuss the case with the patient's health care provider, determine eligibility for treatment under a clinical protocol, and help arrange the referral. Once the patient has been accepted for evaluation, a social worker from the POB will contact the family and provide information on the study, as well as details about travel and lodging. Attending physicians in the POB are also available to provide a second opinion. The patient, family member, or health care provider can contact the POB to talk about a diagnosis or treatment plan. More information about the POB can be found online at http://home.ccr.cancer.gov/oncology/pediatric/.

- **The Neuro-Oncology Branch** offers clinical trials as well as consultations for children with brain tumors. Staff can provide a second opinion for doctors, patients, and family members who are interested in this service. Specialists can either evaluate the patient in person or review the patient's medical records and scans.

  To find out more about this service, and what information is needed, contact the Neuro-Oncology Branch at 301-594-6767 or 866-251-9686 (toll-free) between 9:00 a.m. and 6:00 p.m., Eastern Time. The Branch's website can be found at http://home.ccr.cancer.gov/nob/default.asp.

How does a family find a children's cancer center?

A child's pediatrician or family doctor often can provide a referral to a children's cancer center. Families and health professionals can also call the NCI's Cancer Information Service (CIS) at 800-4-CANCER (800-422-6237) to learn about children's cancer centers that belong to the Children's Oncology Group (COG). All of the cancer centers that participate in these groups have met strict standards of excellence for childhood cancer care. A directory of COG institutions by state is also available online at http://www.curesearch.org/resources/cog.aspx.

How do families cope with practical issues like getting to a treatment center and finding a place to stay near the center?

Many families receive helpful information from their doctors and nurses. Treatment centers often have social work departments that can provide assistance. In addition, various organizations offer support to families, including help with transportation, lodging, and financial assistance.

Chapter 31

Your Cancer Care Hospital Team

Typical members of your health care team may include medical doctors, nurses, and inter-disciplinary team members.

Medical Doctors

Primary Oncologists

A doctor specializing in cancer who is in charge of and responsible for your care, sometimes working in a team with other oncologists. This physician stays in communication with your primary care pediatrician or physician.

Attending Physician

One of a team of doctors responsible for your care. In your hospital, a team of oncologists may work together to care for you on rotating schedules. You may have a primary oncologist but still be seen by other attending physicians while you are in the hospital or clinic. Don't worry—in most hospitals all the doctors work as a team and constantly share information about how you are doing and what you need.

About This Chapter: Reprinted with permission from Teens Living with Cancer, a program of Melissa's Living Legacy Teen Cancer Foundation, © 2013. All rights reserved. The Melissa's Living Legacy Teen Cancer Foundation is a non-profit organization providing resources to help teens with cancer have meaningful, life-affirming experiences throughout all stages of their disease. For additional information, visit www.teenslivingwithcancer.org.

Radiation Oncologist

A doctor who specializes in using radiation to treat cancer. This physician often puts together your radiation treatment plan and may be responsible for your scans and x-rays.

Surgeon

A doctor who performs operations. You may have different types of surgeons involved in your care for different reasons. For example, a general surgeon may insert your central catheter; an orthopedic surgeon may be involved if you have bone cancer; a neurosurgeon may remove your brain tumor, etc.

Oncology Fellow

A doctor who has finished residency training and doing additional training to become a specialist in oncology. A fellow is a fully certified physician who works closely with the attending physicians to make decisions regarding your treatment. The fellow sometimes has more time than your primary doctor to really talk about things that concern you.

Resident

A doctor who has graduated from medical school and is getting more clinical training in the hospital before becoming fully certified. Residents rotate through several specialty areas including oncology, and work with your other doctors. The residents you see in the hospital will change when their rotations end. This is sometimes annoying because you are always seeing new faces during rounds who may not know your medical history. Try to be patient—we all have to learn somewhere.

Anesthesiologist

A doctor who specializes in giving medicines or other agents that prevent or relieve pain, especially during surgery. An anesthesiologist will always be part of your team when you have surgery. For some procedures like bone marrow biopsies, an anesthesiologist may administer some type of anesthesia and monitor your body functions.

Psychiatrists

A psychiatrist is a medical doctor that specializes in providing psychotherapy, or general psychological help. Because they are medical doctors, psychiatrists can also prescribe medication, such as antidepressants or medication to help you sleep.

Radiologist

A physician with advanced training in diagnosing diseases by interpreting x-rays and other types of imaging studies, for example, CT scans and MRIs.

Nurses

Nurse Practitioner Or Advanced Practice Nurse

A registered nurse with additional education and clinical training in Oncology. Nurse Practitioners work with your doctors and do many things including: performing physical examinations and procedures, diagnosing patient problems, ordering labs, tests, and medications, and teaching you about issues related to your care. In some hospitals, you may spend much more time with your nurse practitioner than your doctor. Nurse practitioners usually wear white lab coats like the docs, and not scrubs like the other nurses.

Staff Nurse

A registered nurse who provides the care you require both while you are in the hospital and as an outpatient in the clinic. The nurse may draw your blood, administer chemotherapy and/or medications, teach you about your cancer and treatment, and help arrange follow-up.

Nursing Aides, Patient Care Technicians

The aides in your hospital may have one of several different titles, but they probably all do essentially the same jobs. They often check vitals: blood pressure, temperature, pulse, etc.—and usually have the dubious honor of checking the levels of bodily wastes that you leave behind for closer examination. They might also do things like change your linens, bring in your food trays, and take care of minor problems.

Inter-Disciplinary Team Members

Social Worker

A trained professional who helps you and your family adjust to your illness, access hospital and community resources and deal with problems. Sometimes you may not feel like talking with the social worker about things that are on your mind

They always want to know "How are you feeling?" It's OK if you don't want to talk. If you do, they're available.

Child Life Specialist

A child development expert who offers age-appropriate activities to help meet your social and emotional needs. In some hospitals, child life specialists supervise activity rooms, coordinate activities, and help you deal with difficult procedures and treatments.

Clinical Psychologist

A therapist skilled in administering tests to determine at what level you are functioning intellectually and emotionally. Psychologists can help if you are feeling depressed or sad or having problems dealing with your disease. Psychologists are not medical doctors but have a doctoral degree in psychology and counseling and are referred to as "Dr."

Nutritionists

Registered dietitians are knowledgeable about the nutritional needs of oncology patients. They are nutrition experts who evaluate eating patterns and problems and recommend nutritional options. When you are going through various treatments (chemotherapy, radiation, surgery, etc.) you may not feel like eating. The nutritionist can help you keep your strength up which is very important during treatment.

Chaplains

Members of the clergy (ministers, priests, rabbis, etc.) who are available to help you with your spiritual issues, concerns, or needs.

Physical, Occupational, Speech, And Respiratory Therapists

Individuals with advanced training in their specialty area who may help you with specific problems related to your cancer or its treatment.

Phlebotomists

Individuals who draw your blood when you do not have a central venous catheter like a Broviac or medi-port.

Chapter 32

Cancer Staging

What is staging?

Staging describes the severity of a person's cancer based on the size and/or extent (reach) of the original (primary) tumor and whether or not cancer has spread in the body. Staging is important for several reasons:

- Staging helps the doctor plan the appropriate treatment.

- Cancer stage can be used in estimating a person's prognosis.

- Knowing the stage of cancer is important in identifying clinical trials that may be a suitable treatment option for a patient.

- Staging helps health care providers and researchers exchange information about patients. It also gives them a common terminology for evaluating the results of clinical trials and comparing the results of different trials.

What is the basis for staging?

Staging is based on knowledge of the way cancer progresses. Cancer cells grow and divide without control or order, and they do not die when they should. As a result, they often form a mass of tissue called a tumor. As a tumor grows, it can invade nearby tissues and organs. Cancer cells can also break away from a tumor and enter the bloodstream or the lymphatic system. By moving through the bloodstream or lymphatic system, cancer cells can spread from the primary site to lymph nodes or to other organs, where they may form new tumors. The spread of cancer is called metastasis.

About This Chapter: From "Cancer Staging," National Cancer Institute (NCI; www.cancer.gov), May 5, 2013.

What are the common elements of staging systems?

Staging systems for cancer have evolved over time. They continue to change as scientists learn more about cancer. Some staging systems cover many types of cancer; others focus on a particular type. The common elements considered in most staging systems are as follows:

- Site of the primary tumor and the cell type (such as adenocarcinoma, squamous cell carcinoma)

- Tumor size and/or extent (reach)

- Regional lymph node involvement (the spread of cancer to nearby lymph nodes)

- Number of tumors (the primary tumor and the presence of metastatic tumors, or metastases)

- Tumor grade (how closely the cancer cells and tissue resemble normal cells and tissue)

What is the TNM system?

The TNM system is one of the most widely used cancer staging systems. This system has been accepted by the Union for International Cancer Control (UICC) and the American Joint Committee on Cancer (AJCC). Most medical facilities use the TNM system as their main method for cancer reporting.

The TNM system is based on the size and/or extent (reach) of the primary tumor (T), the amount of spread to nearby lymph nodes (N), and the presence of metastasis (M) or secondary tumors formed by the spread of cancer cells to other parts of the body. A number is added to each letter to indicate the size and/or extent of the primary tumor and the degree of cancer spread.

Primary Tumor (T)

- *TX:* Primary tumor cannot be evaluated

- *T0:* No evidence of primary tumor

- *Tis:* Carcinoma in situ (CIS)—abnormal cells are present but have not spread to neighboring tissue. Although not cancer, CIS may become cancer and is sometimes called pre-invasive cancer.

- *T1, T2, T3, T4:* Size and/or extent of the primary tumor

Regional Lymph Nodes (N)

- *NX:* Regional lymph nodes cannot be evaluated

- *N0:* No regional lymph node involvement

- *N1, N2, N3:* Degree of regional lymph node involvement (number and location of lymph nodes)

Distant Metastasis (M)

- *MX:* Distant metastasis cannot be evaluated

- *M0:* No distant metastasis

- *M1:* Distant metastasis is present

For example, breast cancer classified as T3 N2 M0 refers to a large tumor that has spread outside the breast to nearby lymph nodes but not to other parts of the body. Prostate cancer T2 N0 M0 means that the tumor is located only in the prostate and has not spread to the lymph nodes or any other part of the body.

For many cancers, TNM combinations correspond to one of five stages. Criteria for stages differ for different types of cancer. For example, bladder cancer T3 N0 M0 is stage III, however colon cancer T3 N0 M0 is stage II.

Stage Definition

- *Stage 0:* Carcinoma in situ.

- *Stage I, Stage II, And Stage III:* Higher numbers indicate more extensive disease: Larger tumor size and/or spread of the cancer beyond the organ in which it first developed to nearby lymph nodes and/or tissues or organs adjacent to the location of the primary tumor.

- *Stage IV:* The cancer has spread to distant tissues or organs.

Are all cancers staged with TNM classifications?

Most types of cancer have TNM designations, but some do not. For example, cancers of the brain and spinal cord are staged according to their cell type and grade. Different staging systems are also used for many cancers of the blood or bone marrow, such as lymphomas. The Ann Arbor staging classification is commonly used to stage lymphomas and has been adopted by both the AJCC and the UICC. However, other cancers of the blood or bone marrow, including most types of leukemia, do not have a clear-cut staging system. Another staging system, developed by the International Federation of Gynecology and Obstetrics, is used to stage cancers of the cervix, uterus, ovary, vagina, and vulva. This system is also based on TNM information. Additionally, most childhood cancers are staged using either the TNM system or the staging criteria of the Children's Oncology Group, which conducts pediatric clinical trials; however, other staging systems may be used for some childhood cancers.

Many cancer registries, such as those supported by the National Cancer Institute's Surveillance, Epidemiology, and End Results (SEER) Program, use "summary staging." This system is used for all types of cancer. It groups cancer cases into five main categories:

- **In Situ:** Abnormal cells are present only in the layer of cells in which they developed.

- **Localized**: Cancer is limited to the organ in which it began, without evidence of spread.

- **Regional:** Cancer has spread beyond the primary site to nearby lymph nodes or tissues and organs.

- **Distant:** Cancer has spread from the primary site to distant tissues or organs or to distant lymph nodes

- **Unknown:** There is not enough information to determine the stage.

What types of tests are used to determine stage?

The types of tests used for staging depend on the type of cancer. Tests include the following:

- Physical exams are used to gather information about the cancer. The doctor examines the body by looking, feeling, and listening for anything unusual. The physical exam may show the location and size of the tumor(s) and the spread of the cancer to the lymph nodes and/or to other tissues and organs.

- Imaging studies produce pictures of areas inside the body. These studies are important tools in determining stage. Procedures such as x-rays, computed tomography (CT) scans, magnetic resonance imaging (MRI) scans, and positron emission tomography (PET) scans can show the location of the cancer, the size of the tumor, and whether the cancer has spread.

- Laboratory tests are studies of blood, urine, other fluids, and tissues taken from the body. For example, tests for liver function and tumor markers (substances sometimes found in increased amounts if cancer is present) can provide information about the cancer.

- Pathology reports may include information about the size of the tumor, the growth of the tumor into other tissues and organs, the type of cancer cells, and the grade of the tumor. A biopsy may be performed to provide information for the pathology report.

- Cytology reports also describe findings from the examination of cells in body fluids.

- Surgical reports tell what is found during surgery. These reports describe the size and appearance of the tumor and often include observations about lymph nodes and nearby.

Quick Tip

The doctor most familiar with a patient's situation is in the best position to provide staging information for that person. For background information, PDQ®, the National Cancer Institute's cancer information database, contains cancer treatment summaries that describe the staging of each type of cancer. These are available online:

- Childhood Cancers: http://www.cancer.gov/cancertopics/pdq/pediatrictreatment
- Adult Cancers: http://www.cancer.gov/cancertopics/pdq/adulttreatment

Staging information can also be obtained by calling the National Cancer Institute's Cancer Information Service (CIS) toll-free at 800-4-CANCER (800-422-6237).

CIS information specialists also offer immediate online assistance through LiveHelp at https://livehelp.cancer.gov/app/chat/chat_launch.

Chapter 33

Chemotherapy And Side Effects

Chemotherapy is a general term for medications used to destroy or stop the growth of cancer cells. Your treatment plan will use the best medicine or combination of medicines available to most effectively combat your specific type and stage of cancer.

Why Chemotherapy Medicines Are Used

Chemotherapy medicines are given for several reasons:

- To treat cancers that respond well to chemotherapy

- To decrease the size of tumors for easier and safer removal by surgery

- To enhance the cancer-killing effectiveness of other treatments, such as radiation therapy

- To control the cancer and enhance the patient's quality of life

How Chemotherapy Works

Chemotherapy works by interfering with the ability of cancer cells to divide and duplicate themselves. Chemotherapy can be given through the bloodstream to reach cancer cells all over the body, or it can be delivered directly to specific cancer sites.

Each chemotherapy medicine works to prevent cells from growing, by one of these methods:

- Preventing the copying of cellular components needed for cells to divide

About This Chapter: From "Chemotherapy in Children." The text in this chapter is adapted and reprinted with permission, CureSearch for Children's Cancer, www.curesearch.org. © 2013 CureSearch. All rights reserved.

- Replacing or eliminating essential enzymes or nutrients the cancer cells need to survive

- Triggering cells to self-destruct

Often a combination of drugs will be used, with each medicine attacking the cancer cells in a special way. This decreases the chances that cancer cells will survive, become resistant and continue to grow.

Giving Chemotherapy Medicines To A Patient

Chemotherapy is given in different ways depending on the cancer type and the medicines used:

- Intravenously (IV): Injected into a vein

- Intrathecally (IT): Injected into the spinal canal during a lumbar puncture

- Intramuscular (IM): Injected into a muscle

- Intraperitoneal (IP): Injected into the abdominal cavity

- Intracavitary (IC): Injected into a body cavity

- Subcutaneous (sub.q.): Injected into a port just under the skin

- Oral (PO): As a pill or a liquid to be swallowed

For many patients, the medical team will surgically install a central venous line (catheter) in a vein in the chest (subcutaneous port) or arm before chemotherapy starts. The line will allow treatments to be given and blood samples taken without being "stuck" with a needle. At the end of the treatment, the central line will be removed.

Choosing Chemotherapy Medicines

Many years of research and experience have created successful treatment plans for some types of cancer. For other cancers, research is now underway to find the most effective treatment. Many children and teens are treated according to clinical trial protocols. Each protocol is based on the best available treatment (standard of care) with slight variations that are believed to reduce side effects or improve success. A trial may study two or more different treatment plans, each believed to be effective, with the goal of identifying if one is more effective than the other.

Treatment plans are created using the following guidelines:

- The goal is to maximize the destruction of cancer cells while limiting damage to healthy cells.

- Dosages of the medicines are based on a child's or teen's weight or body surface area.

- The length of treatment depends upon the cancer type and how responsive it is to the chemotherapy.

- Chemotherapy may be stopped if the medicine no longer proves to be effective, or if the child or teen experiences a serious side effect.

- Certain medicines are known to cause permanent side effects after they have been used multiple times. These agents are monitored very closely. Doctors will stop these medicines when the risks of side effects are greater than the potential benefits of continuing treatment.

Tips For Patients And Parents

- Review each medicine with your healthcare team, including all potential side effects.

- Discuss what can be done to prevent, lessen, or treat side effects.

- Understand the tests that will be done to monitor side effects.

- Remember that you are the expert on how you feel. Notify the healthcare team of any changes you notice, or concerns you may have.

Why Does Chemo Cause Side Effects?

Chemotherapy medicines target rapidly dividing cells, including normal ones. Side effects can occur when these normal cells are damaged. Because normal cells are better able to repair the damage or can often be replaced by other healthy cells, side effects are usually temporary.

Factors influencing side effects include:
- The specific chemotherapy medicine
- The dose of the medicine
- The health of the patient

Despite monitoring the effects of chemotherapy very closely, some long-term effects can occur. Some effects may not be known until years after therapy is completed. Therefore, it is important that every patient be followed throughout his or her life by a physician who is aware of the late effects of cancer treatment.

Common Side Effects Of Chemotherapy

Low Red Blood Cell Count (Anemia)

Red blood cells carry oxygen throughout the body. Oxygen enters the lungs with each breath and binds (attaches) to hemoglobin in the red blood cells. Hemoglobin carries the oxygen to all the organs and tissues in the body. Two laboratory tests are done to measure the number and function of red blood cells:

- *A hemoglobin test* shows how much oxygen the red blood cells are able to carry. A normal hemoglobin level is between 12 and 16.

- *A hematocrit* shows the percentage of red blood cells in the blood. A normal hematocrit is between 36 and 50.

Signs Of A Low Red Blood Cell Count: When the hemoglobin count is low, the body is not able to get as much oxygen to go throughout the body.

A person with low hemoglobin may have the following symptoms: tiredness; shortness of breath; headache; fast heart rate; pale skin and/or pale gums; and dizziness.

A blood transfusion may be given if your hemoglobin is too low.

Blood Transfusions: If you need a blood transfusion, the blood given will match your blood type. The blood will be given over several hours into a vein, through a central venous catheter or an IV in the arm. You will be checked during the transfusion for signs of a reaction.

One of the most common concerns about blood transfusions is the risk of getting HIV/AIDS and hepatitis. The risk of getting AIDS or hepatitis from a blood transfusion is very small. All donors are tested for infectious markers in the blood, such as the HIV virus, hepatitis, and others. Blood that tests positive for any disease is thrown away. Although research studies have shown directed donations do not increase blood safety, if it makes you feel more comfortable to receive blood from a family member or friend, such "directed donations" may be available. Blood donations are always welcome, and giving blood is a great way for friends and family to feel like they are helping. For more information about direct donation, ask your health care provider.

Low Platelet Count (Thrombocytopenia)

Platelets stop bleeding in the body by forming clots. When the platelet count is low, you may be at risk for bleeding. A normal platelet count is between 150,000 and 300,000.

Signs Of A Low Platelet Count: If you have a low platelet count, you may see one or more of the following signs:

- Bruising or petechiae (small, red, pinpoint spots on the skin)

- Bleeding from the nose, gums, or central venous access device that doesn't stop after applying pressure for 5 to 10 minutes

- Black stools or vomit (this may mean blood is in the stomach or bowel)

Any child or teen with a low platelet count should not play contact sports (football, rugby), and use a soft toothbrush when brushing teeth to prevent bleeding of the gums.

If you get a nosebleed, sit upright as you apply pressure to the outsides of each nostril, just below the bridge. Pinch the area with your thumb and finger and hold the pressure for 10 minutes. If the bleeding does not stop, call your healthcare provider.

Other Bleeding Issues: In general, you need to be cautious of anything that might cause bleeding.

Low White Blood Cell Count (Neutropenia)

White blood cells fight infection. A normal white blood cell count is between 5,000 and 10,000 cells. A white blood cell count below 1,000 cells increases the risk of infection. In some cases, you may be given a medicine, such as "G-CSF (granulocyte-colony stimulating factor)," to help increase the number of white blood cells in the bone marrow.

Differential: Different types of white blood cells have different jobs. The "differential" is part of the blood count report that shows the breakdown of the various types of white blood cells in your blood count.

- *Neutrophils* help to fight bacterial infections.

- *Lymphocytes* make antibodies to fight infections.

- *Monocytes* help to fight infection by killing and removing bacteria.

- *Basophils* and *eosinophils* respond during an allergic reaction.

The term "ANC," which stands for "absolute neutrophil count," is the total number of neutrophils in your white blood cell count. We often refer to the ANC as the "infection-fighting" count. The lower the ANC drops, the higher the risk of infection. When the ANC drops below 500, the risk of infection is high.

Signs Of Infection: While there are no outward signs of a low white blood cell count, it's important to be aware of the timing of low blood counts following chemotherapy. Call your health care provider right away if you notice any signs of infection, including: fever; chills; cough; trouble breathing; diarrhea; and pain.

If you have a central venous access device (central line or port), check for redness, swelling, pain or pus at the site. A patient with a low ANC may not have redness or pus, but could still have an infection.

Diarrhea

The intestines can be affected by chemotherapy. Proper diet and nutrition can help avoid or reduce these symptoms.

If you have diarrhea tell your healthcare provider the color, amount, and number of times in a day that it occurred. Some ways to help decrease diarrhea include:

- Eat a soft, bland diet (crackers, soup, rice).
- Eat small amounts of food more often, instead of large meals.
- Avoid spicy, fried or fatty foods.
- Avoid food high in fiber (fruits, vegetables, salad).
- Limit high-sugar foods (juice, candy).
- Discuss with your healthcare provider whether milk or milk products should be limited.

Suggestions

- If diarrhea occurs, drink plenty of liquids.
- Try bland foods like rice, noodles with broth, cream of wheat, or canned fruit.
- Milk and milk products can sometimes worsen problems if a child or teen cannot digest milk sugar (lactose), known as lactose intolerance, which can occur after certain types of treatment. It can help to eliminate dairy products or purchase reduced-lactose milk and other products (available at most grocery stores). There are also drops sold at pharmacies that reduce the lactose in milk. A registered dietitian can discuss products that are available to help you.
- Decrease the fiber content in your diet. Eat only cooked vegetables and canned fruits. Omit foods with seeds and tough skins, beans, broccoli, corn, onions, and garlic. Avoid whole grain breads and cereals; instead, offer white bread and refined cereals.

- If you have abdominal cramps, stay away from foods that could cause gas or cramps, such as carbonated drinks, beans, cabbage, broccoli, and cauliflower.

- Avoid fatty foods or foods that are highly spiced if they cause problems.

- Offer smaller amounts of food more often.

Fever

Fever may be a sign of serious infection. Chemotherapy often temporarily destroys white blood cells, which are the body's primary defense against infection. If you have a fever while undergoing chemotherapy treatment, call the doctor right away.

Hair Loss

Some chemotherapy causes hair loss or thinning of the hair. Hair will almost always grow back when treatment is finished, but it may have a different color or texture.

Mouth Sores And Dry Mouth

Cells in the mouth can be affected by chemotherapy and radiation therapy to the head and neck. As such, it's important to keep the mouth and teeth as clean as possible. You will feel more comfortable, and you can help prevent mouth sores or other infections.

General Mouth Care

Brush your teeth with a soft toothbrush after each meal and before bed.

Rinse the mouth with water after brushing. Do not use mouthwashes that contain alcohol. Alcohol dries out the mouth.

If a dry mouth is a problem, suck on sugar-free hard candies or ask your health care provider about mouthwashes or other products for dry mouth.

Caring For Mouth Sores (Stomatitis)

Some chemotherapy medicines and radiation therapy to the head and neck can cause mouth sores. The inside of the mouth may be red or may have sores that can be painful. You may also see white plaques (small raised areas) in the mouth that may be from a fungal infection.

If mouth sores are a problem:

- Drink plenty of fluids.

- Drink fluids with a straw.

- Avoid spicy or acidic foods.

- Take foods that are cold or at room temperature.

- Try soft, tender, or pureed (beaten or blended) foods.

- Avoid dry or coarse foods.

- Cut food into small pieces.

- Rinse the mouth with water or a mouthwash recommended by your healthcare provider several times a day.

- Avoid mouthwash that contains alcohol.

Your healthcare provider may give you a medication to treat a fungal infection in the mouth (thrush), and/or a pain medication if the sores are painful. Call your healthcare provider if the teen or child cannot drink fluids, swallow, or if the teen's or child's medicine does not help take away the pain.

Suggestions

- Avoid food and drinks with extreme temperatures that can hurt the mouth and throat. Lukewarm or room-temperature foods and beverages may be better tolerated.

- Avoid acidic foods and beverages like citrus and tomato juices that can burn the mouth and throat. Fruit nectar, especially pear nectar, may be well tolerated.

- Avoid salty or spicy foods that can burn or sting. Try blander foods instead.

- Try soft foods that are easy to chew, or consider mixing food in a blender with fluid (water, broth, gravy) to make it easier to eat.

- Experiment with liquid nutritional formulas. A registered dietitian can provide suggestions and samples of products to try.

- Encourage using a straw to drink fluids and thinned pureed food instead of a spoon.

- Ask your doctor or nurse about medicine you can take before meals to numb the mouth or throat.

- Avoid commercial mouthwash containing alcohol, which can burn.

Dealing with a Dry Mouth

Radiation therapy to the head or neck area can reduce the flow of saliva and cause a dry mouth, making it harder to chew and swallow foods. Dry mouth can also change the way foods taste.

Suggestions

- Try very sweet or tart foods and beverages (but avoid tart foods if you have a sore mouth or throat).

- Sucking on hard candy, popsicles, or chewing gum can help produce more saliva. Sugar-free candies and gum are better to avoid tooth decay.

- Serve foods with sauces, gravies, or butter to help make them moist and easier to swallow.

- Prepare soft and pureed foods.

- Use lip balm to keep your lips moist.

- Sipping on liquids throughout the day may help keep the mouth moist.

- Ask the doctor about products that can help with a dry mouth.

Nausea And Vomiting

Chemotherapy and radiation therapy can cause nausea, vomiting, and diarrhea. Any of these symptoms can place you at risk for dehydration (loss of fluids in the body).

Medications to help decrease nausea and vomiting are usually given before chemotherapy or radiation. The type and amount of anti-nausea medicine will be based on your treatment plan and reaction to the treatment. It is important to let your healthcare provider know if you have nausea or vomiting at home after chemotherapy, so additional medicine or other types of treatment can be used.

Some ways to help decrease nausea and vomiting include:

- Eat small meals or snacks.

- Eat foods that are easy to digest (crackers, rice, gelatin).

- Sip cool clear liquids.

- Do not eat fried, spicy, or very rich foods.

- Eat in a room that is free from cooking or other smells.

- Rinse your mouth after vomiting.

Nutrition's Role (Advice For Parents And Teens)

- Avoid offering overly sweet or greasy foods, hot and spicy foods, and foods with strong odors.

- Try small amounts of food; it can help to use smaller plates and bowls to avoid overwhelming the teen or child.

- Discourage drinking with meals. Instead, offer liquids 20 to 30 minutes before or after meals.

Table 33.1. Chemotherapy Medications

Medication Name	Also Known As...
5-fluorouracil	5-FU, Efudix
6-mercaptopurine	6-MP, Puri-Nethol, Mercaptopurine
Aldesleukin	Proleukin, IL-2, Interleukin-2, r-serHuIL
Alendronate	Fosamax
Allopurinol sodium	Zyloprim, Aloprim
Amifostine	Ethyol, Ethiofos, Gammaphos
Arsenic trioxide	Trisenox
Bleomycin	Bleo, Blenoxane
Busulfan	Myleran, Busulfex
Carboplatin	Paraplatin, CBDCA
Carmustine	Gliadel Wafer, BCNU, BiCNU, bis-chloronitrosurea
CCNU	Lomustine, Ceenu
Celecoxib	Celebrex
Cisplatin	Cis-diamminedichloroplatinum, Platinol-A
Cladabrine	CDA, Leustatin
Clonazepam	Klonopin, Rivotril
Compound 506U	amino-9, bD -arabinofuranosyl 6- methoxy- 9H-purin
Cyclophosphamide	CTX, Cytoxan
Cyclosporine	Sandimmune, Neoral, Gengraf
Cytarabine	Cytosine arabinoside, AraC, Cytosar
Dactinomycin	Actinomycin-D, Cosmegen
Daunorubicin	Daunomycin, CNR, Cerubidine
Deferoxamine	Desferrioxamine, Desferoxamine, DFO, Desferal
Dexamethasone	Decadron
Dexrazoxane	ADR-529, Zinecard, ICRF-187
Docetaxel	Taxotere
Doxorubicin	Adriamycin
Ecteinascidin	ET-743
Erwinia asparaginase	Erwinase
Etoposide	VP-16, VePeside, Etopophos
Fludarabine	Fludara, F-araAMP
Gemcitabine	Gemzar
Gemtuzumab ozogamicin	Mylotarg
Granulocyte Colony- Stimulating Factor	r-MetHuG-CSF, G-CSF, Filgrastim, Neupogen
Granulocyte Colony- Stimulating Factor, Pegylated	Neulasta, PEG-G-CSF, PEG-filigastim
Granulocyte Macrophage- Colony Stimulating Factor	rhu GM-CSF, GM-CSF, sargramostin, Prokin, Leukine
Hydrocortisone	Cortef, Solu-cortef
Hydroxyurea	HU, Hydrea
Interferon Gamma-1b	Actimmune, gamma interferon, immune interferon, lymphocyte interferon, rIFN-gamma, T-interferon

- Encourage your teen or child to eat and drink slowly. Avoid forcing past his or her point of tolerance.

- Do not offer favorite foods when the teen or child is feeling nauseous. This can "turn off" the child to those foods if they become associated with a feeling of nausea.

Table 33.1. Chemotherapy Medications (continued)

Medication Name	Also Known As...
Interferon-Alpha	alpha-IFN, Intron A, Roferon A
Interleukin-4	IL-4
Isotretinoin	cis-retinoic acid, Accutane
L-Asparaginase E. coli	Elspar, Kidrolase, Crasnitin, Leunase
Leucovorin Calcuim	LCV, Wellcovorin, citrovorum factor, folinic acid
Lymphocyte Immune Globin	Atgam, anti-thymocyte globuline equine
MAB Ch.14.18	
Melphalan	L-Phenylalanine Mustard, L-PAM, L-sarcolysin, Alkeran
Mesna	Mesnex
Methotrexate	MTX, Amethopterin
Methylprednisolone	Solu-medrol
Mitoxantrone	Novantrone, DHAD
Nitrogen mustard	Mechlorethamine hydrochloride, HN2, Mustarge
Oprelvekin	Neumega, Interleukin-11
Paclitaxel	Taxol
Peg-L-Asparaginase	Pegaspargase, Oncaspar, Polyethlene Glycol conjugated L-Asparaginase
Pentostatin	Deoxycoformycin, DCF, Nipent
Prednisone	Deltasone, Meticorten, Liquid Pred
Procarbazine	Matulane, Natulan
PSC-833	Valspodar
R115777	Farnesyl Protein Transferase Inhibitor, Zarnestra
Rasburicase	Elitek, urate oxidase
Rebeccamycin Analogue	BMY-27557-14
Rituximab	Rituxan, IDEC-C2B8
Squalamine Lactate	
Sulindac	Clinoril
Tamoxifen	Nolvadex™, tamoxifen citrate
Temozolomide	Temodar™
Teniposide	VM-26 Vumon®
Thioguanine	6-thioguanine, 6-TG
Thiotepa	Tepa, Tspa
Tirapazamine	
Topotecan	Hycamtin
Trastuzumab	Herceptin
Tretinoin	Vesanoid
Urate Oxidase	Rasburicase, UROX, Elitek
Vinblastine Sulfate	Velban, Exal, Velbe
Vincristine Sulfate	Oncovin, VCR
Vinorelbine	Navelbine

Source: CureSearch

- Avoid giving food for one to two hours before treatment if nausea occurs during radiation therapy or chemotherapy.

- Offer dry crackers, cereal, or toast.

- Clear, cool liquids are refreshing.

- Serve meals and snacks in well-ventilated rooms, since the cooking smells can cause nausea. Cold foods are less aromatic than hot foods and may be better tolerated. Use an exhaust fan in the kitchen when cooking to eliminate odors.

- Avoid taking the lid off of hospital trays in front of the teen or child, as even these odors can be nauseating. Remove the lid outside of the room, and take only the items into the room that the child wants.

- Breakfast foods are often tolerated best, and can be eaten at any time of the day.

- Dress in loose-fitting clothes.

- If nausea and vomiting is severe, try to drink at least some fluids you do not become dehydrated. If the problem continues, call the physician.

Ask your physician about medications that can be used to help control these symptoms, called antiemetics.

Organ Damage

Chemotherapy drugs may affect organs such as the heart, lungs, kidneys, liver, and brain, causing temporary or permanent damage. Some drugs may also affect hearing.

Talk with your healthcare team to understand potential side effects, and to be aware of medical monitoring designed to avoid damage during treatment. You should notify them as soon as there are any changes in your health.

Chemotherapy Medications

It is important to have a basic understanding of the types of chemotherapy that will be used in treatment as well as the most common side effects. Table 33.1 lists the various chemotherapy medications used to treat children's cancer. Talk to your doctor about the specific medications you will receive so you can understand how it is given, how it works, and potential side effects.

Chapter 34

Steroids And Cancer Treatment

When you hear the word steroid you may think of "roid rage" and muscle-bound gym rats with shrunken testicles. But if your doctor prescribed steroids as part of your treatment for cancer or another serious illness, don't worry. It's not "that" kind of steroid.

Your doctor is actually talking about cortisol, a form of steroid that your body produces naturally. It's different from anabolic steroids, which are the illegal muscle-building kind.

How Steroids Help

Although the cortisol-type steroids prescribed for cancer treatment are different from anabolic steroids, you still need to take them under the close supervision of your doctor or medical specialist.

You'll probably get a manmade version of the natural steroid cortisol, such as:

- Cortisone
- Hydrocortisone
- Prednisone
- Methylprednisolone
- Dexamethasone

About This Chapter: "Steroids And Cancer Treatment," October 2012, reprinted with permission from www .kidshealth.org. This information was provided by KidsHealth®, one of the largest resources online for medically reviewed health information written for parents, kids, and teens. For more articles like this, visit www.KidsHealth .org, or www.TeensHealth.org. Copyright © 1995-2013 The Nemours Foundation. All rights reserved.

These can help with your treatment in a variety of ways:

- Reduce nausea associated with chemotherapy and radiation

- Kill cancer cells and shrink tumors as part of chemotherapy

- Decrease swelling

- Reduce allergic reactions (before transfusions, for example)

- Lessen headaches caused by brain tumors

Sometimes, your doctor will recommend steroid treatments just to help you sleep, eat, and feel better.

Doctors can prescribe steroids for cancer treatment several ways:

- By injection

- Through an intravenous (IV) drip

- In liquid or pill form

- As a cream

Side Effects

Steroids used in medical treatments can have some side effects, although they're not as extreme as the side effects from anabolic steroids. Talk to your doctor and ask questions if you're worried.

You may not have any side effects. But if you do, don't worry—they'll only last as long as you're taking the steroids. When you stop your treatment, things will return to normal.

Some of the more common side effects of steroid treatments include:

- Increased appetite

- Weight gain, often in unfamiliar places, like your cheeks or the back of your neck

- Mood swings

- Stomach upset or ulcers

- Osteoporosis (weaker bones)

- Vision problems

- Higher blood pressure

- Increased blood sugar. Sometimes, people develop diabetes temporarily. If you already have diabetes, you'll need to monitor your blood sugar levels more closely.

- For girls, irregular menstruation (missed or late periods)

Less common side effects include bruising more easily, difficulty fighting infections, acne flare-ups, and increased facial hair.

If you develop several of these symptoms, you have a condition called Cushing syndrome. Sometimes it gets better if you make changes in the way you take the steroids. If you're having problems with these side effects, talk to your doctor.

Remember!

You may not have any side effects. If you do, you'll probably find that they're overshadowed by the benefits of the treatment. But check with your doctor about ways to make them easier to live with.

Tips On Taking Steroids For Cancer Treatment

Your doc will give you all the details, of course, but there are some things to remember when taking steroids for cancer treatment. Here are a few:

Don't stop taking the medication without your doctor's guidance. If you notice anything strange while you're being treated with steroids, tell your parents and doctor right away. Don't stop taking the steroid, though. Your body makes less cortisol when you're having steroid treatments, so you need to ease off the medication and give your body a chance to get its own production back up to normal again. If you don't, your body could go through a potentially serious withdrawal. Weaning your body off the medication is easy to do, and your doctor will guide you through it.

Quick Tip

No flush, no foul. If your treatment is done and you have tablets left over, give them to your doctor or a pharmacist. Don't flush them down the toilet or throw them away because they could get into the water supply and cause problems.

Your card—don't leave home without it. A lot of steroid treatments happen in a doctor's office or clinic. But if you're on a long-term steroid treatment and have pills to take at home, your doctor may give you a steroid card or a medical alert bracelet. It's important to keep this card with you (or wear your medical alert bracelet) at all times. If there's an emergency, the card or bracelet will let doctors know you're being treated with steroids—or have been recently, which can change the treatment they need to give you.

Don't "double-up" if you miss a dose. Call your doctor or nurse and ask what to do if you forget to take a tablet.

Chapter 35

Radiation Therapy For Cancer

What is radiation therapy?

Radiation therapy uses high-energy radiation to shrink tumors and kill cancer cells. X-rays, gamma rays, and charged particles are types of radiation used for cancer treatment.

The radiation may be delivered by a machine outside the body (external-beam radiation therapy), or it may come from radioactive material placed in the body near cancer cells (internal radiation therapy, also called brachytherapy).

Systemic radiation therapy uses radioactive substances, such as radioactive iodine, that travel in the blood to kill cancer cells.

About half of all cancer patients receive some type of radiation therapy sometime during the course of their treatment.

Does radiation therapy kill only cancer cells?

No, radiation therapy can also damage normal cells, leading to side effects.

Doctors take potential damage to normal cells into account when planning a course of radiation therapy. The amount of radiation that normal tissue can safely receive is known for all parts of the body. Doctors use this information to help them decide where to aim radiation during treatment.

About This Chapter: Excerpted from "Radiation Therapy for Cancer," National Cancer Institute (NCI), June 30, 2010. Available at: www.cancer.gov. Accessed May 16, 2013.

> ## It's A Fact!
>
> Radiation therapy kills cancer cells by damaging their DNA (the molecules inside cells that carry genetic information and pass it from one generation to the next). Radiation therapy can either damage DNA directly or create charged particles (free radicals) within the cells that can in turn damage the DNA.
>
> Cancer cells whose DNA is damaged beyond repair stop dividing or die. When the damaged cells die, they are broken down and eliminated by the body's natural processes.

Why do patients receive radiation therapy?

Radiation therapy is sometimes given with curative intent (that is, with the hope that the treatment will cure a cancer, either by eliminating a tumor, preventing cancer recurrence, or both). In such cases, radiation therapy may be used alone or in combination with surgery, chemotherapy, or both.

Radiation therapy may also be given with palliative intent. Palliative treatments are not intended to cure. Instead, they relieve symptoms and reduce the suffering caused by cancer.

Some examples of palliative radiation therapy are:

- Radiation given to the brain to shrink tumors formed from cancer cells that have spread to the brain from another part of the body (metastases)

- Radiation given to shrink a tumor that is pressing on the spine or growing within a bone, which can cause pain

- Radiation given to shrink a tumor near the esophagus, which can interfere with a patient's ability to eat and drink

How is radiation therapy planned for an individual patient?

A radiation oncologist develops a patient's treatment plan through a process called treatment planning, which begins with simulation.

During simulation, detailed imaging scans show the location of a patient's tumor and the normal areas around it. These scans are usually computed tomography (CT) scans, but they can also include magnetic resonance imaging (MRI), positron emission tomography (PET), and ultrasound scans.

During simulation and daily treatments, it is necessary to ensure that the patient will be in exactly the same position every day relative to the machine delivering the treatment or doing the imaging. Body molds, head masks, or other devices may be constructed for an individual patient to make it easier for a patient to stay still. Temporary skin marks and even tattoos are used to help with precise patient positioning.

After simulation, the radiation oncologist then determines the exact area that will be treated, the total radiation dose that will be delivered to the tumor, how much dose will be allowed for the normal tissues around the tumor, and the safest angles (paths) for radiation delivery.

The staff working with the radiation oncologist (including physicists and dosimetrists) use sophisticated computers to design the details of the exact radiation plan that will be used. After approving the plan, the radiation oncologist authorizes the start of treatment. On the first day of treatment, and usually at least weekly after that, many checks are made to ensure that the treatments are being delivered exactly the way they were planned.

Radiation can damage some types of normal tissue more easily than others. For example, the reproductive organs (testicles and ovaries) are more sensitive to radiation than bones. The radiation oncologist takes all of this information into account during treatment planning.

If an area of the body has previously been treated with radiation therapy, a patient may not be able to have radiation therapy to that area a second time, depending on how much radiation was given during the initial treatment. If one area of the body has already received the maximum safe lifetime dose of radiation, another area might still be treated with radiation therapy if the distance between the two areas is large enough.

The area selected for treatment usually includes the whole tumor plus a small amount of normal tissue surrounding the tumor. The normal tissue is treated for two main reasons:

- To take into account body movement from breathing and normal movement of the organs within the body, which can change the location of a tumor between treatments

- To reduce the likelihood of tumor recurrence from cancer cells that have spread to the normal tissue next to the tumor (called microscopic local spread)

It's A Fact!

Radiation doses for cancer treatment are measured in a unit called a gray (Gy), which is a measure of the amount of radiation energy absorbed by one kilogram of human tissue. Different doses of radiation are needed to kill different types of cancer cells.

How is radiation therapy given to patients?

Radiation can come from a machine outside the body (external-beam radiation therapy) or from radioactive material placed in the body near cancer cells (internal radiation therapy, more commonly called brachytherapy). Systemic radiation therapy uses a radioactive substance, given by mouth or into a vein, that travels in the blood to tissues throughout the body.

The type of radiation therapy prescribed by a radiation oncologist depends on many factors, including the following:

- Type of cancer.

- Size of the cancer

- The cancer's location in the body

- How close the cancer is to normal tissues that are sensitive to radiation

- How far into the body the radiation needs to travel

- Patient's general health and medical history

- Whether the patient will have other types of cancer treatment

- Other factors, such as the patient's age and other medical conditions

What is external-beam radiation therapy?

External-beam radiation therapy is most often delivered in the form of photon beams (either x-rays or gamma rays). A photon is the basic unit of light and other forms of electromagnetic radiation. It can be thought of as a bundle of energy. The amount of energy in a photon can vary. For example, the photons in gamma rays have the highest energy, followed by the photons in x-rays.

Patients usually receive external-beam radiation therapy in daily treatment sessions over the course of several weeks. The number of treatment sessions depends on many factors, including the total radiation dose that will be given.

One of the most common types of external-beam radiation therapy is called *3–dimensional conformal radiation therapy (3D-CRT)*. 3D-CRT uses very sophisticated computer software and advanced treatment machines to deliver radiation to very precisely shaped target areas.

Many other methods of external-beam radiation therapy are currently being tested and used in cancer treatment. These methods include the following:

Intensity-Modulated Radiation Therapy (IMRT): IMRT uses hundreds of tiny radiation beam-shaping devices, called collimators, to deliver a single dose of radiation. The collimators can be stationary or can move during treatment, allowing the intensity of the radiation beams to change during treatment sessions. This kind of dose modulation allows different areas of a tumor or nearby tissues to receive different dose of radiation.

The goal of IMRT is to increase the radiation dose to the areas that need it and reduce radiation exposure to specific sensitive areas of surrounding normal tissue. Compared with 3D-CRT, IMRT can reduce the risk of some side effects, such as damage to the salivary glands (which can cause dry mouth, or xerostomia), when the head and neck are treated with radiation therapy. However, with IMRT, a larger volume of normal tissue overall is exposed to radiation. Whether IMRT leads to improved control of tumor growth and better survival compared with 3D-CRT is not yet known.

Image-Guided Radiation Therapy (IGRT): In IGRT, repeated imaging scans (CT, MRI, or PET) are performed during treatment. These imaging scans are processed by computers to identify changes in a tumor's size and location due to treatment and to allow the position of the patient or the planned radiation dose to be adjusted during treatment as needed. Repeated imaging can increase the accuracy of radiation treatment and may allow reductions in the planned volume of tissue to be treated, thereby decreasing the total radiation dose to normal tissue.

Tomotherapy: Tomotherapy is a type of image-guided IMRT. A tomotherapy machine is a hybrid between a CT imaging scanner and an external-beam radiation therapy machine The part of the tomotherapy machine that delivers radiation for both imaging and treatment can rotate completely around the patient in the same manner as a normal CT scanner. Tomotherapy machines can capture CT images of the patient's tumor immediately before treatment sessions, to allow for very precise tumor targeting and sparing of normal tissue.

Stereotactic Radiosurgery: Stereotactic radiosurgery (SRS) can deliver one or more high doses of radiation to a small tumor. SRS uses extremely accurate image-guided tumor targeting and patient positioning. Therefore, a high dose of radiation can be given without excess damage to normal tissue.

SRS can be used to treat only small tumors with well-defined edges. It is most commonly used in the treatment of brain or spinal tumors and brain metastases from other cancer types. For the treatment of some brain metastases, patients may receive radiation therapy to the entire brain (called whole-brain radiation therapy) in addition to SRS.

SRS requires the use of a head frame or other device to immobilize the patient during treatment to ensure that the high dose of radiation is delivered accurately.

Stereotactic Body Radiation Therapy: Stereotactic body radiation therapy (SBRT) delivers radiation therapy in fewer sessions, using smaller radiation fields and higher doses than 3D-CRT in most cases. By definition, SBRT treats tumors that lie outside the brain and spinal cord. Because these tumors are more likely to move with the normal motion of the body, and therefore cannot be targeted as accurately as tumors within the brain or spine, SBRT is usually given in more than one dose. SBRT can be used to treat only small, isolated tumors, including cancers in the lung and liver. Many doctors refer to SBRT systems by their brand names, such as the CyberKnife.

Proton Therapy: External-beam radiation therapy can be delivered by proton beams as well as the photon beams described above. Protons are a type of charged particle.

Other Charged Particle Beams: Electron beams are used to irradiate superficial tumors, such as skin cancer or tumors near the surface of the body, but they cannot travel very far through tissue. Therefore, they cannot treat tumors deep within the body.

What is internal radiation therapy?

Internal radiation therapy (brachytherapy) is radiation delivered from radiation sources (radioactive materials) placed inside or on the body. Several brachytherapy techniques are used in cancer treatment. Interstitial brachytherapy uses a radiation source placed within tumor tissue, such as within a prostate tumor. Intracavitary brachytherapy uses a source placed within a surgical cavity or a body cavity, such as the chest cavity, near a tumor. Episcleral brachytherapy, which is used to treat melanoma inside the eye, uses a source that is attached to the eye.

In brachytherapy, radioactive isotopes are sealed in tiny pellets or "seeds." These seeds are placed in patients using delivery devices, such as needles, catheters, or some other type of carrier. As the isotopes decay naturally, they give off radiation that damages nearby cancer cells. If left in place, after a few weeks or months, the isotopes decay completely and no longer give off radiation. The seeds will not cause harm if they are left in the body. Brachytherapy may be able to deliver higher doses of radiation to some cancers than external-beam radiation therapy while causing less damage to normal tissue.

Quick Tip

Patients can discuss different methods of radiation therapy with their doctors to see if any is appropriate for their type of cancer and if it is available in their community or through a clinical trial.

Brachytherapy can be given as a low-dose-rate or a high-dose-rate treatment:

- In low-dose-rate treatment, cancer cells receive continuous low-dose radiation from the source over a period of several days.

- In high-dose-rate treatment, a robotic machine attached to delivery tubes placed inside the body guides one or more radioactive sources into or near a tumor, and then removes the sources at the end of each treatment session. High-dose-rate treatment can be given in one or more treatment sessions.

The placement of brachytherapy sources can be temporary or permanent. For permanent brachytherapy, the sources are surgically sealed within the body and left there, even after all of the radiation has been given off. The remaining material (in which the radioactive isotopes were sealed) does not cause any discomfort or harm to the patient. Permanent brachytherapy is a type of low-dose-rate brachytherapy.

Doctors can use brachytherapy alone or in addition to external-beam radiation therapy to provide a "boost" of radiation to a tumor while sparing surrounding normal tissue.

What is systemic radiation therapy?

In systemic radiation therapy, a patient swallows or receives an injection of a radioactive substance, such as radioactive iodine or a radioactive substance bound to a monoclonal antibody.

Radioactive iodine is a type of systemic radiation therapy commonly used to help treat some types of thyroid cancer. Thyroid cells naturally take up radioactive iodine.

For systemic radiation therapy for some other types of cancer, a monoclonal antibody (a type of protein made in a laboratory) helps target the radioactive substance to the right place. The antibody joined to the radioactive substance travels through the blood, locating and killing tumor cells.

Many other systemic radiation therapy drugs are in clinical trials for different cancer types.

Some systemic radiation therapy drugs relieve pain from cancer that has spread to the bone (bone metastases). This is a type of palliative radiation therapy.

Why are some types of radiation therapy given in many small doses?

Patients who receive most types of external-beam radiation therapy usually have to travel to the hospital or an outpatient facility up to five days a week for several weeks. One dose (a single fraction) of the total planned dose of radiation is given each day. Occasionally, two treatments a day are given.

Most types of external-beam radiation therapy are given in once-daily fractions. There are two main reasons for once-daily treatment:

- To minimize the damage to normal tissue.

- To increase the likelihood that cancer cells are exposed to radiation at the points in the cell cycle when they are most vulnerable to DNA damage.

In recent decades, doctors have tested whether other fractionation schedules are helpful, such as accelerated fractionation, which uses larger daily or weekly doses to reduce the number of weeks of treatments.

Radiation Timing

A patient may receive radiation therapy before, during, or after surgery. Some patients may receive radiation therapy alone, without surgery or other treatments. Some patients may receive radiation therapy and chemotherapy at the same time. The timing of radiation therapy depends on the type of cancer being treated and the goal of treatment (cure or palliation).

Radiation therapy given before surgery is called pre-operative or neoadjuvant radiation. Neoadjuvant radiation may be given to shrink a tumor so it can be removed by surgery and be less likely to return after surgery.

Radiation therapy given during surgery is called intraoperative radiation therapy (IORT). IORT can be external-beam radiation therapy (with photons or electrons) or brachytherapy. When radiation is given during surgery, nearby normal tissues can be physically shielded from radiation exposure. IORT is sometimes used when normal structures are too close to a tumor to allow the use of external-beam radiation therapy.

Radiation therapy given after surgery is called postoperative or adjuvant radiation therapy.

Radiation therapy given after some types of complicated surgery (especially in the abdomen or pelvis) may produce too many side effects; therefore, it may be safer if given before surgery in these cases.

The combination of chemotherapy and radiation therapy given at the same time is sometimes called chemoradiation or radiochemotherapy. For some types of cancer, the combination of chemotherapy and radiation therapy may kill more cancer cells (increasing the likelihood of a cure), but it can also cause more side effects.

Does radiation therapy make a patient radioactive?

External-beam radiation does not make a patient radioactive.

During temporary brachytherapy treatments, while the radioactive material is inside the body, the patient is radioactive; however, as soon as the material is removed, the patient is no longer radioactive. For temporary brachytherapy, the patient will usually stay in the hospital in a special room that shields other people from the radiation.

During permanent brachytherapy, the implanted material will be radioactive for several days, weeks, or months after the radiation source is put in place. During this time, the patient is radioactive. However, the amount of radiation reaching the surface of the skin is usually very low. Nonetheless, this radiation can be detected by radiation monitors and contact with pregnant woman and young children may be restricted for a few days or weeks.

Some types of systemic radiation therapy may temporarily make a patient's bodily fluids (such as saliva, urine, sweat, or stool) emit a low level of radiation. Patients receiving systemic radiation therapy may need to limit their contact with other people during this time, and especially avoid contact with children younger than 18 and pregnant women.

A patient's doctor or nurse will provide more information to family members and caretakers if any of these special precautions are needed. Over time (usually days or weeks), the radioactive material retained within the body will break down so that no radiation can be measured outside the patient's body.

What are the potential side effects of radiation therapy?

Radiation therapy can cause both early (acute) and late (chronic) side effects. Acute side effects occur during treatment, and chronic side effects occur months or even years after treatment ends. The side effects that develop depend on the area of the body being treated, the dose given per day, the total dose given, the patient's general medical condition, and other treatments given at the same time.

Acute radiation side effects are caused by damage to rapidly dividing normal cells in the area being treated. These effects include skin irritation or damage at regions exposed to the radiation beams. Examples include damage to the salivary glands or hair loss when the head or neck area is treated, or urinary problems when the lower abdomen is treated.

Most acute effects disappear after treatment ends, though some (like salivary gland damage) can be permanent. The drug amifostine (Ethyol) can help protect the salivary glands from radiation damage if it is given during treatment.

Fatigue is a common side effect of radiation therapy regardless of which part of the body is treated. Nausea with or without vomiting is common when the abdomen is treated and occurs sometimes when the brain is treated. Medications are available to help prevent or treat nausea and vomiting during treatment.

Late side effects of radiation therapy may or may not occur. Depending on the area of the body treated, late side effects can include the following:

- Fibrosis (the replacement of normal tissue with scar tissue, leading to restricted movement of the affected area)

- Damage to the bowels, causing diarrhea and bleeding

- Memory loss

- Infertility (inability to have a child)

- Rarely, a second cancer caused by radiation exposure

Second cancers that develop after radiation therapy depend on the part of the body that was treated. For example, girls treated with radiation to the chest for Hodgkin lymphoma have an increased risk of developing breast cancer later in life. In general, the lifetime risk of a second cancer is highest in people treated for cancer as children or adolescents.

Whether or not a patient experiences late side effects depends on other aspects of their cancer treatment in addition to radiation therapy, as well as their individual risk factors. Some chemotherapy drugs, genetic risk factors, and lifestyle factors (such as smoking) can also increase the risk of late side effects.

What research is being done to improve radiation therapy?

Doctors and other scientists are conducting research studies called clinical trials to learn how to use radiation therapy to treat cancer more safely and effectively. Clinical trials allow researchers to examine the effectiveness of new treatments in comparison with standard ones, as well as to compare the side effects of the treatments.

Researchers are working on improving image-guided radiation so that it provides real-time imaging of the tumor target during treatment. Real-time imaging could help compensate for normal movement of the internal organs from breathing and for changes in tumor size during treatment.

Researchers are also studying radiosensitizers and radioprotectors, chemicals that modify a cell's response to radiation:

> **Remember!**
>
> When suggesting radiation therapy as part of a patient's cancer treatment, the radiation on-cologist will carefully weigh the known risks of treatment against the potential benefits for each patient (including relief of symptoms, shrinking a tumor, or potential cure). The results of hundreds of clinical trials and doctors' individual experiences help radiation oncologists decide which patients are likely to benefit from radiation therapy.

- Radiosensitizers are drugs that make cancer cells more sensitive to the effects of radiation therapy. Several agents are under study as radiosensitizers. In addition, some anticancer drugs, such as 5-fluorouracil and cisplatin, make cancer cells more sensitive to radiation therapy.

- Radioprotectors (also called radioprotectants) are drugs that protect normal cells from damage caused by radiation therapy. These drugs promote the repair of normal cells exposed to radiation. Many agents are currently being studied as potential radioprotectors.

Chapter 36

What To Expect If You Need Surgery

Even if you're a fan of TV hospital dramas, these shows might also make you nervous about what happens in an operating room. Millions of teens are wheeled into operating rooms (ORs) each year, so it can help to find out what to expect before you get to the hospital.

Depending on the type of surgery you need, you may have inpatient surgery or outpatient surgery (also called ambulatory surgery). Inpatient surgery usually requires that you stay in the hospital for a day or more so the doctors and nurses can monitor your recovery carefully. If you have outpatient surgery, you will go home the same day. This type of surgery may be performed in a hospital or an outpatient surgery clinic and you can go home when the doctor decides you're ready.

What To Expect

If your surgery is not an emergency, it will be planned in advance. You will make a visit to the hospital or outpatient surgery location beforehand. Examples of emergency surgery include a broken elbow and appendicitis. When urgent surgery is required, you will go to the operating room after being diagnosed with a surgical problem.

When you know about your surgery ahead of time, you will arrive at the hospital and a nurse or other hospital employee will begin the pre-surgical process. He or she will begin by asking questions about your medical history, including any allergies you might have and any symptoms or pain you may be having. Girls may be asked if there is any chance of being pregnant. Nurses will also take your vital signs like your heart rate, temperature, and blood pressure.

About This Chapter: "What's It Like To Have Surgery?" August 2010, reprinted with permission from www .kidshealth.org. This information was provided by KidsHealth®, one of the largest resources online for medically reviewed health information written for parents, kids, and teens. For more articles like this, visit www.KidsHealth .org, or www.TeensHealth.org. Copyright © 1995-2013 The Nemours Foundation. All rights reserved.

Soon after you arrive, you'll be given an identification bracelet—a plastic tape with your name and birthdate on it—to wear around your wrist. You'll also be asked about the time you last ate or drank anything. This might seem strange, but it's actually very important to your safety. Having food or liquids in your stomach can lead to vomiting during or after the surgery and cause harmful complications.

You might need to have other tests, like x-rays and blood tests, before your surgery begins.

Before Surgery

Before your operation takes place, you and your family will have a chance to meet with the anesthesiologist—the doctor or certified registered nurse anesthetist (CRNA) who specializes in giving anesthetics, the medications that will help you fall asleep or numb an area of your body so you don't feel the surgery. The anesthesiology staff will have your medical information so you can be given the amount of anesthetic you need for your age, height, and weight.

There are several types of anesthesia. General anesthesia causes you to become completely unconscious during the operation. If you're having general anesthesia, the anesthesiologist or CRNA will be present during the entire operation to monitor your condition and ensure you constantly receive the right doses of medications.

If surgery is done under local anesthesia, you'll be given an anesthetic that numbs only the area of your body to be operated on. You also might be given a medication that makes you drowsy during the procedure.

Before your operation, the nurse or doctor will clean (and shave, if necessary) the area of your body that will be operated on. You'll be asked to take off any jewelry, including barrettes and hair ties, and you'll need to take out contact lenses if you wear them. You'll be given a hospital gown to wear in the operating room.

A nurse will put an IV (intravenous) line in your arm and attach it to thin plastic tubing that is connected to a soft bag of fluid. This line will probably be used to give you anesthetic (if you're having general anesthesia) or provide you with fluids or medicine that may be needed during the operation.

As you're wheeled into a hospital operating room, you may notice that the nurses and doctors are wearing face masks and plastic eyeglasses, as well as paper caps, gowns, and booties over their shoes. Patients are vulnerable to infection during an operation, so this protective gear lowers the chance of infection while you're in the operating room.

The nurse or technician will then place monitoring equipment (sticker-like patches) on your skin to measure your heart rate and blood pressure at regular intervals.

Sometimes medical and nursing students observe surgeries, so don't be surprised if doctors and nurses aren't the only people in the room.

After Surgery

After your surgery is over, you'll be taken to the recovery room, where nurses will monitor your condition very closely for a few hours. Sometimes this room is also called the post-op (post-operative) room or PACU (post-anesthesia care unit). Your parent may be able to visit you here.

Every person has a different surgical experience, but if you've had general anesthesia, it's common to feel groggy, confused, chilly, nauseated, or even sad when you wake up. When the surgery has been completed, the surgeon will let you and your parents know how the procedure went and answer any questions you have.

Once your anesthesia has worn off and you're fully awake, you'll be taken to a regular hospital room if you're staying overnight. If you're having an outpatient procedure, you'll be monitored by nurses in another room until you're able to go home.

If you feel pain after the surgery, the doctors and nurses will make sure you have pain relievers to keep you more comfortable. You may also need to take other medications, such as antibiotics to prevent infection.

Taking The Worry Out Of Your Surgery

The thought of having surgery can be scary. If you're worried, try these tips to help feel more at ease:

- **Ask questions ahead of time.** Your surgeon, anesthesiologist, and nurses will be able to answer your questions about the surgery, how you'll feel afterward, how long it will take to return to your normal activities, what type of scarring you might have, etc. Don't feel embarrassed about asking lots of questions—the more informed you are, the more comfortable you'll feel about having surgery.

Before going into the OR, you may be asked to remove jewelry, including body jewelry like navel rings or tongue studs. That's because jewelry can introduce germs if it's near the area being operated on, or it could interfere with anesthesia or the placement of monitoring equipment. Besides, the safest place for valuables in at home to protect them from being lost or stolen.

Source: Nemours, August 2010.

- **Be sure you're clear on instructions—and ask if you're not.** Your doctor or a nurse will give you instructions on what to do before the surgery (called preoperative instructions) and what you can and can't do afterward (postoperative instructions). For example, your doctor may tell you to stop taking certain medications for a set period of time before surgery. (If you know about your surgery ahead of time, you should let your doctor know well in advance if you are taking any herbal or other non-prescription medications such as ibuprofen as your medical team might instruct you to stop taking them.) And follow your doctor's orders regarding eating before surgery. After surgery, your exercise and activities might be restricted for a while.

- **Practice healthy habits.** Smoking is never a good idea, but it's especially bad news after surgery when your body is trying to recover. Ditch the cigarettes, get plenty of rest, and eat nutritious foods.

Surgery For Cancer

Surgery is a primary treatment method for many types of solid tumors, especially when the cancer has not spread (metastasized) to other parts of your body. This involves surgical removal of all or part of your tumor.

Surgery is rarely used as the only treatment method. It is often preceded by radiation or chemotherapy, with the intent of shrinking your tumor; or followed by radiation or chemotherapy, to destroy any remaining cancer cells and reduce the risk of reoccurrence. The type of surgery you may have will depend on your type of cancer, the location of your tumor, its size, and other factors.

Surgery also plays an important role in the diagnosis of your cancer. Often, cancer can only be correctly identified when cells are viewed under a microscope or tested in a laboratory. This is done through a procedure called a biopsy that takes a small sample of tissue to examine. It may be done under general anesthesia or, as in the case of a bone marrow biopsy, with little or no medication.

Additionally, central lines (Broviacs, Medi-ports, etc.) are surgically implanted, either under local or general anesthesia.

Surgical methods have improved over the years reducing the potential impact to your healthy tissue as well as minimizing the potential side effects and reducing risks. Talk with your medical team about treatment options, including various surgical methods.

Source: "Surgery," reprinted with permission from Teens Living with Cancer, a program of Melissa's Living Legacy Teen Cancer Foundation, © 2013. All rights reserved. The Melissa's Living Legacy Teen Cancer Foundation is a non-profit organization providing resources to help teens with cancer have meaningful, life-affirming experiences throughout all stages of their disease. For additional information, visit www.teenslivingwithcancer.org.

- **Try relaxation techniques.** If you're nervous or anxious, taking a few slow, deep breaths or focusing on an object in the room can help you to tune out stressful thoughts and cope with your anxiety. Think of your favorite place and what you like to do there.

- **Plan ahead**. If you have to miss school because of surgery, talk to your teachers ahead of time and arrange to make up any tests or assignments. Get a friend you trust to take notes for you and drop off homework assignments. By planning ahead, you won't have to spend your recovery time stressing about your grades.

- **Tell a few people.** If you don't feel like sharing the details of your operation, you don't have to—but telling some friends that you'll be out of school for a few days might ensure you'll have some visitors. Your friends might even have some surgery stories of their own to share.

- **Pack a few favorites.** After you're out of the recovery room, you might want the comfort that some favorite CDs, iTunes, books, magazines, or a journal can bring, so make sure that when you're packing your hospital bag, you throw in a few goodies.

Chapter 37

Bone Marrow And Peripheral Blood Cell Transplantation

What are bone marrow and hematopoietic stem cells?

Bone marrow is the soft, sponge-like material found inside bones. It contains immature cells known as hematopoietic or blood-forming stem cells. (Hematopoietic stem cells are different from embryonic stem cells. Embryonic stem cells can develop into every type of cell in the body.) Hematopoietic stem cells divide to form more blood-forming stem cells, or they mature into one of three types of blood cells: white blood cells, which fight infection; red blood cells, which carry oxygen; and platelets, which help the blood to clot. Most hematopoietic stem cells are found in the bone marrow, but some cells, called peripheral blood stem cells (PBSCs), are found in the bloodstream. Blood in the umbilical cord also contains hematopoietic stem cells. Cells from any of these sources can be used in transplants.

What are bone marrow transplantation and peripheral blood stem cell transplantation?

Bone marrow transplantation (BMT) and peripheral blood stem cell transplantation (PBSCT) are procedures that restore stem cells that have been destroyed by high doses of chemotherapy and/or radiation therapy. There are three types of transplants:

- **Autologous Transplants:** Patients receive their own stem cells.

- **Syngeneic Transplants:** Patients receive stem cells from their identical twin.

- **Allogenic Transplants:** Patients receive stem cells from their brother, sister, or parent. A person who is not related to the patient (an unrelated donor) also may be used.

About This Chapter: From "Bone Marrow Transplantation and Peripheral Blood Stem Cell Transplantation," National Cancer Institute (NCI), September 24, 2010. Available at: www.cancer.gov. Accessed May 13, 2013.

What types of cancer are treated with BMT and PBSCT?

BMT and PBSCT are most commonly used in the treatment of leukemia and lymphoma. They are most effective when the leukemia or lymphoma is in remission (the signs and symptoms of cancer have disappeared). BMT and PBSCT are also used to treat other cancers such as neuroblastoma (cancer that arises in immature nerve cells and affects mostly infants and children) and multiple myeloma. Researchers are evaluating BMT and PBSCT in clinical trials (research studies) for the treatment of various types of cancer.

How are the donor's stem cells matched to the patient's stem cells in allogenic or syngeneic transplantation?

To minimize potential side effects, doctors most often use transplanted stem cells that match the patient's own stem cells as closely as possible. People have different sets of proteins, called human leukocyte-associated (HLA) antigens, on the surface of their cells. The set of proteins, called the HLA type, is identified by a special blood test.

In most cases, the success of allogenic transplantation depends in part on how well the HLA antigens of the donor's stem cells match those of the recipient's stem cells. The higher the number of matching HLA antigens, the greater the chance that the patient's body will accept

Why Transplantation Is Used To Treat Cancer

One reason bone marrow and peripheral blood stem cell transplantation are used in cancer treatment is to make it possible for patients to receive very high doses of chemotherapy and/or radiation therapy. To understand more about why BMT and PBSCT are used, it is helpful to understand how chemotherapy and radiation therapy work.

Chemotherapy and radiation therapy generally affect cells that divide rapidly. They are used to treat cancer because cancer cells divide more often than most healthy cells. However, because bone marrow cells also divide frequently, high-dose treatments can severely damage or destroy the patient's bone marrow. Without healthy bone marrow, the patient is no longer able to make the blood cells needed to carry oxygen, fight infection, and prevent bleeding. BMT and PBSCT replace stem cells destroyed by treatment. The healthy, transplanted stem cells can restore the bone marrow's ability to produce the blood cells the patient needs.

In some types of leukemia, the graft-versus-tumor (GVT) effect that occurs after allogenic BMT and PBSCT is crucial to the effectiveness of the treatment. GVT occurs when white blood cells from the donor (the graft) identify the cancer cells that remain in the patient's body after the chemotherapy and/or radiation therapy (the tumor) as foreign and attack them. (A potential complication of allogenic transplant called graft-versus-host disease is discussed in this chapter.)

the donor's stem cells. In general, patients are less likely to develop a complication known as graft-versus-host disease (GVHD) if the stem cells of the donor and patient are closely matched.

Close relatives, especially brothers and sisters, are more likely than unrelated people to be HLA-matched. However, only 25 to 35 percent of patients have an HLA-matched sibling. The chances of obtaining HLA-matched stem cells from an unrelated donor are slightly better, approximately 50 percent. Among unrelated donors, HLA-matching is greatly improved when the donor and recipient have the same ethnic and racial background. Although the number of donors is increasing overall, individuals from certain ethnic and racial groups still have a lower chance of finding a matching donor. Large volunteer donor registries can assist in finding an appropriate unrelated donor.

Because identical twins have the same genes, they have the same set of HLA antigens. As a result, the patient's body will accept a transplant from an identical twin. However, identical twins represent a small number of all births, so syngeneic transplantation is rare.

How is bone marrow obtained for transplantation?

The stem cells used in BMT come from the liquid center of the bone, called the marrow. In general, the procedure for obtaining bone marrow, which is called "harvesting," is similar for all three types of BMTs (autologous, syngeneic, and allogenic). The donor is given either general anesthesia, which puts the person to sleep during the procedure, or regional anesthesia, which causes loss of feeling below the waist. Needles are inserted through the skin over the pelvic (hip) bone or, in rare cases, the sternum (breastbone), and into the bone marrow to draw the marrow out of the bone. Harvesting the marrow takes about an hour.

The harvested bone marrow is then processed to remove blood and bone fragments. Harvested bone marrow can be combined with a preservative and frozen to keep the stem cells alive until they are needed. This technique is known as cryopreservation. Stem cells can be cryopreserved for many years.

How are PBSCs obtained for transplantation?

The stem cells used in PBSCT come from the bloodstream. A process called apheresis or leukapheresis is used to obtain PBSCs for transplantation. For four or five days before apheresis, the donor may be given a medication to increase the number of stem cells released into the bloodstream. In apheresis, blood is removed through a large vein in the arm or a central venous catheter (a flexible tube that is placed in a large vein in the neck, chest, or groin area). The blood goes through a machine that removes the stem cells. The blood is then returned to the donor and the collected cells are stored. Apheresis typically takes four to six hours. The stem cells are then frozen until they are given to the recipient.

How are umbilical cord stem cells obtained for transplantation?

Stem cells also may be retrieved from umbilical cord blood. For this to occur, the mother must contact a cord blood bank before the baby's birth. The cord blood bank may request that she complete a questionnaire and give a small blood sample.

Cord blood banks may be public or commercial. Public cord blood banks accept donations of cord blood and may provide the donated stem cells to another matched individual in their network. In contrast, commercial cord blood banks will store the cord blood for the family, in case it is needed later for the child or another family member.

After the baby is born and the umbilical cord has been cut, blood is retrieved from the umbilical cord and placenta. This process poses minimal health risk to the mother or the child. If the mother agrees, the umbilical cord blood is processed and frozen for storage by the cord blood bank. Only a small amount of blood can be retrieved from the umbilical cord and placenta, so the collected stem cells are typically used for children or small adults.

How does the patient receive the stem cells during the transplant?

After being treated with high-dose anticancer drugs and/or radiation, the patient receives the stem cells through an intravenous (IV) line just like a blood transfusion. This part of the transplant takes one to five hours.

Are any special measures taken when the cancer patient is also the donor (autologous transplant)?

The stem cells used for autologous transplantation must be relatively free of cancer cells. The harvested cells can sometimes be treated before transplantation in a process known as "purging" to get rid of cancer cells. This process can remove some cancer cells from the harvested cells and minimize the chance that cancer will come back. Because purging may damage some healthy stem cells, more cells are obtained from the patient before the transplant so that enough healthy stem cells will remain after purging.

What happens after the stem cells have been transplanted to the patient?

After entering the bloodstream, the stem cells travel to the bone marrow, where they begin to produce new white blood cells, red blood cells, and platelets in a process known as "engraftment." Engraftment usually occurs within about two to four weeks after transplantation. Doctors monitor it by checking blood counts on a frequent basis. Complete recovery of immune function takes much longer, however—up to several months for autologous transplant recipients and one to two years for patients receiving allogenic or syngeneic transplants. Doctors evaluate the results of various blood tests to confirm that new blood cells are being produced and that the cancer has not returned. Bone marrow aspiration (the removal of a small sample of bone marrow through a needle for examination under a microscope) can also help doctors determine how well the new marrow is working.

What are the possible side effects of BMT and PBSCT?

The major risk of both treatments is an increased susceptibility to infection and bleeding as a result of the high-dose cancer treatment. Doctors may give the patient antibiotics to prevent or treat infection. They may also give the patient transfusions of platelets to prevent bleeding and red blood cells to treat anemia. Patients who undergo BMT and PBSCT may experience short-term side effects such as nausea, vomiting, fatigue, loss of appetite, mouth sores, hair loss, and skin reactions.

Potential long-term risks include complications of the pretransplant chemotherapy and radiation therapy, such as infertility (the inability to produce children); cataracts (clouding of the lens of the eye, which causes loss of vision); secondary (new) cancers; and damage to the liver, kidneys, lungs, and/or heart.

Are any risks associated with donating bone marrow or PBSCs?

Bone Marrow Donation: Because only a small amount of bone marrow is removed, donating usually does not pose any significant problems for the donor. The most serious risk associated with donating bone marrow involves the use of anesthesia during the procedure.

The area where the bone marrow was taken out may feel stiff or sore for a few days, and the donor may feel tired. Within a few weeks, the donor's body replaces the donated marrow; however, the time required for a donor to recover varies. Some people are back to their usual routine within two or three days, while others may take up to three to four weeks to fully recover their strength.

PBSC Donation: Apheresis usually causes minimal discomfort. During apheresis, the person may feel lightheadedness, chills, numbness around the lips, and cramping in the hands. Unlike bone marrow donation, PBSC donation does not require anesthesia. The medication that is given to stimulate the mobilization (release) of stem cells from the marrow into the bloodstream may cause bone and muscle aches, headaches, fatigue, nausea, vomiting, and/or difficulty sleeping. These side effects generally stop within two to three days of the last dose of the medication.

With allogenic transplants, GVHD sometimes develops when white blood cells from the donor (the graft) identify cells in the patient's body (the host) as foreign and attack them. The most commonly damaged organs are the skin, liver, and intestines. This complication can develop within a few weeks of the transplant (acute GVHD) or much later (chronic GVHD). To prevent this complication, the patient may receive medications that suppress the immune system. Additionally, the donated stem cells can be treated to remove the white blood cells that cause GVHD in a process called "T-cell depletion." If GVHD develops, it can be very serious and is treated with steroids or other immunosuppressive agents. GVHD can be difficult to treat, but some studies suggest that patients with leukemia who develop GVHD are less likely to have the cancer come back. Clinical trials are being conducted to find ways to prevent and treat GVHD.

The likelihood and severity of complications are specific to the patient's treatment and should be discussed with the patient's doctor.

What is a "mini-transplant"?

A "mini-transplant" (also called a non-myeloablative or reduced-intensity transplant) is a type of allogenic transplant. This approach is being studied in clinical trials for the treatment of several types of cancer, including leukemia, lymphoma, multiple myeloma, and other cancers of the blood.

A mini-transplant uses lower, less toxic doses of chemotherapy and/or radiation to prepare the patient for an allogenic transplant. The use of lower doses of anticancer drugs and radiation eliminates some, but not all, of the patient's bone marrow. It also reduces the number of cancer cells and suppresses the patient's immune system to prevent rejection of the transplant.

Unlike traditional BMT or PBSCT, cells from both the donor and the patient may exist in the patient's body for some time after a mini-transplant. Once the cells from the donor begin to engraft, they may cause the GVT effect and work to destroy the cancer cells that were not eliminated by the anticancer drugs and/or radiation. To boost the GVT effect, the patient may be given an injection of the donor's white blood cells. This procedure is called a "donor lymphocyte infusion."

What is a "tandem transplant"?

A "tandem transplant" is a type of autologous transplant. This method is being studied in clinical trials for the treatment of several types of cancer, including multiple myeloma and germ cell cancer. During a tandem transplant, a patient receives two sequential courses of high-dose chemotherapy with stem cell transplant. Typically, the two courses are given several weeks to several months apart. Researchers hope that this method can prevent the cancer from recurring (coming back) at a later time.

How do patients cover the cost of BMT or PBSCT?

Advances in treatment methods, including the use of PBSCT, have reduced the amount of time many patients must spend in the hospital by speeding recovery. This shorter recovery time has brought about a reduction in cost. However, because BMT and PBSCT are complicated technical procedures, they are very expensive. Many health insurance companies cover some of the costs of transplantation for certain types of cancer. Insurers may also cover a portion of the costs if special care is required when the patient returns home.

There are options for relieving the financial burden associated with BMT and PBSCT. A hospital social worker is a valuable resource in planning for these financial needs. Federal government programs and local service organizations may also be able to help.

The National Cancer Institute (NCI) offers a service, Cancer Information Service (CIS), that can provide patients and their families with additional information about sources of financial assistance at 800-422-6237 (800-4-CANCER). NCI is part of the National Institutes of Health.

National Marrow Donor Program

The National Marrow Donor Program® (NMDP), a federally funded nonprofit organization, was created to improve the effectiveness of the search for donors. The NMDP maintains an international registry of volunteers willing to be donors for all sources of blood stem cells used in transplantation: bone marrow, peripheral blood, and umbilical cord blood.

The NMDP website contains a list of transplant centers that perform allogenic transplants. The list includes descriptions of the centers as well as their transplant experience, survival statistics, research interests, pretransplant costs, and contact information. The website is at: http://marrow.org/Patient/Transplant_Planning/Choosing_a_Transplant_Center/U_S_ _Transplant_Centers.aspx [note: there are two underscores after the S before Transplant]

Contact the National Marrow Donor Program at 800-627-7692 (800-MARROW2) for the Be The Match Registry or 888-999-6743 for Be The Match Patient Services. The program can be contacted by email at patientinfo@nmdp or visited online at http://www.bethematch.org.

What are the costs of donating bone marrow, PBSCs, or umbilical cord blood?

Persons willing to donate bone marrow or PBSCs must have a sample of blood drawn to determine their HLA type. This blood test usually costs $65 to $96. The donor may be asked to pay for this blood test, or the donor center may cover part of the cost. Community groups and other organizations may also provide financial assistance. Once a donor is identified as a match for a patient, all of the costs pertaining to the retrieval of bone marrow or PBSCs is covered by the patient or the patient's medical insurance.

A woman can donate her baby's umbilical cord blood to public cord blood banks at no charge. However, commercial blood banks do charge varying fees to store umbilical cord blood for the private use of the patient or his or her family.

Where can people get more information about clinical trials of BMT and PBSCT?

Clinical trials that include BMT and PBSCT are a treatment option for some patients. Information about ongoing clinical trials is available from NCI's CIS at 800-422-6237 (800-4-CANCER) or on NCI's website at http://www.cancer.gov/clinicaltrials.

Chapter 38

Cancer And Complementary Health Therapies

People with cancer want to do everything they can to combat the disease, manage its symptoms, and cope with the side effects of treatment. Many turn to complementary health practices, including natural products—such as botanical (herbal) and other dietary supplements—and mind and body therapies—such as acupuncture, massage, and yoga.

About Complementary Health Practices

The term *complementary health practices* refers to a group of diverse medical and health care systems, practices, and products whose origins come from outside of mainstream medicine. It includes natural products, such as dietary supplements, herbs, and probiotics, as well as mind and body practices, such as meditation, acupuncture, and massage.

Some complementary health practices are beginning to find a place in cancer treatment—not as cures but as complementary approaches that may help patients feel better.

Use Of Complementary Health Practices For Cancer

Many people who have been diagnosed with cancer use complementary health practices. In 2002 and 2007, the National Health Interview Survey (NHIS) included comprehensive questions on the use of complementary health practices by Americans. According to the 2007 NHIS, more than one-third of adults (about 38 percent) had used some form of complementary health practice. A special analysis of 2002 NHIS data found that use was more prevalent among people with

About This Chapter: Excerpted from "Cancer And Complementary Health Practices," National Center for Complementary and Alternative Medicine (NCCAM), March 2012.

a prior diagnosis of cancer. About 40 percent of cancer survivors reported using these practices; 18 percent had used multiple practices. Rates of use for cancer survivors were similar to rates for people with other chronic illnesses such as arthritis, asthma, inflammatory bowel disease, irritable bowel syndrome, or ulcers. The most popular practices among cancer survivors were herbal and other natural products (20 percent), deep breathing (14 percent), and meditation (9 percent).

Other surveys also find that use of complementary health practices is common among people who have been diagnosed with cancer, although estimates of use vary widely. Studies have found that cancer patients who use these practices usually do not expect them to cure their disease. Rather, they hope to boost their immune system, relieve pain, or manage the side effects they are experiencing from the disease or its treatment. Few cancer patients say they use complementary health practices because they are disappointed with their standard treatment. Their motivation is more likely to be a perceived benefit from the practice, a desire to feel more in control of their health, or a strong belief in the practice.

Surveys also indicate that use of vitamin and mineral supplements is widespread among cancer patients and survivors, but many health care providers are unaware that their cancer patients are using these supplements.

What The Science Says

To date, relatively little is known about the safety and effectiveness of complementary health practices that people may use for cancer. However, some of these practices have undergone careful evaluation, and many more studies are being carried out every year. In 2009, the Society for Integrative Oncology issued evidence-based clinical practice guidelines for health care providers to consider when incorporating complementary health practices in the care of cancer patients.

Remember!

Before using any complementary health practice, people who have been diagnosed with cancer should talk with the health care providers who treat their condition—to make sure that all aspects of their cancer care work together. Be aware that some dietary supplements can interfere with standard cancer treatments.

Tell all your health care providers about any complementary health practices you use. Give them a full picture of what you do to manage your health. This will help ensure coordinated and safe care.

Source: NCCAM, March 2012.

Complementary Health Practices For Cancer Prevention

Vitamin And Mineral Supplements: Although researchers continue to investigate the possible role of vitamin and mineral supplements in preventing cancer, available evidence does not support taking these supplements for this purpose:

- A 2007 review of clinical trials looking at the effectiveness of multivitamin/mineral supplements for cancer prevention found that few such trials have been conducted, and that the results of most large-scale trials have been mixed. According to the National Cancer Institute, the following supplements have been studied but have not been shown to lower the risk of cancer: vitamins B6, B12, E, and C; beta-carotene; folic acid; and selenium.

- Two large-scale studies—the Alpha-Tocopherol, Beta-Carotene (ATBC) Cancer Prevention Trial and the Beta-Carotene and Retinol Efficacy Trial (CARET)—found evidence that supplements containing beta-carotene increased the risk of lung cancer among smokers.

- An independent review of data from the Selenium and Vitamin E Cancer Prevention Trial (SELECT), funded by the National Cancer Institute, the National Center for Complementary and Alternative Medicine (NCCAM), and other agencies at the National Institutes of Health (NIH), showed that selenium and vitamin E supplements, taken either alone or together, did not prevent prostate cancer. A 2011 updated analysis from this trial concluded that vitamin E supplements significantly increased the incidence of prostate cancer in healthy men. At an average follow-up of seven years, the researchers observed that the incidence of prostate cancer was increased by 17 percent in men who received the vitamin E supplement alone compared with those who received placebo. There was no increased incidence of prostate cancer when vitamin E and selenium were taken together.

- A 2003 Agency for Healthcare Research and Quality (AHRQ) review found little evidence of cancer prevention benefits from three antioxidants (vitamins C and E and coenzyme Q10).

- A 2008 review of 20 clinical trials found no convincing evidence that antioxidant supplements prevent gastrointestinal cancer, but did find indications that some might actually increase overall mortality. The review looked at beta-carotene, selenium, and vitamins A, C, and E. Selenium alone demonstrated some preventive benefits.

- Higher intake of calcium may be associated with reduced risk of colorectal cancer, but the National Cancer Institute has concluded that the available evidence does not support taking calcium supplements to prevent colorectal cancer.

Green Tea: A 2009 review of 51 studies with more than 1.6 million participants found "insufficient and conflicting" evidence regarding an association between green tea consumption and cancer prevention.

Complementary Health Practices For Cancer Treatment

Botanical Supplements: A 2008 review of the research literature concluded that some botanical supplements used in Ayurvedic medicine and traditional Chinese medicine may have a role in cancer treatment. However, scientific evidence is limited—much of the research on botanicals and cancer treatment is in the early stages. The review also notes that botanicals can have side effects and can interact with cancer drugs, blood thinners and other prescription drugs, and each other.

Medical Marijuana

Cannabis, also known as marijuana, is a plant grown in many parts of the world. The use of *Cannabis* for medicinal purposes dates back to ancient times. By federal law, possessing *Cannabis* is illegal in the United States, where it is a controlled substance that requires special licensing for its use.

Though federal law prohibits the use of *Cannabis,* currently 17 states and the District of Columbia permit its use for certain medical conditions.

Cannabinoids are active chemicals in *Cannabis* that cause drug-like effects throughout the body, including the central nervous system and the immune system. They can be taken by mouth, inhaled, or sprayed under the tongue.

Cannabis and cannabinoids have been studied in the laboratory and the clinic for relief of pain, nausea and vomiting, anxiety, and loss of appetite. They may have benefits in treating the symptoms of cancer or the side effects of cancer.

Two cannabinoids—dronabinol and nabilone—are approved by the U.S. Food and Drug Administration (FDA) for the prevention or treatment of chemotherapy-related nausea and vomiting

Cannabis has been shown to kill cancer cells in the laboratory and to affect the immune system. However, there is no evidence that the effects of *Cannabis* on the immune system help the body fight cancer.

At this time, there is not enough evidence to recommend that patients inhale or ingest *Cannabis* as a treatment for cancer-related symptoms or side effects of cancer therapy.

Cannabis is not approved by the FDA for use as a cancer treatment.

Source: Excerpted from "PDQ® Cancer Information Summary. National Cancer Institute; Bethesda, MD. Cannabis and Cannabinoids (PDQ): Patient version. Updated 03/2013. Available at: www.cancer.gov. Accessed May 18, 2013.

Vitamin And Mineral Supplements: It is unclear whether the use of vitamin and mineral supplements by people who have been diagnosed with cancer is beneficial or harmful. For example, taking a daily multivitamin might improve the nutritional status of patients who cannot eat a healthful diet, but there is concern that some supplements might interfere with cancer treatment or increase the risk of a recurrence. Related studies have been inconsistent or inconclusive.

Antioxidants: While some research has reported benefits from taking antioxidants for cancer, there is not enough scientific evidence to support their use by cancer patients. A 2003 AHRQ review of cancer-related research on three antioxidants (vitamins C and E and co-enzyme Q10) found little scientific evidence of cancer treatment benefits. Patients' use of antioxidants while undergoing chemotherapy or radiation therapy has not been well studied. However, a 2008 review of published research suggests that antioxidant supplements may decrease the effectiveness of chemotherapy and radiation therapy.

Complementary Health Practices For Cancer Symptoms And Side Effects

Acupuncture: Studies have found acupuncture to be useful in managing chemotherapy-associated vomiting in some cancer patients. Although some early studies have shown beneficial effects, research on acupuncture for cancer pain control and for management of other cancer symptoms is limited. A 2008 evidence-based review of clinical options for managing nausea and vomiting in cancer patients noted electroacupuncture as an option to be considered.

Hypnosis, Massage, Meditation, And Yoga: Various studies also suggest possible benefits of hypnosis, massage, meditation, and yoga in helping cancer patients manage side effects and symptoms of the disease. For example, a study of 380 patients with advanced cancer concluded that massage therapy may offer some immediate relief for these patients, and that simple touch therapy (placing both hands on specific body sites)—which can be provided by family members and volunteers—may also be helpful. The study was conducted at 15 hospices in the Population-based Palliative Care Research Network.

Botanicals: A 2008 review of the research literature on botanicals and cancer concluded that although several botanicals have shown promise for managing side effects and symptoms such as nausea and vomiting, pain, fatigue, and insomnia, the scientific evidence is limited (the reviewers did not find sufficient evidence to recommend any specific treatment), and many clinical trials have not been well designed. As with use for cancer treatment, use of botanicals for symptom management raises concerns about interactions with cancer drugs, other drugs, and other botanicals.

NIH Research On Complementary Health Practices For Cancer

NCCAM funds numerous laboratory studies and clinical trials related to cancer. Recent NCCAM-supported clinical trials have been investigating the following:

- Massage for swelling of the arms and legs (lymphedema) related to breast cancer treatment

- Tai chi for physical fitness and stress in cancer survivors

- Yoga and qi gong for fatigue in breast cancer survivors

In addition to NCCAM-funded research on cancer, the National Cancer Institute conducts many studies through its Office of Cancer Complementary and Alternative Medicine (OCCAM), some of which are cofunded with NCCAM. Additional information on OCCAM is available at www.cancer.gov/cam.

Safety: Some Precautions For Cancer Patients

- **Dietary Supplements:** Some dietary supplements can interfere with cancer treatments; for example, the herb St. John's wort may cause certain anticancer drugs not to work as well as they should, and high doses of vitamins (even vitamin C) may affect how chemotherapy and radiation work. There are also general safety cautions about dietary supplements to be aware of; for example, some products may contain ingredients that are not on the label.

- **Acupuncture:** Complications from acupuncture are very rare, as long as the acupuncturist uses sterile needles and proper procedures. Because chemotherapy and radiation therapy weaken the body's immune system, cancer patients who are undergoing these therapies should be sure that the acupuncturist follows strict clean-needle procedures. The acupuncturist should use new disposable (single-use) needles for each patient.

- **Massage Therapy:** Although massage therapy appears to be generally safe, cancer patients should consult the health care provider who treats their cancer before they have a massage that involves deep or intense pressure. Any direct pressure over a tumor usually is discouraged.

Source: NCCAM, March 2012.

If You Have Been Diagnosed With Cancer And Are Considering A Complementary Health Practice

- Cancer patients need to make informed decisions about using complementary health practices. NCCAM and the National Cancer Institute have written a brochure that can help: "Thinking About Complementary and Alternative Medicine: A Guide for People with Cancer." It's available online at www.cancer.gov/cancertopics/thinking-about-CAM.

- Gather information about the complementary health product or therapy that interests you, and then discuss it with your health care providers. If you have been diagnosed with cancer, it is especially important to talk with your health care providers before you use any complementary health practice. Some practices may interfere with standard treatment or may be harmful when used along with standard treatment. Examples of questions to ask include:

  - What is known about the benefits and risks of this complementary health product or therapy? Do the benefits outweigh the risks?

  - What are the potential side effects?

  - Will this complementary health practice interfere with conventional treatment?

  - Can you refer me to a practitioner who provides the complementary health product or therapy?

- Do not use any health product or therapy that has not been proven safe and effective as a replacement for conventional cancer care or as a reason to postpone seeing your health care provider about any medical problem.

- Tell all your health care providers about any complementary health practices you use. Give them a full picture of what you do to manage your health. This will help ensure coordinated and safe care. For tips about talking with your health care providers about complementary and alternative medicine, see NCCAM's Time to Talk campaign at nccam.nih.gov/timetotalk.

Chapter 39

Cancer Clinical Trials

What are clinical trials, and why are they important?

Clinical trials are research studies that involve people. These studies test new ways to prevent, detect, diagnose, or treat diseases. People who take part in cancer clinical trials have an opportunity to contribute to scientists' knowledge about cancer and to help in the development of improved cancer treatments. They also receive state-of-the-art care from cancer experts.

Are there different types of cancer clinical trials?

Yes. Cancer clinical trials differ according to their primary purpose. They include the following types:

- Treatment trials test the effectiveness of new treatments or new ways of using current treatments in people who have cancer. The treatments tested may include new drugs or new combinations of currently used drugs, new surgery or radiation therapy techniques, and vaccines or other treatments that stimulate a person's immune system to fight cancer. Combinations of different treatment types may also be tested in these trials.

- Prevention trials test new interventions that may lower the risk of developing certain types of cancer. Most cancer prevention trials involve healthy people who have not had cancer; however, they often only include people who have a higher than average risk of

About This Chapter: Excerpted from "Cancer Clinical Trials," National Cancer Institute (NCI), February 22, 2013. Available at: www.cancer.gov. Accessed May 19, 2013.

developing a specific type of cancer. Some cancer prevention trials involve people who have had cancer in the past; these trials test interventions that may help prevent the return (recurrence) of the original cancer or reduce the chance of developing a new type of cancer.

- Screening trials test new ways of finding cancer early. When cancer is found early, it may be easier to treat and there may be a better chance of long-term survival. Cancer screening trials usually involve people who do not have any signs or symptoms of cancer. However, participation in these trials is often limited to people who have a higher than average risk of developing a certain type of cancer because they have a family history of that type of cancer or they have a history of exposure to cancer-causing substances (such as cigarette smoke).

- Diagnostic trials study new tests or procedures that may help identify, or diagnose, cancer more accurately. Diagnostic trials usually involve people who have some signs or symptoms of cancer.

- Quality of life (also called supportive) care trials focus on the comfort and quality of life of cancer patients and cancer survivors. New ways to decrease the number or severity of side effects of cancer or its treatment are often studied in these trials. How a specific type of cancer or its treatment affects a person's everyday life may also be studied.

Who sponsors clinical trials?

Government agencies, such as the National Cancer Institute (NCI) and other parts of the National Institutes of Health (NIH), the Department of Defense, and the Department of Veterans Affairs, sponsor and conduct clinical trials. In addition, organizations or individuals, including physicians, academic medical centers, foundations, volunteer groups, and biotechnology and pharmaceutical companies, also sponsor cancer clinical trials.

NCI sponsors a large number of clinical trials each year, and it has developed a variety of programs to make cancer clinical trials widely available in the United States and elsewhere. [See Chapter 53 for information on specific sponsors.]

Where do cancer clinical trials take place?

Cancer clinical trials take place in cities and towns across the United States and in other countries. They take place in doctors' offices, cancer centers and other medical centers, community hospitals and clinics, and veterans' and military hospitals. A single trial may take place at one or two specialized medical centers only or at hundreds of offices, hospitals, and centers.

Who manages clinical trials?

Each clinical trial is managed by a research team that can include doctors, nurses, research assistants, data analysts, and other specialists. The research team works closely with other health professionals, including other doctors and nurses, laboratory technicians, pharmacists, dietitians, and social workers, to provide medical and supportive care to people who take part in a clinical trial.

The research team closely monitors the health of people taking part in the clinical trial and gives them specific instructions when necessary. To ensure the reliability of the trial's results, it is important for the participants to follow the research team's instructions. The instructions may include keeping logs or answering questionnaires. The research team may also seek to contact the participants regularly after the trial ends to get updates on their health.

What are eligibility criteria, and why are they important?

Every clinical trial has a protocol, or action plan, that describes what will be done in the trial, how the trial will be conducted, and why each part of the trial is necessary. The protocol also includes guidelines for who can and cannot participate in the trial. These guidelines, called eligibility criteria, describe the characteristics that all interested people must have before they can take part in the trial. Eligibility criteria can include age, sex, medical history, and current health status. Eligibility criteria for cancer treatment trials often include the type and stage of cancer, as well as the type(s) of cancer treatment already received.

Enrolling people who have similar characteristics helps ensure that the outcome of a trial is due to the intervention being tested and not to other factors. In this way, eligibility criteria help researchers obtain the most accurate and meaningful results possible.

How is the safety of clinical trial participants protected?

National and international regulations and policies have been developed to help ensure that research involving people is conducted according to strict scientific and ethical principles. In these regulations and policies, people who participate in research are usually referred to as "human subjects."

Clinical trials that are conducted or supported by agencies of the U.S. federal government or that evaluate new drugs or medical devices that are subject to regulation by the U.S. Food and Drug Administration (FDA) must be reviewed and approved by an Institutional Review Board (IRB). The IRB reviews all aspects of a clinical trial to make sure that the rights, safety, and well-being of trial participants will be protected. The IRB must also review ongoing trials at least yearly and, based on those reviews, can decide whether the trial should continue as initially planned or if changes should be made to improve participant protection. An IRB can stop a clinical trial if the researchers are not following the protocol or if the trial appears to be causing unexpected harm to the study participants.

What is informed consent?

Informed consent is a process through which people 1) learn the important facts about a clinical trial to help them decide whether or not to take part in it, and 2) continue to learn new information about the trial that helps them decide whether or not to continue participating in it.

Adolescents And Young Adult Cancer

Survival of children with cancer has climbed dramatically in the last five decades, with five-year survival rates of less than 10 percent 50 years ago and almost 80 percent today. At the same time, progress in treating adolescents and young adults (AYAs) has stagnated, with five-year survival rates staying constant at about 70 percent over the last 30 years.

Researchers attribute this lack of progress in part to the fact that relatively few AYAs participate in clinical trials, which have allowed pediatric oncologists to make such rapid advances in treatment for children. One of the main reasons that so few AYAs participate in clinical trials is that, even at major cancer centers, there are few clinical trials available to this age group.

For example, a 2007 study by Dr. Peter Shaw, head of the AYA oncology program at the Children's Hospital of Pittsburgh, and his colleagues found that, of the new patients diagnosed at their institution over a five-year period, 38 percent of all children younger than 15 joined a trial, compared with 27 percent of older adolescents. Fifty-seven percent of the older group did not enroll in a trial because there were none available to them, wrote Dr. Shaw and his colleagues.

"Too little is known about AYA cancers, in large part because the patients are not on clinical trials," commented Dr. Nita Seibel, of the Clinical Investigations Branch in NCI's Cancer Therapy Evaluation Program. "And if the patients are not on these trials, then researchers cannot gather information about their treatment and survival, nor do they have tumor samples to try to understand the biology of their disease."

Across the country, researchers are testing innovative ways to enroll more AYAs in clinical trials—and in the right clinical trials—using expanded access, patient navigation, community outreach, and collaborations between academic and community doctors.

Treating Them Like Children

Several years ago, retrospective studies from researchers across the United States began hinting that, for many types of cancer, patients between the ages of 18 and 39 might do better when given pediatric treatment regimens than when given adult regimens.

During the first part of the informed consent process, people are given detailed information about a trial, including information about the purpose of the trial, the tests and other procedures that will be required, and the possible benefits and harms of taking part in the trial. Besides talking with a doctor or nurse, potential trial participants are given a form, called an informed consent form, that provides information about the trial in writing. People who agree to take part in the trial are asked to sign the form. However, signing this form does not mean that a person must remain in the trial. Anyone can choose to leave a trial at any time—either before it starts or at any time during the trial or during the follow-up period. It is important for people who decide to leave a trial to get information from the research team about how to leave the trial safely.

In a 2008 study in Blood, Dr. Wendy Stock, director of the leukemia program at the University of Chicago, and her colleagues looked at survival for more than 300 patients between the ages of 16 and 20 with acute lymphoblastic leukemia (ALL) who had been treated either in pediatric trials through the Children's Cancer Group (now part of the Children's Oncology Group; COG) or in adult ALL trials through the Cancer and Leukemia Group B (CALGB).

"We found that there was a significant difference in outcome favoring the treatment that the pediatricians were using," said Dr. Stock. Similar results have been seen in retrospective studies from France, the United Kingdom, and the Netherlands.

A separate retrospective study published in 2010 by researchers from St. Jude Children's Research Hospital showed a jump in cure rates for older adolescents with ALL who received a pediatric regimen that used drugs that are not traditionally given to older patients because of concerns about side effects.

Another trial is testing whether a pediatric regimen for Ewing sarcoma is effective in young adults. The study is recruiting through NCI's Cancer Trials Support Unit, a program that provides doctors access to cooperative group cancer trials when they or their medical centers are not members of a cooperative group. Most AYAs with cancer are not treated at academic medical centers but are seen by local oncologists, most of whom do not normally have direct access to cooperative group trials.

"It's not the first thought of most medical oncologists to reach out to a pediatric oncologist when the patient is in their late teens to early adulthood," said Dr. Shaw. "They may just think of [the patient] as a regular adult with cancer and not think that [he or she] would be eligible for a pediatric trial. Two miles away or even two buildings over, there might be a pediatric oncologist who's an investigator for a national COG study that could enroll their patient, and they just don't know to ask."

Source: Excerpted from "Clinical Trials Offer A Path To Better Care For AYAs With Cancer," written by Sharon Reynolds, *NCI Cancer Bulletin*, July 26, 2011, National Cancer Institute.

The informed consent process continues throughout a trial. If new benefits, risks, or side effects are discovered during the course of a trial, the researchers must inform the participants so they can decide whether or not they want to continue to take part in the trial. In some cases, participants who want to continue to take part in a trial may be asked to sign a new informed consent form.

What does a trial's "phase" mean?

New interventions are often studied in a stepwise fashion, with each step representing a different "phase" in the clinical research process.

- **Phase 0:** These trials represent the earliest step in testing new treatments in humans. In a phase 0 trial, a very small dose of a chemical or biologic agent is given to a small number of people (approximately 10-15) to gather preliminary information about how the agent is processed by the body and how the agent affects the body. The people who take part in these trials usually have advanced disease, and no known, effective treatment options are available to them.

- **Phase I:** Also called phase 1, these trials are conducted mainly to evaluate the safety of chemical or biologic agents or other types of interventions (such as a new radiation therapy technique). They help determine the maximum dose that can be given safely (also known as the maximum tolerated dose) and whether an intervention causes harmful side effects. Phase I trials enroll small numbers of people (20 or more) who have advanced cancer that cannot be treated effectively with standard (usual) treatments or for which no standard treatment exists.

- **Phase II:** Also called phase 2, these trials test the effectiveness of interventions in people who have a specific type of cancer or related cancers. They also continue to look at the safety of interventions. Phase II trials usually enroll fewer than 100 people but may include as many as 300.

- **Phase III:** Also called phase 3, these trials compare the effectiveness of a new intervention, or new use of an existing intervention, with the current standard of care (usual treatment) for a particular type of cancer. Phase III trials also examine how the side effects of the new intervention compare with those of the usual treatment. If the new intervention is more effective than the usual treatment and/or is easier to tolerate, it may become the new standard of care.

  Phase III trials usually involve large groups of people (100 to several thousand), who are randomly assigned to one of two treatment groups. In the control group, everyone receives usual treatment for their type of cancer. In the investigational or experimental group, everyone receives the new treatment or new use of an existing treatment. Trial participants are assigned to their individual groups by random assignment, or randomization. Randomization is usually done by a computer program to ensure that human choices or other factors do not influence study results. In most cases, studies will move into phase III testing only after it has shown promise in phase I and phase II trials.

- **Phase IV:** Also called phase 4, these trials further evaluate the effectiveness and long-term safety of drugs or other treatment. They usually take place after the treatment has been approved by the FDA for standard use. Several hundred to several thousand people may take part in a phase IV trial. These trials are also known as post-marketing surveillance trials. They are generally sponsored by drug companies.

What are some of the possible benefits of taking part in a clinical trial?

The benefits of participating in a clinical trial include the following:

- Participants have access to promising new approaches that are generally not available outside of a clinical trial.

- The approach being studied may be more effective than standard therapy. If it is more effective, trial participants may be the first to benefit from it.

- Participants receive regular and careful medical attention from a research team that includes doctors, nurses, and other health professionals.

- Results of the trial may help other people who need cancer treatment in the future.

- Participants are helping scientists learn more about cancer.

What are some of the potential risks associated with taking part in a clinical trial?

The potential risks or participating in a clinical trial include the following:

- New drugs or procedures being studied may not be better than standard therapy, or it may have harmful side effects that doctors do not expect or that are worse than those associated with standard therapy.

- Participants may be required to make more visits to the doctor than they would if they were not in a clinical trial and/or may need to travel farther for those visits.

- Health insurance may not cover all patient care costs in a trial.

Part Four
Cancer Survivorship

Chapter 40

Cancer Fatigue

Fatigue is the most common side effect of cancer treatment. Cancer treatments such as chemotherapy, radiation therapy, and biologic therapy can cause fatigue in cancer patients. Fatigue is also a common symptom of some cancers. Patients describe fatigue as feeling tired, weak, worn-out, heavy, slow, or that they have no energy or get-up-and-go. Fatigue in cancer patients may be called cancer fatigue, cancer-related fatigue, and cancer treatment-related fatigue.

Fatigue can decrease a patient's quality of life. It can affect all areas of life by making the patient too tired to take part in daily activities, relationships, social events, and community activities. Patients may miss work or school, spend less time with friends and family, or spend more time sleeping. In some cases, physical fatigue leads to mental fatigue and mood changes. This can make it hard for the patient to pay attention, remember things, and think clearly.

Causes Of Fatigue

Doctors do not know all the reasons cancer patients have fatigue. Many conditions may cause fatigue at the same time. Fatigue in cancer patients may be caused by the following:

- Cancer treatment with chemotherapy, radiation therapy, and some biologic therapies
- Anemia (a lower than normal number of red blood cells)
- Hormone levels that are too low or too high
- Trouble breathing or getting enough oxygen
- Heart trouble

About This Chapter: PDQ® Cancer Information Summary. National Cancer Institute; Bethesda, MD. Fatigue (PDQ): Patient version. Updated 05/2/2013. Available at: www.cancer.gov. Accessed May 19, 2013.

- Infection

- Pain

- Stress

- Loss of appetite or not getting enough calories and nutrients

- Dehydration (loss of too much water from the body, such as from severe diarrhea or vomiting)

- Changes in how well the body uses food for energy

- Loss of weight, muscle, and/or strength

- Medicines that cause drowsiness

- Problems getting enough sleep

- Being less active

- Other medical conditions

Fatigue is common in people with advanced cancer who are not receiving cancer treatment.

How cancer treatments cause fatigue is not known. Doctors are trying to better understand how cancer treatments such as surgery, chemotherapy, and radiation therapy cause fatigue. Some studies show that fatigue is caused by:

- The need for extra energy to repair and heal body tissue damaged by treatment

- The build-up of toxic substances that are left in the body after cells are killed by cancer treatment

- The effect of biologic therapy on the immune system

- Changes in the body's sleep-wake cycle

When they begin cancer treatment, many patients are already tired from medical tests, surgery, and the emotional stress of coping with the cancer diagnosis. After treatment begins, fatigue may get worse. Patients who are older, have advanced cancer, or receive more than one type of treatment (for example, both chemotherapy and radiation therapy) are more likely to have long-term fatigue.

Different cancer treatments have different effects on a patient's energy level. The type and schedule of treatments can affect the amount of fatigue caused by cancer therapy.

It's A Fact!

Fatigue related to cancer is different from fatigue that healthy people feel. When a healthy person is tired by day-to-day activities, their fatigue can be relieved by sleep and rest. Cancer-related fatigue is different. Cancer patients get tired after less activity than people who do not have cancer. Also, cancer-related fatigue is not completely relieved by sleep and rest and may last for a long time. Fatigue usually decreases after cancer treatment ends, but patients may still feel some fatigue for months or years.

Fatigue Caused By Chemotherapy

Patients treated with chemotherapy usually feel the most fatigue in the days right after each treatment. Then the fatigue decreases until the next treatment. Fatigue usually increases with each cycle. Some studies have shown that patients have the most severe fatigue about mid-way through all the cycles of chemotherapy. Fatigue decreases after chemotherapy is finished, but patients may not feel back to normal until a month or more after the last treatment. Many patients feel fatigued for months or years after treatment ends.

Fatigue during chemotherapy may be increased by the following:

- Pain

- Depression

- Anxiety

- Anemia. Some types of chemotherapy stop the bone marrow from making enough new red blood cells, causing anemia (too few red blood cells to carry oxygen to the body).

- Lack of sleep caused by some anticancer drugs

Fatigue Caused By Radiation Therapy

Many patients receiving radiation therapy have fatigue that keeps them from being as active as they want to be. After radiation therapy begins, fatigue usually increases until mid-way through the course of treatments and then stays about the same until treatment ends. For many patients, fatigue improves after radiation therapy stops. However, in some patients, fatigue will last months or years after treatment ends. Some patients never have the same amount of energy they had before treatment.

Fatigue Caused By Biologic Therapy

Biologic therapy often causes flu-like symptoms. These symptoms include being tired physically and mentally, fever, chills, muscle pain, headache, and not feeling well in general. Some patients may also have problems thinking clearly. Fatigue symptoms depend on the type of biologic therapy used.

Fatigue Caused By Surgery

Fatigue is often a side effect of surgery, but patients usually feel better with time. However, fatigue caused by surgery can be worse when the surgery is combined with other cancer treatments.

Fatigue Caused By Anemia

Anemia is a common cause of fatigue. Anemia affects the patient's energy level and quality of life. Anemia may be caused by the cancer, cancer treatments, or a medical condition not related to the cancer.

The effects of anemia on a patient depend on the following:

- How quickly the anemia occurs
- The patient's age
- The amount of plasma (fluid part of the blood) in the patient's blood
- Other medical conditions the patient has

Fatigue Related To Nutrition

Side effects related to nutrition may cause or increase fatigue. The body's energy comes from food. Fatigue may occur if the body does not take in enough food to give the body the energy it needs. For many patients, the effects of cancer and cancer treatments make it hard to eat well. In people with cancer, three major factors may affect nutrition:

- A change in the way the body is able to use food. A patient may eat the same amount as before having cancer, but the body may not be able to absorb and use all the nutrients from the food. This is caused by the cancer or its treatment.

- A decrease in the amount of food eaten because of low appetite, nausea, vomiting, diarrhea, or a blocked bowel.

- An increase in the amount of energy needed by the body because of a growing tumor, infection, fever, or shortness of breath.

Emotions And Fatigue

Anxiety and depression are the most common psychological causes of fatigue in cancer patients. The emotional stress of cancer can cause physical problems, including fatigue. It's common for cancer patients to have changes in moods and attitudes. Patients may feel anxiety and fear before and after a cancer diagnosis. These feelings may cause fatigue. The effect of the disease on the patient's physical, mental, social, and financial well-being can increase emotional distress.

About 15 percent to 25 percent of patients who have cancer get depressed, which may increase fatigue caused by physical factors. The following are signs of depression:

- Feeling tired mentally and physically
- Loss of interest in life
- Problems thinking
- Loss of sleep
- Feeling a loss of hope

Some patients have more fatigue after cancer treatments than others do.

Attention Fatigue

During and after cancer treatment, patients may find they cannot pay attention for very long and have a hard time thinking, remembering, and understanding. This is called attention fatigue. Sleep helps to relieve attention fatigue, but sleep may not be enough when the fatigue is related to cancer. Taking part in restful activities and spending time outdoors may help relieve attention fatigue.

Sleep-Related Fatigue

Some people with cancer are not able to get enough sleep. The following problems related to sleep may cause fatigue:

- Waking up during the night
- Not going to sleep at the same time every night
- Sleeping during the day and less at night
- Not being active during the day

Poor sleep affects people in different ways. For example, the time of day that fatigue is worse may be who have trouble sleeping may feel more fatigue in the morning. Others may have severe fatigue in both the morning and the evening.

Medicines And Fatigue

Patients may take medicines for cancer symptoms, such as pain, or conditions other than the cancer. These medicines may cause the patient to feel sleepy. Opioids, antidepressants, and antihistamines have this side effect. If many of these medicines are taken at the same time, fatigue may be worse.

Assessing Fatigue

There is no test to diagnose fatigue, so it is important for the patient to tell family members and the health care team if fatigue is a problem. To assess fatigue, the patient is asked to describe how bad the fatigue is, how it affects daily activities, and what makes the fatigue better or worse. The doctor will look for causes of fatigue that can be treated.

The assessment process may include a physical exam, rating the level of fatigue, answering a series of questions, and undergoing blood tests to check for anemia. A fatigue assessment is repeated at different times to see if there are patterns of fatigue.

A fatigue assessment is repeated to see if there is a pattern for when fatigue starts or becomes worse. Fatigue may be worse right after a chemotherapy treatment, for example.

Treatment Of Fatigue

Treatment of fatigue depends on the symptoms and whether the cause of fatigue is known. When the cause of fatigue is not known, treatment is usually given to relieve symptoms and teach the patient ways to cope with fatigue.

Treatment Of Anemia

Treating anemia may help decrease fatigue. When known, the cause of the anemia is treated. When the cause is not known, treatment for anemia is supportive care and may include the following:

- **Change In Diet:** Eating more foods rich in iron and vitamins may be combined with other treatments for anemia.

- **Transfusions Of Red Blood Cells:** Transfusions work well to treat anemia. Possible side effects of transfusions include an allergic reaction, infection, graft-versus-host disease, immune system changes, and too much iron in the blood.

- **Medicine:** Drugs that cause the bone marrow to make more red blood cells may be used to treat anemia-related fatigue in patients receiving chemotherapy.

Treatment Of Pain

If pain is making fatigue worse, the patient's pain medicine may be changed or the dose may be increased. If too much pain medicine is making fatigue worse, the patient's pain medicine may be changed or the dose may be decreased.

Treatment Of Depression

Fatigue in patients who have depression may be treated with antidepressant drugs. Psychostimulant drugs may help some patients have more energy and a better mood, and help them think and concentrate. The use of psychostimulants for treating fatigue is still being studied. The U.S. Food and Drug Administration has not approved psychostimulants for the treatment of fatigue. Psychostimulants have side effects, especially with long-term use.

Increasing Energy And Learning to Cope

Treatment of fatigue may include teaching the patient ways to increase energy and cope with fatigue in daily life.

Exercise

Exercise (including walking) may help people with cancer feel better and have more energy. The effect of exercise on fatigue in cancer patients is being studied. One study reported that breast cancer survivors who took part in enjoyable physical activity had less fatigue and pain and were better able to take part in daily activities. In clinical trials, some patients reported the following benefits from exercise:

- More physical energy

- Better appetite

- More able to do the normal activities of daily living

- Better quality of life

- More satisfaction with life

- A greater sense of well-being

- More able to meet the demands of cancer and cancer treatment

Moderate activity for three to five hours a week may help cancer-related fatigue. You are more likely to follow an exercise plan if you choose a type of exercise that you enjoy.

Schedule Of Activity And Rest

Changes in daily routine make the body use more energy. A regular routine can improve sleep and help the patient have more energy to be active during the day. A program of regular times for activity and rest help to make the most of a patient's energy. A health care professional can help patients plan an exercise program and decide which activities are the most important to them. The following sleep habits may help decrease fatigue:

- Lying in bed for sleep only

- Taking naps for no longer than one hour

- Avoiding noise (like television and radio) during sleep

Talk Therapy

Therapists use talk therapy (counseling) to treat certain emotional or behavioral disorders. This kind of therapy helps patients change how they think and feel about certain things. Talk therapy may help decrease a cancer patient's fatigue by working on cancer-related factors that make fatigue worse, such as:

- Stress from coping with cancer

- Fear that the cancer may come back

- Feeling hopeless about fatigue

- Lack of social support

- A pattern of sleep and activity that changes from day to day

Fatigue After Cancer Treatment Ends

Fatigue continues to be a problem for many cancer survivors long after treatment ends and the cancer is gone. Studies show that some patients continue to have moderate-to-severe fatigue years after treatment. Long-term therapies such as tamoxifen can also cause fatigue. In children who were treated for brain tumors and cured, fatigue may continue after treatment.

The causes of fatigue after treatment ends are different than the causes of fatigue during treatment. Treating fatigue after treatment ends also may be different from treating it during cancer therapy.

Since fatigue may greatly affect the quality of life for cancer survivors, long-term follow-up care is important.

Chapter 41

Cancer Pain

Types And Causes Of Cancer Pain

Causes Of Cancer Pain

Most cancer pain is caused by the tumor pressing on bones, nerves, or other organs in your body. Sometimes pain is related to your cancer treatment. For example, some chemotherapy drugs can cause numbness and tingling in your hands and feet or a burning sensation at the place where they are injected. Radiotherapy can cause skin redness and irritation.

Acute And Chronic Pain

Cancer pain can be acute or chronic. Acute pain is due to damage caused by an injury and tends to only last a short time. For example, having an operation can cause acute pain. The pain goes when the wound heals. In the meantime, painkillers will usually keep it under control.

Chronic pain is pain caused by changes to nerves. Nerve changes may occur due to cancer pressing on nerves or due to chemicals produced by a tumor. It can also be caused by nerve changes due to cancer treatment. The pain continues long after the injury or treatment is over and can range from mild to severe. It can be there all the time and is also called persistent pain. Chronic pain can be difficult to treat, but painkillers or other pain control methods can successfully control it in about 95 out of every 100 people (95 percent).

About This Chapter: This chapter includes "Types and Causes of Cancer Pain," "What Painkillers Are," and "Other Ways of Treating Cancer Pain." Reprinted with permission from CancerHelp UK, the patient information website of Cancer Research UK: http://www.cancerresearchuk.org/cancerhelp. © Cancer Research UK, 2013. All rights reserved.

Quick Tip

Remember that some pain may have nothing to do with your cancer. You may have the general aches and pains that everyone gets from time to time.

Source: "Types and Causes of Cancer Pain," © Cancer Research UK, 2013.

Pain that is not well controlled can develop into chronic pain. So it is important to take painkillers that you are prescribed. Trying to put up with the pain can make it harder to control in the future.

If you have chronic cancer pain, you may have times when the pain is not controlled by the medicines you are taking. This is called breakthrough pain. If you are taking regular painkillers but still get pain at times, let your doctor or nurse know. They can prescribe extra top up doses of painkillers for you to take when you need them.

Sometimes pain can come on quickly, for example when you need to have a dressing changed or move around. This type of pain is called incident pain.

Pain can greatly affect your quality of life. Chronic pain can make it hard for you to do everyday things such as bathing, shopping, cooking, sleeping and eating. This may be hard for your close friends and relatives to understand.

Types Of Cancer Pain

Doctors talk about and describe pain in different ways. They may talk about acute and chronic pain. Or they may talk about the body tissue your pain comes from. It is extremely important for your doctor to find out the type and cause of your pain so that they can treat it in the right way. Different types of pain need different treatment. Types of pain include:

- Nerve pain
- Bone pain
- Soft tissue pain
- Phantom pain
- Referred pain

Nerve Pain

Nerve pain is caused by pressure on nerves or the spinal cord, or by damage to nerves. It is also called neuropathic pain. People often describe nerve pain as burning or as a feeling of something crawling under their skin. It can be difficult to describe exactly how it feels. It can sometimes be more difficult to treat than other types of pain.

Some people have long-term nerve pain after surgery. Nerves are cut during surgery and they take a long time to heal because they grow very slowly. Some people may have pain around their scar for two years or more after their surgery. It does usually go eventually. Nerve pain can also occur after other cancer treatments such as radiotherapy or chemotherapy.

Bone Pain

Cancer can spread into the bone and cause pain. The cancer may affect one specific area of bone or several areas. The cancer cells within the bone damage the bone tissue and cause the pain. You may also hear bone pain called somatic pain. People often describe this type of pain as aching, dull or throbbing.

Soft Tissue Pain

Soft tissue pain means pain from a body organ or muscle. For example, you may have pain in your back caused by tissue damage to the kidney. You can't always pinpoint this pain, but it is usually described as sharp, aching or throbbing. Soft tissue pain is also called visceral pain.

Phantom Pain

Phantom pain means pain in a part of the body that has been removed. For example, pain in an arm or leg that has been removed due to sarcoma or osteosarcoma. Or pain in the breast area after removal of the breast (mastectomy). Phantom pain is very real and people sometimes describe it as unbearable.

Doctors are still trying to understand why phantom pain happens. One theory is that the thinking part of your brain knows that you have had a part of your body removed but the feeling part of your brain can't understand this. Other possible causes of phantom pain are poor pain control at the time of surgery.

Between six and seven out of ten people (60 to 70 percent) who have had an arm or leg removed feel phantom pain. About one third of women who have had a breast removed to treat breast cancer feel phantom breast pain. The pain usually lessens after the first year but some people can still feel phantom pain after a year or more. In most people it will go away after a few months. It is as though your brain has to realize that part of your body has gone. It is important to let your doctor or specialist nurse know about phantom pain because it can be controlled with painkillers.

Referred Pain

Sometimes pain from an organ in the body may be felt in a different part of the body. This is called referred pain. For example, a swollen liver may cause pain in the right shoulder, even though the liver is under the ribs on the right side of the body. This is because the liver presses on nerves that end in the shoulder.

How Much Pain You Might Have

The amount of pain you have with cancer depends on:

- The type of cancer you have

- Where it is

- The stage of your cancer

- Whether the cancer or treatment has damaged any nerves

If you have pain it is very important to let your medical team know straight away. If you try to put up with the pain, this can lead to nerve changes that may make the pain harder to control in the future.

What Painkillers Are

Painkillers

Painkillers are also called analgesics or analgesia. There are many different types and strengths of painkillers suitable for different types of pain. If you have mild pain you usually have simple painkillers, such as paracetamol [acetaminophen]. If you have moderate pain you usually have treatment with opioid painkillers, such as codeine. If you have ongoing or severe pain you usually have morphine type opioid painkillers.

An experienced doctor or nurse can judge which type of painkiller is best for you.

The important thing is that you have the right type of painkiller for your pain and the right dose. You might also have anti-inflammatory drugs such as ibuprofen (Nurofen) [Advil or Motrin] alongside any of the other painkillers. Or antidepressants or anti-epileptic drugs to help with nerve pain.

Many people use complementary methods of pain control alongside painkillers.

Taking Painkillers

If you are taking painkillers to control pain, it is very, very important that you take them regularly as prescribed by your doctor. Some people try to take as few as possible by spacing them out. Then you may be in pain before you take your next tablet. This is not good pain control. The idea is that you should take your next dose before you are in pain again.

If your pain is not controlled, you can get nerve changes that make the pain more difficult to control in the future. So it is important to take painkillers regularly enough to keep the pain under control. It is better for your body, and your quality of life, to take a regular dose rather than to swing between taking nothing at all and then taking a large dose because you have severe pain.

If You Still Have Pain

There are many different painkillers for mild, moderate and severe pain. It is important to help your doctor or nurse get your dose right by giving honest, detailed information about your pain and how well your painkillers are working. If your painkillers are not controlling your pain, there are plenty of others to try. Or you may need to have a slightly higher dose. You could also try some of the other ways of controlling pain described below.

Other Ways Of Treating Cancer Pain

Cancer Treatments

Cancer treatments can help to reduce pain by shrinking a tumor and reducing pressure on nerves or surrounding tissues. This is called palliative treatment. It won't cure the cancer, but can reduce or get rid of symptoms. Treatments used in this way include:

- Chemotherapy
- Radiotherapy
- Hormone therapy
- Biological therapy
- Radiofrequency ablation

You may have some side effects from palliative cancer treatments. But the aim is to make you feel better, so your cancer specialist will try to choose treatments that have as few side effects as possible.

You may be able to cut down on your painkillers after cancer treatments. But the treatments can take a while to work. It can take several weeks to get the full benefit. So you will need to carry on taking your painkillers in the meantime.

Chemotherapy or biological therapies can shrink many types of cancer to reduce symptoms such as pain.

Hormone treatments can shrink some types of advanced cancer such as breast cancer, prostate cancer, womb [uterine] cancer, and kidney cancer.

Radiotherapy can give very good long lasting pain control for certain types of cancer pain such as bone pain. The treatment kills the cancer cells so that the tumor shrinks. The affected bone then begins to heal and strengthen itself. The pain may ease to some extent or may go completely. When treated with radiotherapy, about three out of ten people (30 percent) with pain from cancer that has spread to the bones will have no pain within a month. Another four out of ten people (40 percent) will have pain that is half as bad as it was. Radiotherapy is often used to treat bones that have fractured because they have been weakened by cancer (pathological fracture). Radiotherapy can also reduce pain caused by spinal cord compression.

Radiofrequency ablation uses heat made by radio waves to kill cancer cells. The electrical energy heats up the tumor and kills the cancer cells. You have RFA through a probe that goes through your skin into the tumor. It is quite a new treatment and at the moment only a few specialist centers offer it. But some research has shown that it can control pain caused by some types of cancer.

Surgery

In some situations surgery can be used to control pain. A surgeon may carry out an operation to take away as much of a tumor as possible. This is called debulking. It can relieve pain by relieving pressure. It may also prevent complications developing, such as a blocked bowel.

Injecting Painkillers Into The Fluid Around The Spine

This may be called an epidural, intrathecal anesthetic or spinal anesthetic. To give painkillers in this way a small tube (called a catheter) is put into your back and into the area around the spinal cord. The painkiller is continuously injected through the tube into your spine. If you are having a big operation for your cancer this may be the best way to control your pain. It will give good pain control for up to 24 hours after your surgery.

This type of pain control is not a first choice to treat non-surgical cancer pain. But it can help some people whose pain is not controlled by other ways of giving painkillers, such as tablets or injections. This method can give excellent pain control but it needs a highly experienced doctor (anesthetist) to do the procedure and highly trained nurses to watch you very closely afterwards. Not all hospitals, hospices or pain clinics are able to provide this service.

Sometimes a small pump is put into the fluid around the spinal cord. It is in your back area just below the waist. Painkillers can be injected into the pump every few weeks. This type of treatment is usually used where other methods of pain control have not worked. You can stay at home with the pump. It is called an implanted intrathecal pump.

Nerve Blocks

If you have pain that is difficult to treat, your doctor may suggest a nerve block. This is a way of killing or deadening a nerve to stop it causing pain. There are not usually many side effects to nerve blocks. You may have low blood pressure afterwards. The low blood pressure can make you feel light headed if you stand up too quickly. But this usually gets better over a few days. There are different types of nerve block, named after the nerves that are treated.

The celiac plexus (pronounced seel-ee-ak pleck-sus) is a complicated web of nerves at the back of the abdomen. It can be responsible for ongoing pain in people with pancreatic cancer and some other types of cancer. To block the pain, the doctor injects alcohol into the celiac plexus. You will have a small injection of local anesthetic first to numb your skin. You may then have a CT scan or ultrasound scan so that your doctor can check that the needle is in exactly the right place. Then they put a long needle in through your chest to the coeliac plexus. Or you may have the needle put into the nerves through the stomach wall during an endoscopy.

Some research has shown that up to nine out of ten people (90 percent) with abdominal cancers can get short and long term pain relief with a celiac nerve block. Up to six out of 10 people (60 percent) have diarrhea after this treatment, but this usually gets better within a couple of days. A very small number of people have severe, ongoing diarrhea after this treatment.

Your doctor may think it is better to cut the nerves causing the pain, rather than just inject them. This is a small operation and you may have it done during other surgery, such as bypass surgery. You may have a medicine to make you drowsy. You then have a local anesthetic and the anesthetist pushes a thin needle into the nerve. The needle has a laser or radiofrequency probe at the tip, which cuts the nerve. The anesthetist may use ultrasound or a CT scan during the procedure, to make sure the needle is in the right place.

Pressure on the splanchnic nerves can cause continuing pain in some types of cancer. The splanchnic nerves send signals from the spinal cord to the organs in the chest and abdomen. Cutting the splanchnic nerve is called splanchnicectomy (pronounced splank-nik-ectomy). It can reduce pain for many people.

Another type of nerve block is called thoracoscopic sympathectomy. This means the doctor uses a thoracoscope to reach the nerves in the chest. This is a tube with a camera, eyepiece and light that enables the surgeon to look inside the body. It is similar to an endoscope. You will have either a general anesthetic or a sedative. You have a few small cuts (incisions) made between your neck and breastbone. The surgeon uses the thoracoscope to look inside your body and find nerves that are part of a chain called the sympathetic nerve chain. The surgeon then uses a laser or radiofrequency probe at the tip of the thorascope to block this chain of nerves.

Strengthening Painful Bones

If cancer spreads to the bones it often causes pain. Cancer in the bones can make them weak and more likely to break. This type of break is called a pathological fracture. Doctors have developed ways of treating bones affected by cancer, by using special cement to strengthen them. These relatively new techniques are:

- Percutaneous cementoplasty
- Vertebroplasty and kyphoplasty

Percutaneous Cementoplasty

Cementoplasty means using a special cement to strengthen and support bone. Percutaneous means under the skin, and describes how the cement is put into the bone. Doctors use the cement to fill parts of bone that have been destroyed by cancer and are causing pain. It can help to relieve pain and make the bone more stable. It has also improved walking for some people.

You have this minor operation either under a general anesthetic or when you are drowsy after taking a sedative. Using x-rays to guide the way, the doctor puts a needle into the skin and injects the cement into the bone.

You are most likely to have percutaneous cementoplasty to help control symptoms of secondary bone cancer. You are less likely to have this treatment for a cancer that started in the bone (primary bone cancer). The U.K. National Institute for Health and Clinical Excellence (NICE) has issued guidance on percutaneous cementoplasty. NICE says that it can be used as part of U.K. National Health Service (NHS) treatment but only if other ways of treating your pain have not worked.

Vertebroplasty And Kyphoplasty

These are forms of cementoplasty. In vertebroplasty, bone cement is injected into damaged bones in the spine (vertebrae). The treatment eases pain and helps to support the spine.

Balloon kyphoplasty is similar to vertebroplasty and treats fractures of the spine. For kyphoplasty, little balloons are put into the spine. They are slowly inflated so that the spine goes back to as near its normal height as possible. Then special cement is injected into the space created by the balloon to strengthen the bone. Trials have shown that this technique can help to relieve pain and restore some height.

NICE has issued guidance on vertebroplasty for treating fractures in people with painful conditions of the spine, including tumors. They say that it should only be considered if other ways of treating your pain don't work. NICE has approved balloon kyphoplasty for use in the NHS as a treatment for collapsed bones in the spine.

Electrical Nerve Stimulation

TENS stands for transcutaneous electrical nerve stimulation. TENS may temporarily help pain that is in one area of the body. But more studies are needed in people with cancer pain to know this for sure. Small pads are stuck onto the skin and they release a small electrical charge. This causes a tingling feeling in the skin. By stimulating the nerves that run up the spine to the brain, TENS blocks nerves carrying the pain messages. TENS can be worth a try as it is easy to use and has few side effects. You can ask your doctor or specialist nurse if it may be helpful for your type of pain.

What about acupuncture?

There is not yet enough evidence to show for sure that acupuncture can relieve cancer pain. But some research studies have shown that acupuncture can reduce muscle pain or bone pain for some people. It makes the body release pain relieving chemicals. It can work very well when cancer pain is causing muscle spasms that make the pain worse.

Source: "Other Ways of Treating Cancer Pain." © Cancer Research UK, 2013.

Other Ways of Reducing Pain

There are many ways that you and your family can help to control your pain. You may have noticed that your pain seems worse if you are anxious or worried. It often seems worse at night if you cannot sleep and there is nothing else to distract you. Here are some things to try that can help relieve your pain:

- Change your position at least every two hours to prevent stiffness and sore skin.

- Hot or cold packs can help relieve pain but wrap them in a soft towel to prevent them damaging your skin.

- Watching TV, reading, or chatting can help to take your mind off your aches and pains.

- Relaxation: Use tapes or listen to some calming music and think of somewhere beautiful you would like to be.

- Breathing: Try to breathe slowly and deeply when you are tense.

- Massage: Ask your family or friends to give gentle massage to your back, hands, or feet, or treat yourself to a professional massage.

- Aromatherapy, hypnotherapy, acupuncture, and reflexology may all help—some cancer support groups can tell you where to find these services in your area.

- Talking to someone about your pain, perhaps a counselor, can help to relieve stress and tension and make it easier to cope.

These may help you to take some control over your pain and make it seem better for a time. If you can't sleep, learning relaxation exercises can be very helpful. Remember not to get too tired. Visitors are a wonderful distraction, but it is often better to see people for short periods of time when you are not well.

Chapter 42

What Will Happen To My Body During Cancer Treatment?

Losing your hair can be one of the most obvious signs that you are being treated for cancer. It is not an easy thing for a lot of people. Here are some ideas about how to deal with it.

Is my hair going to fall out?

Not everyone who gets treated for cancer loses their hair, but most people do. It happens differently for everyone. Some people do not lose very much hair, and other people lose all of it. Sometimes, it just helps to know what to expect or at least to know a little more about why it happens.

How come cancer treatment makes people lose their hair?

Cancer treatment kills any cells that grow really fast. That is because cancer cells grow fast, and your treatments are meant to kill cancer cells. But there are other cells in your body that grow fast too—like hair, skin, and nails. So treatment can affect all of those.

What many teens and young adults don't realize is that your treatment can affect all the hair on your body, not just the hair on your head. This includes hair on your face (like your eyebrows and lashes), armpits, pubic area, and legs. Is there any good news? At least losing your hair does not hurt!

When will I lose my hair?

It depends on your body and your treatment. Hair loss usually starts about two weeks after treatment begins. You may notice a bunch of hair in the shower drain or clumps of hair on your pillow in the morning. Your hair might come out in clumps, or it might just start breaking off.

How can I deal with losing my hair?

Some teens and young adults would rather just shave their heads or cut their hair short right when they start losing their hair. Other teens and young adults just let it fall out on its own.

Another thing that might help is to think about what you are going to look like without any hair. This is one way to get ready for this temporary change. You also might want to go shopping with a friend, parent, or caregiver and try on various hats, wigs, scarves, or bandanas to see what will make you feel comfortable.

Some people try to have fun with it—here are some things you can try:

- Throw a hair-shaving party. Your friends and family can shave their heads, too.

- Dye your hair or cut it in whatever style you want.

- Find things to put on your hair (hats or wigs) that make you feel good and that suit your style. If you would rather just go bald, be sure to wear sunscreen when you go outside.

- You can lose a lot of body heat through your head. So even if you do not wear a hat, wig, bandana, or scarf for looks, you might want to have one handy for keeping warm.

- Your head can sometimes be very tender, and it can be hard to lie down on your pillow. Some teens and young adults find that rubbing lotion or oil onto their scalp makes their head feel less sensitive. Always use fragrance-fee and hypoallergenic lotions and oils.

When will my hair grow back?

For most teens and young adults, your hair will start to grow back about six weeks after you finish treatment. At first, hair usually grows back thin and fuzzy. Some people's hair grows back a different texture or even a different color. So do not be surprised if you suddenly have curly hair if it was straight before, or brown instead of blond.

What other ways will treatment affect my body?

Chemo and radiation can also change the way your skin and nails look. Some treatments might make you gain weight or look puffy. There might also be some long-term effects from treatment. Some people might have trouble having kids later in life.

We do not know right away exactly how changes will affect your body. Here are some things to get prepared for, and some things you can do to help make yourself more comfortable during these changes.

Skin And Nails

Just like hair, skin and nails grow fast. So cancer treatment can also do strange things to your skin and nails. For example:

- Your skin might become really dry, itchy, and red.

- Your skin might change color. You might notice your skin getting a little darker along the veins used for chemo.

- Your nails might become brittle or cracked. They might also turn yellow or change to a darker color.

Here are some things you can do to keep your skin and nails in good shape during treatment:

- Only use products that are for sensitive skin, fragrance-free, or hypoallergenic. This includes lotion, make-up, shampoo, deodorant, soap, laundry detergent, etc.

- Drink lots of fluids. This helps your skin stay hydrated.

- Put lotion on your skin right after a shower, while you are still a little wet. The lotion will help hold in the extra moisture.

- Use lip balm around your cuticles to help prevent cracking and bleeding.

Weight Gain And Steroids

If your treatment includes steroids, you will probably gain some weight. The steroids that are part of your treatment are not the muscle-building kind. But they are great at killing cancer cells and can help with nausea and allergic reactions. They can make you really hungry.

You might gain weight in places that you do not expect. Sometimes, steroids can give you a swollen face, big cheeks, or a fatty hump at the back of your neck. These things will go away when you stop taking steroids.

Chapter 43

After Cancer Treatment Ends

Medical Considerations

Keeping Your Past In the Rear View Mirror

Part of embracing your survivorship is learning to optimize your life-long health. While you may be cured or in remission from your cancer, it's important to be in tune with your current health, as well as your history. You'll need to get good follow-up care and be aware of the potential late effects of your cancer treatments.

It's not uncommon for survivors to just want to put their diagnosis behind them and not talk about their cancer. Even if it's uncomfortable, you must discuss your cancer diagnosis and treatment with your doctor. Now is the time in life to take responsibility for your survivorship. Your long-term health depends on it.

Holding Worries At Bay

Getting follow-up care can cause young survivors some stress. Anxiety over the cancer returning or beginning to see new late effects is normal. Keep in mind, only a small number of survivors incur serious late effects. Research is ongoing and has the potential to reduce or prevent many late effects if you experience them. Practicing preventive medicine and maintaining a healthy lifestyle are your best defenses for reducing your overall risks. But more than anything, stay educated. The body of information about childhood cancer is continually growing. Keep informed using our Late Effects Assessment Tool at beyondthecure.org.

About This Chapter: The text in this chapter is reprinted with permission from "Keeping Your Past in the Rear View Mirror," *The View from Up Here: Your Guide to Surviving Childhood Cancer,* © 2013 The National Children's Cancer Society (www.thenccs.org). All rights reserved.

The 411 On Late Effects

As the number of childhood cancer survivors continues to grow, so does the available information about late effects. The Institute of Medicine (2003) defines late effects as "complications, disabilities or adverse outcomes that are a result of the disease process, the treatment or both."

Many factors affect your risk for late effects. These include your diagnosis, your age at the time of diagnosis, gender, treatments, and complications, as well as family history, health prior to diagnosis, and your overall health. Some late effects are more visible, such as the amputation of a limb or the removal of an eye. Others will require testing to diagnose and may occur during childhood or adolescence. They can also be triggered by an unrelated disease or may just occur as you age.

Studies have shown that two-thirds of young adult survivors report one or more chronic late effects and of that group, one-third report severe or life-threatening late effects. Medical late effects can occur in any organ or system of the body and vary with each person depending on the diagnosis and the treatment received.

Medical History: Knowledge Is Power

Knowing your medical history is the key to maintaining good health and achieving the best possible quality of life. As you gradually take on more responsibility for your health information, you also become better able to determine whether a symptom may be linked to side effects of therapy.

Keep accurate, well-written medical records. The following information should be included:

- Previous and current medications

- Place of treatment

- Names and numbers of treatment providers

- Your specific diagnosis, including stage and location of cancer

- Date of diagnosis

- Dates and duration of treatment

- Number of relapses and dates of relapses

- Copies of any pertinent x-rays, MRIs, and CT scans

- Your specific treatment: (not all treatments will apply to you)

1. **Chemotherapy:** Drug, dosage total, frequency, and modality

2. **Surgery:** Date and type, including placement of central line catheters

3. **Radiation:** Area and total dosage

4. **Date and type—autologous, related, or unrelated allogenic—of bone marrow or stem cell transplant** as well as treatments in preparation for any transplants, if applicable

5. **Any complications and/or side effects during treatment and follow-up recommendations**

Follow Up And Follow Through

About two years after you've completed treatment, your status will change from "cancer patient" to "cancer survivor." It is still very important that you maintain oncology follow-up visits, get yearly physicals and regular examinations to maintain good health. Reviewing information on late effects with your healthcare team can lessen feelings of anxiety and prevent over-testing down the road.

Follow-up visits may include routine check-ups with other sub-specialists, as well as annual visits to a late effects clinic. These annual visits give you access to a multi-disciplinary team at a major medical center. The team may include a physician specializing in long-term follow-up care, a nurse, psychologist, a dietitian, a school liaison, a social worker, or other specialists. You'll receive comprehensive care in one setting and may participate in research that will benefit future cancer patients.

Make An Appointment With Organization

Whether you go to a late effects clinic or your primary physician, be sure your doctor is aware of your cancer history. Your physician should be assessing your current health status, tracking your progress on previously identified problems, as well as screening you for new problems.

When making medical appointments, keep these things in mind:

1. **Share all your medical history.** Any new doctor or medical provider will need copies of your records.

2. **Ask questions.** Express any concerns you have about potential late effects of treatments.

3. **Discuss any physical changes.** Share your concerns, no matter how small.

4. **Schedule yearly check-ups.** Physical exams should include blood count, urinalysis, and any other relevant exams.

5. **Screen for other cancers.** These include cancers of the breast, cervix, and colorectal as recommended by your doctor.

6. **Monitor for conditions related to your treatment.** Watch for symptoms or problems. Upon review, your doctor may recommend additional testing.

Tools For Survival

Keeping teen and young adult survivors informed is a role we take very seriously. On the Beyond the Cure website, beyondthecure.org, you'll find a Late Effects Assessment Tool which allows you and other survivors to develop a risk profile based on the treatment you received. This interactive tool provides results listing the potential medical issues you may face and offers strategies for maintaining your overall health.

By creating a risk profile, you will have additional information to discuss with your physician. If you are not attending a late effects clinic, be sure your doctor is aware of your cancer and the Long-term Follow-Up Guidelines created by the Children's Oncology Group at survivorshipguidelines.org.

The Real Weight Of An Ounce Of Prevention

Along with your annual physical examinations, you should practice preventive medicine. Get regular dental exams and follow-up on any tests that are relevant to your diagnosis. This can vary from person to person. For example, if you had long-term steroid use or radiation delivered around your eyes, you may need regular eye exams to test for cataracts. Certain medications and chemotherapy drugs can have late effects as well. Stay proactive with your health and stay in communication with your doctor to reduce your long-term risks.

From Childhood Cancer Survivor To Adulthood

Part of becoming a responsible adult survivor entails learning to take control of your own health. As you move away from the oncology setting, you'll find that many doctors aren't aware of all the potential late effects of childhood cancer or what follow-up care is necessary. You will need to become your own advocate. Sometimes, new healthcare providers will need to be educated.

To ease the transition to an adult care setting, it helps to begin initiating more healthcare responsibilities at home. Track your own medical information in a journal. Maintain a thorough treatment summary so you will have accurate details. Take charge of making and keeping your own medical appointments. Keep track of your medications and when you need to order medical supplies. The more responsibility you take, the more empowered you will feel about your own health.

As a young adult, think about the obstacles that may prevent you from attending follow-up appointments. Are you afraid of a recurrence? Do you want to put the cancer treatment behind you? Get in touch with the feelings behind these obstacles and discuss them with your healthcare provider, your social worker, or family.

Treatment Ends, Questions Begin

The end of your cancer treatment is a celebrated time, but it's also common to feel some apprehension and confusion. Finding answers to the following questions will help you maintain your long-term health:

- When should check-ups occur and how often?
- What tests are required at follow-up visits?
- What is your doctor's experience with long-term cancer survivors?
- Is there a long-term follow-up clinic you can attend?
- What are the signs of a relapse or a second cancer?
- What are the potential late effects from the treatment you received?
- What are the current recommendations or tests for your particular type of cancer?
- What are the symptoms of potential late effects?
- Is there a special diet you should be following?
- Are there special tests to check your heart, lungs, eyes, teeth, bones, and hormones?
- How and when can you reach your healthcare provider with questions?
- Who should you contact with questions related to fertility, activity, psychosocial issues, or concerns about school and/or your job?

Finding And Paying For Care

One of the biggest responsibilities you'll face in an adult healthcare setting is locating and paying for your healthcare services. Services may not be easily accessible and you will have to advocate for your healthcare needs. These suggestions will help you find the best medical treatment available.

1. **Look for a long-term follow-up clinic in your area.** Find a list of clinics at beyondthe cure.org.

2. **Find a primary care physician to meet your everyday needs.** Look for a doctor with knowledge of the late effects from the treatment of childhood cancer. Ask your oncologist for a recommendation or contact the American Medical Association (AMA) at 800-621-8335. Be aware, some doctors will need educating on these issues.

3. **Understand your insurance coverage.** Discuss your coverage and healthcare financing with your parents before leaving home. Whatever you do, don't let your policy lapse.

Transitioning into adulthood is tough for everyone. As a cancer survivor, you face more issues in maintaining your health. Your best tools are your own persistence and determination. Being well-educated and using your own initiative to overcome any healthcare barriers will help you maintain good health and peace of mind.

Healthy Living After Cancer

As a survivor, lifestyle can play an important role in your long-term health. Some cancer diagnoses and treatments carry a greater risk of developing certain diseases later in life. Practicing good health habits can reduce these risks and also lessen some late effects. While some risks are beyond your control, there are a lot of lifestyle changes you can make that promote better overall health.

You may feel invincible because you survived cancer. Take pride in your strength, but realize that your survival is also the result of the decisions you made during treatment. Now it's important to arm yourself against the late effects that may occur after treatment. The best thing you can do for your health now is to make good choices. Avoid risky behavior and surround yourself with the people who share your values and make smart choices for healthy living.

Smoking Kills

Tobacco use and smoking is the single most preventable cause of death in the United States. Statistics show that one million teens will start smoking each year and one-third will eventually die from their addiction. The best thing you can do to maintain your health is to never smoke or use any form of smokeless tobacco. If you currently smoke, make a pledge to quit.

Stay away from second-hand smoke, too. Non-smokers who live or work with smokers experience a 30 to 50 percent greater risk for lung cancer. That makes second-hand smoke the number one preventable risk factor for serious and chronic diseases of non-smokers in our country. Avoid exposure to tobacco whenever you can.

Tobacco is highly addictive, so quitting is difficult. But studies show that smokers who quit before age 50 will cut their risk of dying in half over the next five years. If you have trouble quitting, get help. To learn more about quitting smoking, call the Center for Disease Control and Prevention at 800-232-4636 or the National Cancer Institute at 800-4-CANCER.

There's Nothing Wrong With Eating Right

What you eat has a direct impact on your health. Although childhood cancer isn't directly related to diet, eating a balanced diet is key to any healthy lifestyle. A policy study from the American Institute of Cancer Research reports that of the 12 common adult cancers, about 35 percent of cases in the USA are preventable through a healthy diet, being physically active, and maintaining a healthy weight.

A healthy diet should include a variety of fruits, vegetables, nuts, and beans. Limit your intake of red meat and processed foods that are high in sugar, low in fiber, or high in fat. Watch the salty foods, too, and cut back on processed foods high in salt.

Move It Along, Folks

Exercise provides great physical and mental benefits for the body. Regular physical activity has been proven to reduce the incidence of colorectal cancer, coronary disease, osteoporosis, diabetes, and possibly breast cancer. Exercise also improves mood, boosts self-esteem, stimulates the immune system, and reduces the symptoms of pain, diarrhea, and constipation.

Start a workout plan that has a consistent level of limited to moderate activity and do it several times a week. USDA guidelines recommend that adults should have 60 minutes of moderate to vigorous activity, most days of the week. Moderate activity is considered exercise that raises your heart rate.

Diet and physical activity together will help you maintain a healthy weight that your doctor defines as normal for your height. Research shows there is an increased risk of obesity with certain types of childhood cancer. Think of weight as a long-term health goal. Once you reach your optimum weight, limit weight gain throughout adulthood to less than 11 pounds. Avoid frequent weight fluctuations. The American Institute for Cancer Research offers great nutritional guidelines for maintaining a healthy weight on their website at aicr.org.

Tips To Eat By

Maintaining a healthy diet can be overwhelming at first. But these simple tips will help you ensure the foods you put in your body will do right by you.

1. **Limit your salt intake.** Use other herbs and spices like paprika, garlic powder, thyme, and oregano to flavor food. High salt intake may contribute to high blood pressure in some people.

2. **Stay away from fat.** Only 20–25 percent of your total calories each day should come from fat. Less than one-third of these calories from fat should be from an animal source.

3. **Avoid fast food.** It's high in fat, calories, and sodium.

4. **Drink skim milk.** Substitute whole milk with fat free, Vitamin D fortified milk.

5. **Use low-fat varieties of dairy products:** Eat only moderate amounts of cheese.

6. **Skip the butter:** Opt for olive oil and canola oil in cooking.

7. **Eat enough protein:** As you eat less meat, add other protein sources such as soy products and beans.

8. **Monitor your health with your doctor:** Discuss any changes in your weight, appetite, or problems with digestion. Ask if there are specific nutritional needs related to your diagnosis or treatment.

9. **Don't be misled by restaurant portion sizes.** Servings are much larger than one person needs, so don't eat everything on your plate. Take leftovers home.

Even if you're in good health and feeling great, talk to your doctor before beginning any workout program. Certain chemotherapies used in treating childhood cancer can lead to increased risk of heart disease, so your doctor will need to be aware of your activity level to assess your risk. Remember, you can build your own late effects assessment at beyondthecure.org to proactively care for yourself as a survivor.

A Toast To Being Alcohol Free

As you begin mapping out your way to healthy living, you're bound to run into some challenges. Alcohol may be one of them. Alcohol provides a lot of calories without any nutrition. Evidence also suggests that drinking large amounts of alcohol increases your risk of several types of cancer and other chronic conditions. It's easy to see why drinking isn't recommended as part of a healthy lifestyle.

The legal drinking age is 21, yet a staggering 70 percent of American high school seniors have consumed some form of alcohol within the last month. Studies show that the sooner a person starts drinking, the more likely they are to have alcohol-related problems in adulthood.

If you are of legal drinking age and choose to drink, do it in moderation. Don't justify a night of heavy drinking by not drinking alcohol several days in advance. In fact, many studies show that binge drinking is more dangerous than moderate alcohol consumption. Part of being a responsible survivor is making healthy choices about everything you put in your body.

Find Your Safe Place In The Sun

We all enjoy a little sunshine, but too much sun exposure can cause serious health problems. Melanoma is a serious form of skin cancer, and it's the most common form of cancer in Americans aged 25–29. Everyone experiences some burning and damage from the sun, but taking these preventive steps will help you minimize further skin damage:

1. **Use a minimum of SPF 15.** Apply 15–20 minutes before sun exposure. Broad spectrum SPF 15 will block out 93 percent of UVA & UVB rays, which are the more dangerous burning rays.

2. **Apply sunscreen every two hours.** Apply a thick layer and reapply after swimming.

3. **Check the date on the package.** Sunscreen has a shelf life of two years.

4. **Limit your time in the sun.** Avoid peak hours of damaging rays between late morning and early afternoon.

5. **Shade yourself in peak hours.** Wear a hat with a wide brim or carry an umbrella to create extra shade.

6. **Wear sunglasses.** Protect your eyes from exposure to UV light.

7. **Avoid reflective surfaces.** Water, sand, and concrete can increase your risk of burning rays.

8. **Don't use indoor tanning beds.** They contain the same dangerous UV rays as natural sun exposure.

Keep an eye out for changes in moles on your body. While most moles are harmless, alert your doctor if any moles change color, shape, or size, or suddenly appear out of nowhere. Pay attention to moles with irregular borders or any moles that bleed or are itchy. A change of a couple millimeters in a single mole can actually make the difference between life and death.

If you have already been exposed to radiation treatment, you are at a higher risk for skin cancer and should limit your sun exposure as much as possible. Be sure to keep an eye on moles in areas of your body that have received radiation therapy. You can't ever be too careful with skin cancer.

Emotional Challenges

Healing Your Mind As Well As Your Body

It's easy to understand the physical healing that you must endure with a cancer diagnosis. But childhood cancer affects you emotionally, too. Throughout your life, you may experience heightened feelings, both positive and negative. Often, you'll be able to incorporate these feelings into your life and hopefully draw courage and inspiration from them.

Even Emotions Have Growing Pains

Some survivors experience post-traumatic growth, (Tedeschi and Calhoun, 2004) which can be expressed in many different ways. You may gain a greater appreciation for life and every new experience. Cancer can give many people personal strength, spiritual development and better interpersonal relationships. Facing your fears and triumphing is what being a survivor is all about.

Experiencing post-traumatic growth doesn't mean you have overcome the stress of your cancer experience. Surviving your diagnosis and treatment at a young age brings with it a roller coaster of emotions. Many survivors experience depression, anxiety and fear. And long after the end of treatment, some survivors experience post-traumatic stress.

When times get tough, it's important to learn how to handle stress and emotional challenges that come with your diagnosis. Good coping skills can help you integrate the cancer experience into your life, instead of being ruled by it.

Holding On As The Ride Gets Bumpy

The end of treatment is indeed a joyous time. Certainly, it is a cause for celebration, but you may also begin to feel anxious. Losing constant contact with your healthcare team may be frightening.

Friends and family who provided support during your treatment may not understand that the cancer is still part of your life. It's easy to feel alone.

You may also fear potential late effects, a relapse, or have some physical changes that are causing anxiety. Sometimes, survivors experience greater anxiety because it is finally safe to allow yourself to feel everything you held back during treatment.

Feelings of stress and anxiety are common. Finding ways to cope and relieve these feelings will help you maintain a healthier lifestyle.

1. **Move your body.** Exercise at least 30 minutes, four times a week with your doctor's approval.

2. **Eat healthy.** The good foods you put in your body will have a positive impact on your emotions and your physical health.

3. **Avoid alcohol and drugs.** These can mask your true feelings and cause other health complications.

4. **Avoid stimulants.** Caffeine and decongestants can interfere with your sleep.

5. **Get lots of sleep.** Get at least eight hours a day.

6. **Start a hobby.** Find something you like to do alone, such as knitting or painting. Or, involve others by joining a book club or sports team.

7. **Talk about your concerns.** Join a support group or discuss things with a friend, counselor or clergy member.

8. **Learn to pace yourself.** Set priorities for yourself that include making time for activities that you like to do.

9. **Relax.** Learn techniques such as deep breathing or meditation that will allow you to unwind when you're feeling tense.

Fear of recurrence is very real and can be intense for many survivors. When these fears take over, take a moment to determine your actual risk of recurrence. Think how you can be proactive about reducing your risk of the cancer returning. Have your potential problems evaluated by a medical professional. And always talk with someone about your concerns. Don't leave things bottled up.

Whatever you do, don't let these fears keep you from living a happy and healthy life.

Post-Traumatic Stress After Cancer

Survivors who are treated at a young age may not be fully aware of how their cancer experience has affected them. Some choose to ignore their feelings and just move on with life. Studies show that unresolved feelings of helplessness and anxiety may increase the risk of post-traumatic stress disorder (PTSD).

When The Bad Feelings Don't Get Better

At the anniversary of your diagnosis, you may find that you experience disappointment, tiredness, and loneliness. Lots of survivors have these feelings. It's important that you learn to distinguish between "normal" levels of sadness and a more serious case of depression. Symptoms of depression include loss of interest in most activities; changes in eating and sleeping habits; nervousness; tiredness; sluggishness; worthlessness; poor concentration; too much sleep or difficulty sleeping at all.

It is common for survivors to experience these symptoms in the years following cancer treatment. Generally, they lessen with time. If you have feelings that persist or they are beginning to affect your relationships or your ability to work, seek help. Don't hesitate to use these resources to get the guidance you need:

- The National Association of Social Workers (naswdc.org): 202-408-8600
- American Counseling Association (counseling.org): 800-347-6647
- National Suicide Prevention Lifeline: 800-273-TALK (800-273-8255)
- 911

Symptoms of PTSD include:

- Recurring and distressing dreams or recollections about the event

- Inability to recall important aspects of the trauma

- Heightened arousal, such as nausea or increased heart rate, which is triggered by reminders of the original experience

- Feelings of detachment from others

- Sleep disturbances

- Irritability or outbursts of anger

- Difficulty concentrating

- Intrusive, unwanted thoughts

- Avoidance of stress-inducing settings and situations

If you are worried that you are experiencing PTSD, contact a professional counselor or one of your hospital social workers. For a list of specialists and support groups in your area, contact the American Cancer Society at 800-ACS-2345 or CancerCare at 800-813-HOPE.

Reaching Out For Support

Connecting with people who have shared similar cancer experiences and emotions can be helpful in the healing process. A childhood cancer support group is a great place to talk about your fears and emotions. Survivors share information, provide emotional support and inspiration to boost one another's sense of self-worth. Sometimes, sharing your experience makes you feel like you're helping others, which gives you a chance to grow and heal.

Is a support group a good option for you? You'll need to be comfortable sharing your feelings, be interested in learning about others' experiences, and enjoy being part of a group dynamic. The setting gives you a platform to provide helpful information to others and to reach out to other survivors in need of emotional healing. Every support group has a unique make-up and the focus of the meetings can be different from one week to the next depending on who attends. Be sure to attend a group at least twice before deciding whether or not to join.

Online support groups are another way to go. You can talk about your feelings and concerns and still maintain a feeling of anonymity. Consider becoming part of the NCCS online community at theNCCS.org.

Support is where you find it. If you're not comfortable in a group setting, reach out to a psychologist, social worker, psychiatrist, or clergy member. Talk to your family and friends and explain how they can help you. Or, extend your support to others. It can relieve your isolation and allow you to feel empowered and more in control. More than anything, draw on your own strengths. Read books by other survivors and reach inside to find the strength and support that got you through this incredible journey.

Chapter 44

Cancer And Your Friendships

Cancer can affect your friendships. Some relationships may grow stronger, and others may fade. It often helps to understand how your friends feel and learn to tell them how you feel. This chapter has information to help you understand:

- What your friends may be thinking

- How to talk with your friends

- Ways your friends can help

- How to accept changes

What Your Friends May Be Thinking

Your friends may have never had a friend with cancer, and some may not know how to react. Your friends may be thinking:

- If they are avoiding you, they may not know what to say or worry about saying the wrong thing.

- If they avoid mentioning your cancer, they may be afraid of upsetting you.

- If they aren't calling you, it may be because they think you won't feel like talking.

- If they aren't inviting you to be a part of activities, they may think you won't be able to go or they may feel guilty about having fun when you're sick.

- If they aren't visiting you, they may think you don't want visitors or worry about any potential awkward moments during the visit.

Don't be afraid to take the lead and call your friends or invite them over. Plan activities that you feel comfortable doing, and your friends will probably have a better understanding of what you are able to do with them.

Talking With Your Friends

Because your friends probably don't know much about cancer, you can begin by explaining your cancer and treatment. First, decide what you want your friends to know. You may want to tell your good friends a lot, but just tell your casual friends or people at school something simple like, "I have cancer, but I'm getting treatment and will be OK." Your friends might not bring up your cancer, so discuss it when you feel ready. The more open you are with your friends, the more opportunities they have to be supportive and accepting.

If you're nervous about talking with your friends, decide ahead of time what you want to say. Remember that you are in charge of what you tell people, so you don't have to tell anyone until you're ready, and you don't have to say more than you want. Answer your friends' questions with as much information as you are comfortable giving.

Ways Your Friends Can Help

Your friends may want to help you, but some may not know how. Be honest about what you need and what they can do to help.

- Ask them to keep calling you, even if you don't always feel like talking.

- Ask them to keep inviting you to things. Even if you can't always go, you'll go when you can.

- If you can't go out, ask some friends over to watch a movie or just hang out together.

- Ask friends to visit you in the hospital—give them a heads up on what to expect, especially if you look a little different.

- If you can't see your friends, ask them to keep in touch online or through texting, instant messaging, phone, or e-mail.

- Tell your friends that sometimes all you need is for them to listen.

- Remind them that even though you may look different on the outside, you're still the same on the inside.

Accepting Changes

Your friendships are likely to change, but many changes will be positive. You may be closer to some of your friends and find it easier to talk about important things. You may also find that the experience of cancer changes you somewhat—you may become more serious about school or want to help other people. You may make new friends whose interests are more like yours. You may also make friends with other teens with cancer who are more likely to understand your experiences.

Despite your best efforts, some friendships could fade. You may lose some friends but strengthen relationships with others or make new friends.

What about boyfriends and girlfriends?

Many young people say that they feel "different" from their friends when they have been through cancer treatment.

It can be hard to feel confident when you have lost your hair and are not your usual weight. Making new friends when you look different or can't do everything that other people can do, can feel like a big challenge.

It's the same when it comes to girlfriends and boyfriends. It's good to remember that almost everyone you meet will also feel that there are parts of themselves or their background that they would like to change.

A lot of the people you meet will feel that they couldn't have coped with your illness and the treatment you've had. It's up to you who you tell about your illness, but remember that often the people, who you are open with, will feel much more able to tell you about their own worries.

Having had cancer doesn't stop you having normal relationships and getting married just like your friends.

Source: "What about boyfriends and girlfriends?" Reprinted with permission from www.teenagecancertrust.org. © 2013 Teenage Cancer Trust. All rights reserved.

Chapter 45

Cancer And Your Education

Learning To Embrace Your New Educational Needs

When a teen or child gets cancer, they and their parents have to adjust their thinking about school attendance and their needs for learning. Treatments can cause many absences, so be sure to discuss attendance plans with your school and your teachers as quickly as possible. Some hospitals have school liaisons that will assist with all areas of education. These people work with you and your parents throughout treatment to maintain some educational consistency. That also means you should be included in any meetings regarding your learning.

You and your parents will need to re-inform teachers and administrators at the beginning of every new school year in order to keep everyone up-to-date on your educational needs.

Enroll In The School Of Flexibility

Parents may feel an instinct to shelter their child while they are sick, but kids should attend school whenever possible. Research shows that long-term survivors who attended school during treatment had better social skills, more self-confidence, and were also less likely to have academic problems than kids who were in tutoring programs at home.

The reality is tough; many children with cancer have to miss school frequently due to treatment, complications, or a compromised immunity. For this reason, many schools offer Homebound Tutoring or private tutoring to students who must be absent from school over an extended period.

About This Chapter: The text in this chapter is adapted and reprinted with permission from "School: Learning to Embrace Their New Educational Needs," *The Other Side of the Mountain: A Parent's Guide to Surviving Childhood Cancer,* © 2013 The National Children's Cancer Society (www.thenccs.org). All rights reserved.

If you do a homebound program, you would remain enrolled in school and be expected to return as soon as you are able.

Programs are administered in different ways so it's important to find out what your school can provide. Most students benefit from intermittent home tutoring, meaning they attend school when they are able, and are tutored at home when they are not. This process can be discussed and arranged through a school counselor. Intermittent instruction, however, may not be right for every child or available in every district.

Sometimes, you may need to be hospitalized. While you are an inpatient, the hospital's educational coordinator can help with academics. Many coordinators will also help when you are an outpatient.

Missing School Without Missing Out

Unfortunately, by missing school, kids also miss the important socialization lessons that school provides. There are ways to help you stay involved while you are at home:

1. Attend special days and parties. Work with the school to allow you to be there for activities like Halloween, Valentine's Day, or classroom functions.

2. Interact with classmates. Encourage friends to send cards, letters, and pictures. You can even set up a collection box at school to make it easy for people to stay in touch with you.

3. E-mail is another great way to keep in touch. Keep in touch through social media or other free websites. You can set up a Facebook account and regularly post updates on your progress. Please note: Facebook does not allow young children to have their own account so parents will need to closely manage and monitor any activity. A personal website can be established on caringbridge.org to stay connected with family and friends.

4. Use video conferencing to interact. Skype is a free video conferencing service that's easy to use. Web cameras are becoming a standard component of many computers. Web cams can also be purchased separately and are an inexpensive and simple way to add video conferencing to your existing system.

5. Invite friends to visit and play. It's important you continue being a kid.

When School Isn't An Option

There are some children who need to avoid school altogether during treatment. If that is the case with you, consider homeschooling. When a child is home schooled, there is no official connection to public or private schools. It's legal in all 50 states and Canada, but each state has its own laws regarding the process. To find out the laws in your state, visit homeschool.com.

What most children survivors want is to be treated normally. To make this happen, you and your parents will need to educate your school community. Your treatment may last more than one school year, so you may need to present this information at the start of each grade.

Before returning to school, you and your parents should discuss these things with teachers and your principal:

1. Your health in detail. Parents: Talk about your or your child's diagnosis, treatment plan, as well as low blood counts and risk of infection.

2. Central line issues. Tell them if you (or your child) have a Port-A-Cath or Broviac.

3. When to contact parents. Parents: Stress the importance of calling you if your child has a fever and of informing you if anyone in school has contracted an infectious disease such as chicken pox.

4. Any immunization restrictions. Discuss with the school nurse what is expected if there is an outbreak of a disease for which the teen or child has not been adequately immunized.

5. Future absences. Talk about who will pick up and return schoolwork when you are absent from school.

6. Accommodations for your special needs. Consider whether you will need permission or a special pass to go to the nurse or restroom when necessary.

7. Who will administer your medication at school, if needed.

8. If there are issues preventing you from completing assignments on time. Mention if there are side effects of treatment or if you have chronic fatigue.

9. If there are areas in which you are falling behind. Set up tutors if necessary.

10. Arrangements for your (your child's) condition. Discuss if there are activities you cannot participate in or if extra time will be needed to move between classrooms.

11. Classroom seating. Talk to teachers about your (your child's) placement in the classroom if they need to accommodate for hearing and visual problems.

12. Side effects caused by treatment. Find out if the school is equipped for a wheelchair or walker and if handicapped parking spots are available. Discuss whether special permission is required to wear a hat or a scarf to school.

Take It Easy, And Adjust Accordingly

Going back to school can trigger a variety of emotional responses. Parents: Stay in contact with your child's teachers and communicate regularly about changes in academic and social behaviors. It's helpful to have a teacher, counselor, or school nurse to oversee your child's adjustment back into school.

The transition back to school will be easier if you and your family make the following decisions about your condition:

1. What do you want to share? Consider how much information about your diagnosis and treatment you are willing to let the school community know.

2. How will you provide this information? Will you give a presentation to the class? Parents: Will you talk to school administrators? Or will you ask someone from the hospital to lead the discussion?

3. When should the discussion take place? Discussions should occur prior to your (or your child's) return to school after diagnosis/treatment and following any new developments that could impact performance.

4. Who should the teachers and the teen's peers contact with questions? Who would you like to handle questions? Consider how you will handle rumors should they start.

Smart Planning For College

Many childhood cancer survivors will eventually head off to college. Rest assured that the same courage and determination that got you through cancer treatment will serve you well in college. There are many things to consider when choosing a school. If you require regular follow-up care, be sure the school is located near a reliable hospital with respected doctors to continue overseeing their care. If you require special accommodations, find out if the school will provide them. Inquire if the school has an office that serves students with disabilities.

Here are some helpful questions to ask:

- Does the school have an office that serves students with disabilities, including a full-time staff (Student Disability Services-SDS)?

- How long has the program been running?

- What type of support does the SDS Office offer?

- Are the counselors or staff specially trained in working with learning disabilities?

- Is there any threat that the office will close before you finish college?

- Do they have an ADA/504 coordinator?

- Who should parents contact if they have questions during the school year?

- Who counsels students during registration, orientation, and course selection?

- Is tutoring available, and are the tutors professors or students?

- Is tutoring automatic or does it need to be requested?

- Does the college have an established grievance policy?

- Has it published a notice of nondiscrimination?

- Does the college faculty receive any disability awareness training?

- How are classroom accommodations requested?

Cost

Of course, the cost of a college education can be staggering. Financial aid may be available for you, and your guidance counselor can help you with the process. As a cancer survivor, you may also be able to apply for special scholarships for childhood cancer survivors. The National Children's Cancer Society's (NCCS') Beyond the Cure Scholarship Program makes college scholarships available to survivors of childhood cancer who have been diagnosed before the age of 18. To learn more about the program and other scholarships available to survivors, visit beyondthecure.org.

Applications Made Easier

Keeping comprehensive files that include academic records, special education services, and any additional support you (or your child) have received will be helpful during the admission process. Here are some additional questions to ask:

- Does the college offer early enrollment?

- Is additional time provided for students to meet with professors and learn the location of classes?

- Can students take longer to graduate?

Leaving Home Without Anxiety Following

You may have done well in the high school setting, but sometimes, the transition to college life can be a bigger adjustment. If you have experienced any limitations, make college decisions that contribute to your educational growth and success.

327

1. Be realistic about the college completion timeframe. Think carefully about course requirements, course sizes, course waiver provisions, and course curriculums. Parents: Encourage your child to take five to six years to graduate if necessary.

2. Choose instructors with teaching styles that complement your learning style. If you learn best in class discussions, ask advisors to help choose professors who encourage class participation.

4. Consider health insurance coverage. Parents: Will your child continue your healthcare coverage or be covered through the university?

5. Get acquainted with other students with disabilities. It can be helpful to learn from others the type of problems you may face, and to hear suggestions for overcoming the challenges you may encounter.

An Education In Life

You and your family are childhood cancer survivors. As you consider these important aspects of your educational growth, remind yourself of the journey you have shared together. The things you have learned throughout your climb will enrich all aspects of your life, not just your education. Your cancer experience has provided you with lessons of strength and emotional growth that can't be learned in books. Celebrate your amazing achievements.

Chapter 46

Late Effects: Chronic Problems That Can Result After Cancer And Treatment

What are late effects?

The cancer itself or the treatment of cancer may cause health problems for childhood cancer survivors months or years after successful treatment has ended. Cancer treatments may harm the body's organs, bones, or tissues and cause health problems later in life. These health problems are called late effects. Treatments that may cause late effects include surgery, chemotherapy, radiation therapy, or stem cell transplant.

While most late effects are not life-threatening, they may cause serious problems that affect health and quality of life. Late effects in childhood cancer survivors are both physical and emotional.

Late effects in childhood cancer survivors may affect the following:

- Organs, tissues, and body function

- Growth and development

- Mood, feelings, and actions

- Thinking, learning, and memory

- Social and psychological adjustment

- Risk of second cancers

About This Chapter: Excerpted from PDQ® Cancer Information Summary. National Cancer Institute; Bethesda, MD. Late Effects of Treatment For Childhood Cancer (PDQ): Patient version. Updated 4/4/2013. Available at: www.cancer.gov. Accessed May 20, 2013.

The risk of late effects depends on many things, including the following:

- Type of cancer and where it is in the body
- The type and amount of treatment
- The child's age when treated
- Genetic factors and health problems the child had before the cancer
- Being exposed to substances in the environment that cause cancer

What late effects are related to the heart and blood vessels?

Heart and blood vessel late effects may include the following:

- Abnormal heartbeat
- Weakened heart muscle
- Inflamed heart or sac around the heart
- Damage to the heart valves
- Coronary artery disease (hardening of the heart arteries)
- Congestive heart failure
- Chest pain or heart attack
- Blood clots or stroke
- Carotid artery disease
- Trouble breathing

The following may increase the risk of heart and blood vessel late effects:

- Being female
- Being young at the time of treatment (the younger the child, the greater the risk)
- Having other risk factors for heart disease, such as a family history of heart disease, being overweight, smoking, or having high blood pressure, high cholesterol, or diabetes

Childhood cancer survivors who were treated with both radiation to the chest and chemotherapy using anthracyclines are at greatest risk. New treatments that decrease the amount of radiation give and use lower doses of chemotherapy may decrease the risk of heart and blood vessel late effects.

What late effects are related to the central nervous system?

Childhood cancer survivors who received radiation, intrathecal chemotherapy, or surgery to the brain or spinal cord are at risk of late effects to the brain and spinal cord. These include the following:

- Headaches

- Loss of coordination and balance

- Seizures

- Loss of the myelin sheath that covers nerve fibers in the brain

- Movement disorders that affect the legs and eyes or the ability to speak and swallow

- Nerve damage in the hands or feet

- Stroke

- Hydrocephalus

- Loss of bladder and/or bowel control

Survivors may also have late effects that affect thinking, learning, and behavior. Possible signs of brain and spinal cord late effects include headaches, loss of coordination, and seizures.

It's A Fact!

Regular follow-up by health professionals who are experts in finding and treating late effects is important for the long-term health of childhood cancer survivors. Follow-up care will be different for each person who has been treated for cancer. The type of care will depend on the type of cancer, the type of treatment, genetic factors, and the person's general health and health habits.

It is important that childhood cancer survivors have an exam at least once a year. The exams should be done by a health professional who is familiar with the survivor's risk for late effects and can recognize the early signs of late effects. Blood and imaging tests may also be done.

Long-term follow-up may improve the health and quality of life for cancer survivors and also helps doctors study the late effects of cancer treatments so that safer therapies for newly diagnosed children may be developed.

Late Effects And Educational Concerns

Possible effects of cancer treatment involving the brain and spinal cord can include the following:

- Problems with memory
- Problems with paying attention
- Trouble with solving problems
- Trouble with organizing thoughts and tasks
- Ability to learn and use new information slows down
- Trouble learning to read, write, or do math
- Trouble coordinating movement between the eyes, hands, and other muscles
- Delays in normal development
- Social withdrawal

Other conditions may cause the same symptoms. Talk to your doctor if any of these problems occur.

What are late effects are related to emotional and social issues?

Survivors of childhood cancer may have anxiety and depression related to physical changes, the way they look, or the fear of cancer coming back. This may cause problems with personal relationships, education, employment, and health. Survivors with these problems may be less likely to live independently as adults.

Yearly follow-up exams for childhood cancer survivors should include screening and treatment for possible psychological distress.

Some childhood cancer survivors have post-traumatic stress disorder.

Being diagnosed and treated for a life-threatening disease may be traumatic. This trauma may cause post-traumatic stress disorder (PTSD). PTSD is defined as having certain behaviors following a stressful event that involved death or the threat of death, serious injury, or a threat to oneself or others. In general, childhood cancer survivors show low levels of PTSD, depending in part on the coping style of patients and their parents.

Teens who are diagnosed with cancer may reach fewer social milestones or reach them later in life than teens not diagnosed with cancer. Social milestones include having a first boyfriend, getting married, and having a child. They may also have trouble getting along with other people or feel like they are not liked by their peers.

Cancer survivors in this age group have reported being less satisfied with their health and their lives in general compared with others of the same age who did not have cancer. Teens and young adults who have survived cancer need special programs that provide psychological, educational, and employment support.

What late effects are related to the teeth and jaws?

Childhood cancer survivors who received radiation to the head and neck or certain chemotherapy drugs are at risk of late effects to the teeth and jaws. These include the following:

- Teeth that are not normal
- Tooth decay (including cavities) and gum disease
- Salivary glands do not make enough saliva
- Jaw bones do not fully form
- Death of the bone cells in the jaw
- Possible signs of late effects of the teeth and jaws include tooth decay
- Teeth are small or do not have a normal shape
- Missing permanent teeth
- Permanent teeth come in at a later than normal age
- More tooth decay (cavities) and gum disease than normal
- Dry mouth
- Jaw pain
- Jaws do not open and close the way they should

Treatment for these and other childhood cancers may cause the late effect of problems with teeth and jaws:

- Head and neck cancers
- Hodgkin lymphoma
- Leukemia that has spread to the brain and spinal cord
- Nasopharyngeal cancer
- Neuroblastoma

Radiation to the head and neck and certain chemotherapy drugs increase the risk of late effects to the teeth and jaws.

Quick Tip

Regular dental care is very important for survivors of childhood cancer. A dental check-up is suggested every six months. Also a dental cleaning and fluoride treatment is suggested every six months.

What late effects are related to the digestive tract?

Digestive tract late effects include the following:

- A narrowing of the esophagus or intestine

- Blocked bowel (chronic)

- Bowel perforation (a hole in the intestine)

- Intestine is not able to absorb nutrients from food

- Infection of the intestines

- Trouble swallowing or feeling like food is stuck in your throat

- Heartburn

- Fever with severe pain in the abdomen and nausea

- Pain in the abdomen

- A change in bowel habits (constipation or diarrhea)

- Nausea and vomiting

- Frequent gas pains, bloating, fullness, or cramps

- Weight loss for no known reason

Treatment for rhabdomyosarcoma, Wilms tumor, and other childhood cancers may cause digestive tract side effects. Radiation therapy to the abdomen and surrounding areas may damage the blood vessels. Pelvic surgery, surgery to remove the bladder, or abdominal laparotomy may also cause digestive tract late effects. Chemotherapy with alkylating agents may increase the risk, as well as stem cell transplant and a history of chronic graft-versus-host disease.

What late effects are related to the liver and bile ducts?

Liver and bile duct late effects include the following:

- Liver doesn't work the way it should or stops working
- Gallstones
- Hepatitis B or C infection
- Liver damage caused by veno-occlusive disease/sinusoidal obstruction syndrome (VOD/SOS)
- Liver fibrosis (an overgrowth of connective tissue in the liver) or cirrhosis
- Fatty liver with insulin resistance (a condition in which the body makes insulin but cannot use it well)
- Liver failure

Certain chemotherapy drugs and radiation to the liver or bile ducts increase the risk of late effects. These include cancers treated with a stem cell transplant, Wilms tumor, and acute lymphoblastic anemia (ALL).

Quick Tip

Childhood cancer survivors with liver late effects should take care to protect their health, including:

- Having a healthy weight
- Not drinking alcohol
- Getting vaccines for hepatitis A and hepatitis B viruses

What late effects are related to the pancreas?

Pancreatic late effects include the following:

- **Insulin Resistance:** A condition in which the body does not use insulin the way it should. Insulin is needed to help control the amount of glucose (a type of sugar) in the body. Because the insulin does not work the way it should, glucose and fat levels rise.

- **Diabetes Mellitus:** A disease in which the body does not make enough insulin or does not use it the way it should. When there is not enough insulin, the amount of glucose in the blood increases and the kidneys make a large amount of urine.

What late effects are related to the thyroid?

Thyroid late effects may include the following:

- Hypothyroidism (not enough thyroid hormone)
- Hyperthyroidism (too much thyroid hormone)
- Goiter
- Lumps in the thyroid

The risk of thyroid late effects may be increased in childhood cancer survivors after treatment with radiation therapy to the brain and spinal cord or head and neck, total-body irradiation (TBI) as part of a stem cell transplant, chemotherapy, and radioactive iodine therapy for neuroblastoma.

The risk also is increased in females, in survivors who were a young age at the time of treatment, in survivors who had a higher radiation dose, and as the time since diagnosis and treatment gets longer.

What late effects are related to the neuroendocrine system?

Neuroendocrine late effects may include the following:

- Low levels of pituitary hormones, including growth hormones
- Puberty at a later age than normal or early puberty
- Pituitary gland disorders
- Hypothalamus disorders

A low level of growth hormone is the most common side effect of radiation to the brain in childhood cancer survivors. The higher the radiation dose and the longer the time since treatment, the greater the risk of this late effect. A low level of growth hormone in childhood results in adult height that is shorter than normal. Low growth hormone levels may be treated with growth hormone replacement therapy.

Quick Tip

Childhood cancer survivors who get enough exercise and have a normal amount of anxiety have a lower risk of obesity.

Treatment for acute lymphoblastic leukemia (ALL), brain and spinal cord tumors, nasopharyngeal cancer, cancers treated with total-body irradiation (TBI) before a stem cell transplant, and radiation therapy to the hypothalamus increase the risk of neuroendocrine system late effects.

What late effects are related to metabolic syndrome?

Metabolic syndrome is more likely to occur after treatment for certain childhood cancers. Metabolic syndrome is a group of medical conditions that includes having too much fat around the abdomen and two of the following:

- High blood pressure
- High levels of triglycerides and low levels of high-density lipoprotein cholesterol (considered "good" cholesterol) in the blood
- High levels of glucose (sugar) in the blood

Childhood cancer survivors who received radiation to the brain or had a stem cell transplant are at risk for metabolic syndrome. Metabolic syndrome may cause low levels of growth hormone, which helps promote growth and control metabolism. This may cause the survivor to be shorter than normal.

What late effects are related to body weight?

The risk of obesity may increase with the following:

- Being diagnosed with cancer when aged five to nine years
- Being female
- Not doing enough physical activity to stay at a healthy body weight
- Taking an antidepressant called paroxetine

Treatment for acute lymphocytic leukemia (ALL), brain tumors (especially craniopharyngiomas, and cancers treated with total-body irradiation (TBI) as part of a stem cell transplant increase the risk of obesity in cancer survivors. Radiation therapy to the brain and surgery that damage the hypothalamus or pituitary gland may also increase the risk of obesity.

What late effects are related to the spleen?

Spleen late effects may increase the risk of very serious bacterial infections. Children who have had their spleen removed may need antibiotics to prevent infection. The risk of spleen late effects increases after surgery to remove the spleen, high-dose radiation therapy to the spleen, stem cell transplant, and graft-versus-host disease during or after treatment.

What late effects are related to the bones?

Bone and joint late effects may include the following:

- Swelling over a bone or bony part of the body

- Pain in a bone or joint

- Redness or warmth over a bone or joint

- Joint stiffness or trouble moving normally

- A bone that breaks for no known reason or breaks easily

- Short stature (being shorter than normal)

- One side of the body looks higher than the other side or the body tilts to one side

- Always sitting or standing in a slouching position or having the appearance of a hunched back

Treatment for acute lymphoblastic leukemia (ALL), bone cancer, brain and spinal cord tumors, osteosarcoma, retinoblastoma, soft tissue sarcoma, Wilms tumor, and cancers treated with a stem cell transplant increase the risk of bone and joint late effects, as do surgery, chemotherapy, and radiation therapy. Risk may be increased in childhood cancer survivors who receive anticancer therapy that includes methotrexate or corticosteroids or glucocorticoids such as dexamethasone.

What late effects are related to the reproductive system?

Testicles: Testicular late effects may cause infertility or a low sperm count. Low sperm counts may be temporary or permanent. This depends on the radiation dose and schedule, the area of the body treated, and the age when treated.

The risk of testicular late effects may be increased in childhood cancer survivors who receive surgery, such as the removal of a testicle, part of the prostate, or lymph nodes in the abdomen. Chemotherapy with alkylating agents, such as cyclophosphamide, procarbazine, and ifosfamide, radiation therapy to the abdomen or pelvis, and total-body irradiation (TBI) before a stem cell transplant may also increase risk.

Treatment for acute lymphoblastic leukemia (ALL), Hodgkin lymphoma, osteosarcoma, sarcoma, testicular cancer, and Wilms tumor may cause testicular late effects.

Ovaries: Ovarian late effects may include early menopause, changes in menstrual periods, infertility, and puberty that does not begin. The risk may be increased in childhood cancer survivors who were treated with both an alkylating agent and radiation therapy to the abdomen.

Ovarian late effects may be caused by treatment for Hodgkin lymphoma.

Chemotherapy with alkylating agents, such as cyclophosphamide, mechlorethamine, cisplatin, ifosfamide, lomustine, and especially procarbazine may increase risk, along with radiation therapy to the abdomen or pelvis. In survivors who had radiation to the abdomen, damage to the ovaries depends on the radiation dose, age at the time of treatment, and whether all or part of the abdomen received radiation.

In survivors who had total-body irradiation (TBI) before a stem cell transplant, the damage to the ovaries is greatest in those who had not reached puberty at the time of treatment. The risk may also be greater in survivors who were age 13 to 20 years at the time of treatment.

Fertility And Reproduction: Childhood cancer survivors may have late effects that affect pregnancy including increased risk of high blood pressure, miscarriage or stillbirth, low birthweight babies, early labor and/or delivery, delivery by Cesarean section, and abnormal position of the fetus.

In boys, the risk of infertility increases with radiation therapy to the testicles. In girls, it increases with radiation therapy to the pelvis, including the ovaries and uterus.

Methods that may be used to help childhood cancer survivors have children include the following:

- Freezing the eggs or sperm before cancer treatment in patients who have reached puberty

- Testicular sperm extraction (the removal of a small amount of tissue containing sperm from the testicle

- Intracytoplasmic sperm injection (an egg is fertilized with one sperm that is injected into the egg outside the body)

- In vitro fertilization (IVF) (eggs and sperm are placed together in a container, giving the sperm the chance to enter an egg)

What late effects are related to the lungs?

These symptoms may be caused by lung late effects:

- Dyspnea (shortness of breath), especially when being active

- Wheezing when you breathe

- Dry cough

- Radiation pneumonitis (inflamed lung caused by radiation therapy)

- Pulmonary fibrosis (the build-up of scar tissue in the lung)

Lung late effects are more likely to occur after treatment for Hodgkin lymphoma, Wilms tumor, or cancers treated with total-body irradiation (TBI) or certain chemotherapy drugs before a stem cell transplant.

The risk of health problems that affect the lungs increases after treatment with the following:

- Surgery to remove all or part of the lung

- Certain chemotherapy drugs, such as bleomycin, busulfan, lomustine, dactinomycin, or doxorubicin

- Radiation therapy to the chest

- Total-body irradiation (TBI) or certain chemotherapy drugs before a stem cell transplant

The risk of lung late effects may be increased in childhood cancer survivors who had infections or graft-versus-host disease after a stem cell transplant, lung disease, such as asthma, before cancer treatment, and cigarette smoking.

What late effects are related to the senses?

Ears: Hearing loss is the most common sign of hearing late effects in childhood cancer survivors. The risk of may be increased after treatment with either of the following:

- Certain chemotherapy drugs, such as cisplatin or high-dose carboplatin

- Radiation therapy to the brain

- Risk may also be increased in childhood cancer survivors who were young at the time of treatment (the younger the child, the greater the risk) or received radiation therapy to the brain and chemotherapy at the same time

Treatment for brain tumor, head and neck cancers, neuroblastoma, retinoblastoma, other childhood cancers may cause hearing late effects.

Eyes: Eye late effects may include the following:

- Having a small eye socket that affects the shape of the child's face as it grows

- Loss of vision

- Vision problems, such as cataracts or glaucoma

- Not being able to make tears

- Damage to the optic nerve and retina

- Eyelid tumors

The risk of eye problems or vision loss may be increased in childhood cancer survivors after treatment with any of the following:

- Therapy to the brain, eye, or eye socket

- Surgery to remove the eye

- Total-body irradiation (TBI) as part of a stem cell transplant

- Certain chemotherapy drugs, such as busulfan

- Corticosteroids

- Stem cell transplant and a history of chronic graft-versus-host disease

Treatment for retinoblastoma, rhabdomyosarcoma, and other tumors of the eye, brain tumors, and head and neck cancers may cause eye and vision late effects.

What late effects are related to the kidneys?

Kidney late effects in childhood cancer survivors may include the following:

- Damage to the parts of the kidney that filter and clean the blood

- Damage to the parts of the kidney that remove extra water from the blood

- Loss of electrolytes, such as magnesium, calcium, or potassium, from the body

- Hypertension (high blood pressure)

The following may also increase the risk of kidney late effects:

- Having cancer in both kidneys

- Age at the time of treatment. Older children treated with cisplatin and carboplatin are at greater risk. Younger children (5 years and younger) treated with ifosfamide are at greater risk.

- Having a genetic syndrome that increases the risk of kidney problems, such as Denys-Drash syndrome or WAGR syndrome

- Having an abnormal genitourinary system (in men)

Risk may also increase after treatment with the chemotherapy drugs including cisplatin, carboplatin, ifosfamide and methotrexate, radiation therapy to the middle of the back, surgery to remove part or all of a kidney, or stem cell transplant.

What late effects are related to second cancers?

Childhood cancer survivors have an increased risk of a second cancer later in life.

A different primary cancer that occurs at least two months after cancer treatment ends is called a second cancer. A second cancer may occur months or years after treatment is completed. The type of second cancer that occurs depends in part on the original type of cancer and the cancer treatment.

Patients who have been treated for cancer need regular screening tests to check for a second cancer. It is important for patients who have been treated for cancer to be checked for a second cancer before symptoms appear. This is called screening for a second cancer and may help find a second cancer at an early stage. When abnormal tissue or cancer is found early, it may be easier to treat. By the time symptoms appear, cancer may have begun to spread.

It is important to remember that your doctor does not necessarily think you have cancer if he or she suggests a screening test. Screening tests are given when you have no cancer symptoms.

Healthy Habits

Good health habits are important for survivors of childhood cancer.

The quality of life enjoyed by cancer survivors may be improved by behaviors that promote health and well-being. These include a healthy diet, exercise, and regular medical and dental checkups. These self-care behaviors are especially important for cancer survivors because of their risk of treatment-related health problems. Healthy behaviors may make late effects less severe and lower the risk of other diseases.

Avoiding behaviors that are damaging to health is also important. Smoking, excess alcohol use, illegal drug use, sun exposure, or not being physically active may worsen treatment-related organ damage and possibly increase the risk of second cancers.

Chapter 47

Can I Have Children After Cancer Treatment?

You may be thinking, "Someday, I'd like to be a parent. How will my cancer treatment affect my ability to have children?"

Chemotherapy, radiation, and other treatments can be very effective at doing their job. But what makes them good at fighting cancer or other illnesses also can cause side effects: As these treatments attack harmful cells, they may affect some healthy cells too.

Your doctor has probably talked about whether you'll have any side effects from your cancer treatment. Side effects like reduced fertility all depend on your diagnosis, the type of treatment you're getting, and the doses of medications or radiation. Everyone is different, so it's best to bring any questions or worries up with your medical team.

Which Treatments Can Affect Fertility?

Your doctor can tell you if there's a chance that cancer treatment might affect your reproductive organs. It helps to be aware of what might happen so you can deal with the possibilities, both physically and emotionally.

Here's how some cancer treatments can affect fertility:

About This Chapter: "Can I Have Children After Cancer Treatment?" May 2012, reprinted with permission from www.kidshealth.org. This information was provided by KidsHealth®, one of the largest resources online for medically reviewed health information written for parents, kids, and teens. For more articles like this, visit www.KidsHealth.org, or www.TeensHealth.org. Copyright © 1995-2013 The Nemours Foundation. All rights reserved.

Chemotherapy

Some chemotherapy drugs are more likely to lead to infertility than others. Cytoxan (known generically as cyclophosphamide) is part of a group of chemo drugs called alkylating agents. These are more likely to affect the reproductive organs when given at higher doses.

Other chemotherapy drugs and combinations of drugs also may affect your fertility. Because there are so many different chemotherapy drugs, it's best to ask your doctor or nurse if the drugs you are taking put you at risk for fertility problems.

Sometimes, medications are used to put the gonads "to rest" during chemotherapy, so that they may be less likely to be damaged during treatment.

Radiation Treatments

Radiation treatments also can damage sperm and eggs, whether they are aimed directly or scattered. If radiation is focused on or near the pelvic area, it can damage a girl's ovaries or reduce sperm count in guys. These changes may gradually go away after treatment is stopped, but can be permanent.

Depending on the type and target area of treatment, it may be possible to shield the testes or ovaries from damage, or even move the ovaries out of the path of radiation (this is called transposition).

Some cancer treatments involve radiation to the head as a way to kill cancer cells that may be in the central nervous system. Sometimes this can injure the parts of the brain (and the pituitary gland) that make hormones that control puberty and the menstrual cycle. If that happens, doctors can give these hormones to a patient so he or she can have normal pubertal development, sexual function, and fertility.

Surgery

For patients who need surgery for cancer, doctors may sometimes need to remove part of the reproductive organs. It all depends on where the cancer is.

Getting The Facts

Start by asking your doc lots of questions. Don't hesitate to raise any concerns. Above all, don't worry that fertility isn't a topic for your doctor. It may seem like your doc is focused only on getting rid of the cancer. But getting better is about more than just killing cancer cells. Your future quality of life is part of the healing process.

> ## Three Questions To Ask Your Doctor About Fertility
>
> 1. Is this treatment likely to affect my fertility?
> 2. Can doctors do something to protect my fertility during treatment?
> 3. After treatment, how will I know if my fertility has been affected?

Ask your doctor about all your options. Then come up with a plan together. If you don't feel comfortable talking to your doctor about fertility, find someone on your medical team—like a nurse or social worker—to talk to instead.

Options For Preserving Fertility

In some cases, it may be possible to preserve (or "bank") some of your sperm or eggs. The technical term for this process is cryopreservation, and it happens in a special facility that can freeze and save sperm, eggs, or ovarian tissue. When you're ready to have children, your sperm or eggs can be unfrozen and used to try to have a baby.

For males, sperm banking has been around for a long time and is a pretty common procedure, although not all hospitals offer it. You may have to go to a clinic that specializes in sperm banking.

For younger teens and boys, a more experimental procedure called sperm aspiration may be possible. This process removes immature sperm cells for later use in in vitro fertilization (which means that the sperm is used to fertilize the egg outside of the woman's uterus and the fertilized embryo is then transferred to uterus). Talk to your doctor about your options.

For females, it's a little trickier. Doctors can attempt to freeze eggs or ovarian tissue, but many of the techniques are still experimental and not all hospitals or clinics have access to the technology. Ask your doctor about the options available for you.

In some situations, your doctor may tell you that it isn't a good idea to bank your sperm or eggs, because using them later could put you at risk of re-introducing cancer cells into your body.

Dealing With Feelings

Build A Positive Self-Image: It's normal for people—even adults—to be afraid of the side effects that go with cancer treatment. Such feelings can be particularly difficult for teens. Coping with the side effects of cancer treatment at a time when you're developing your own identity can make everything seem even more complicated.

Sexuality is an important part of a person's identity (even if you're not yet ready to have sex). But sexuality has little to do with fertility. People who can't have kids are just as feminine or masculine as people who can. And fertility has nothing to do with a person's ability to give and receive love. In fact, some cancer survivors develop qualities that may make them more attractive to others, like a greater passion for life and the desire to make the most of their experiences.

Find Support: You're not alone. Other teens have gone through what you're feeling now, and you can connect and share experiences through online networks and cancer blogs. It also may help to find a support group or counselor who can help you work through the feelings you're bound to have during your treatment.

Stay Positive: Many people who were told that cancer treatments could lead to infertility have gone on to have children. Others go on to become parents through adoption or other methods. By thinking about the many different options for parenthood, you can be realistic and positive at the same time. Planning for the future helps you heal. And, if you are having sex, you'll still need to use condoms to protect against HIV and other sexually transmitted diseases (STDs).

Right now, you're focused on recovering—and on the treatments that can save your life. But it's also natural to think about your future. Talk to your health care team, parents, and friends about your options, your plans, and your feelings.

Note-Taking: Not Just For School

By now, you're probably used to taking a notepad and pen to each visit with your medical team, so you don't forget important information about your treatment. But it also helps to take your notebook to meetings with counselors or support groups so you can keep track of ideas and tips for the rest of your life.

Part Five
When A Loved One Has Cancer

Chapter 48

When Your Parent Has Cancer

You've Just Learned That Your Parent Has Cancer

You've just learned that one of the most important people in your life has cancer. Do you feel shocked, numb, angry, or afraid? Do you feel like life is unfair? One thing is certain—you don't feel good. For now, try to focus on these facts:

- **Many people survive cancer:** There are about 12 million cancer survivors living in the United States today. That's because scientists are discovering new and better ways to find and treat cancer. During this really tough time, it will help you to have hope.

- **You're not alone:** Right now it might seem that no one else in the world feels the way you do. In a way you're right. No one can feel exactly like you do. But it might help to know that many teens have a parent who has cancer. Talking to others may help you sort out your feelings. Remember, you are not alone.

- **You're not to blame:** Cancer is a disease with various causes, many of which doctors don't fully understand. None of these causes has anything to do with what you've done, thought, or said.

- **Balance is important:** Many teens feel like their parent's cancer is always on their mind. Others try to avoid it. Try to strike a balance. You can be concerned about your parent and still stay connected with people and activities that you care about.

- **Knowledge is power:** It can help to learn more about cancer and cancer treatments. Sometimes what you imagine is actually worse than the reality.

About This Chapter: Excerpted from "When Your Parent Has Cancer: A Guide For Teens," National Cancer Institute (NCI), February 2012.

Your Feelings

As you deal with your parent's cancer, you'll probably feel all kinds of things. Many other teens who have a parent with cancer have felt the same way you do now. Some of these emotions are listed below. Think about people you can talk with about your feelings.

Feelings You May Have

Scared

- My world is falling apart.
- I'm afraid that my parent might die.
- I'm afraid that someone else in my family might catch cancer. (They can't.)
- I'm afraid that something might happen to my parent at home, and I won't know what to do.

It's normal to feel scared when your parent has cancer. Some of your fears may be real. Others may be based on things that won't happen. And some fears may lessen over time.

Guilty

- I feel guilty because I'm healthy and my parent is sick.
- I feel guilty when I laugh and have fun.

You may feel bad about having fun when your parent is sick. However, having fun doesn't mean that you care any less. In fact, it will probably help your parent to see you doing things you enjoy.

Remember!

- Nothing you did, thought, or said caused your parent to get cancer.
- You can't catch cancer from another person.
- Scientists are discovering new and better ways to find and treat cancer.
- Many people survive cancer.

Angry

- I am mad that my mom or dad got sick.

- I am upset at the doctors.

- I am angry at God for letting this happen.

- I am angry at myself for feeling the way I do.

Anger often covers up other feelings that are harder to show. Try not to let your anger build up.

Neglected

- I feel left out.

- I don't get any attention.

- No one ever tells me what's going on.

- My family never talks anymore.

When a parent has cancer, it's common for the family's focus to change. Some people in the family may feel left out. Your parent with cancer may be using his or her energy to get better. Your well parent may be focused on helping your parent with cancer. Your parents don't mean for you to feel left out. It just happens because so much is going on.

Lonely

- No one understands what I'm going through.

- My friends don't come over anymore.

- My friends don't seem to know what to say to me anymore.

For now, try to remember that these feelings won't last forever.

Embarrassed

- I'm sometimes embarrassed to be out in public with my sick parent.

- I don't know how to answer people's questions.

Many teens who feel embarrassed about having a parent with cancer say it gets easier to deal with over time. What you're feeling is normal There is no one "right" way to feel. And you're not alone—many other teens in your situation have felt the same way. Some have said that having a parent with cancer changes the way they look at things in life. Some even said that it made them stronger.

Dealing With Your Feelings

A lot of people are uncomfortable sharing their feelings. They ignore them and hope they'll go away. Other people choose to act cheerful when they're really not. They think that by acting upbeat they won't feel sad or angry anymore. This may help for a little while, but not over the long run. Actually, holding your feelings inside can keep you from getting the help you need.

Try these tips:

- Talk with family and friends who you feel close to. You owe it to yourself.

- Write down your thoughts in a journal.

- Join a support group to talk with other teens who are facing some of the same things you are. Or meet with a counselor.

It is probably hard to imagine right now, but, if you let yourself, you can grow stronger as a person through this experience.

Does this sound like you?

Many kids think that they need to protect their parents by not making them worry. They think that they have to be perfect and not cause any trouble because one of their parents is sick. If you feel this way, remember that no one can be perfect all the time. You need time to vent, to feel sad, and to be happy. Try to let your parents know how you feel—even if you have to start the conversation.

During Treatment

In addition to getting one or more cancer treatments, your parent will also get tests to find out how well the cancer is responding to treatment.

Things To Look For

Some treatments may make your parent more likely to get an infection. This happens because cancer treatment can affect the white blood cells, which are the cells that fight infection. An infection can make your mom or dad sicker. So your parent may need to stay away from crowded places or people who have an illness that he or she could catch (such as a cold, the flu, or chicken pox).

You may need to:

- Wash your hands often with soap and water, or use a hand sanitizer, to keep from spreading germs.

- Avoid bringing home friends who are sick or have a cold.

- Stay away from your parent if you are sick or have a fever.

Talk with your parent if you aren't sure what to do.

The Waiting

It's hard to wait to see whether the treatment will work. Your parent's doctor may try one treatment, then another. One day your parent may feel a lot better. The next day or week he or she may feel sick again. Treatment can go on for months or sometimes years. This emotional roller coaster is hard on everyone.

Who Can Answer My Questions?

Ask your parent or other trusted adults any questions that you have. Ask your dad or mom if it is okay to go with them to their appointment.

Perhaps your parent can arrange for you to talk with their doctor, nurse, or social worker to learn more. It will help to bring a list of questions with you.

When you talk with them, don't hesitate to:

- Ask what new words mean. Ask for information to be explained in another way, if what the doctor says is confusing.

- Ask to see a model or a picture of what the doctor is talking about. Ask what videos or podcasts you can watch to learn more.

- Ask about support groups for young people that meet online or in your community.

Want to visit?

If your parent is in the hospital, you may be nervous about visiting. Learn ahead of time how your parent is doing and what to expect. Remember that they are still the same person, even though they are sick. Don't be afraid to ask your parent questions and share your thoughts. You can also call, write, and e-mail them.

What Your Parent May Be Feeling

Knowing what your parent may be feeling could help you figure out how to help, or at least to understand where he or she is coming from. You may be surprised to learn that they are feeling a lot of the same things you are:

- **Sad Or Depressed:** People with cancer sometimes can't do things they used to do. They may miss these activities and their friends. Feeling sad or down can range from a mild case of the blues to depression, which a doctor can treat.

- **Afraid:** Your parent may be afraid of how cancer will change his or her life and the lives of family members. He or she may be scared about treatment. Your parent may even be scared that he or she will die.

- **Anxious:** Your parent may be worried about a lot of things. Your mom or dad may feel stressed about going to work or paying the bills. Or he or she may be concerned about looking different because of treatment. And your mom or dad is probably very concerned about how you are doing. All these worries may upset your parent.

- **Angry:** Cancer treatment and its side effects can be difficult to go through. Anger sometimes comes from feelings that are hard to show, such as fear or frustration. Chances are your parent is angry at the disease, not at you.

- **Lonely:** People with cancer often feel lonely or distant from others. They may find that their friends have a hard time dealing with their cancer and may not visit. They may be too sick to take part in activities they used to enjoy. They may feel that no one understands what they're going through.

- **Hopeful:** There are many reasons for your parent to feel hopeful. Millions of people who have had cancer are alive today. People with cancer can lead active lives, even during treatment. Your parent's chances of surviving cancer are better today than ever before.

All these feelings are normal for people living with cancer. You might want to share this list with your mom or dad.

Changes In Your Family

Changing Routines And Responsibilities

Whatever your family situation, chances are that things have changed since your parent got sick.

> **Does this sound like your home?**
> - Are you doing more chores?
> - Are you spending more time with relatives or friends?
> - Are you home alone more?
> - Are you asked to help make dinner or do the laundry?
> - Are you looking after younger brothers or sisters more?
> - Do you want to just hang out with your friends when you are needed at home?

Let your parents know if you feel that there is more to do than you can handle. Together, you can work it out.

Touching Base When Things Are Changing

Families say that it helps to make time to talk together, even if it's only for a short time each week. Talking can help your family stay connected.

Here are some things to consider when talking with different family members:

Brothers And Sisters

If you are the oldest child, your brothers or sisters may look to you for support. Help them as much as you can. It's okay to let them know that you're having a tough time, too.

If you are looking to your older brother or sister for help, tell them how you are feeling. They can help, but won't have all the answers. Try saying something like the following:

- "I'm doing the best job I can."
- "How can we work together to get through this?"
- "I know, it's tough for me too."

Your Parent Who Is Well

Expect your parent to feel some stress, just as you do. Your parent may snap at you. He or she may not always do or say the right thing. Lend a hand when you can. Try saying something like the following:

- "How are you doing?"
- "Is there anything I can do to help you out?"

Your Parent With Cancer

Your mom or dad may be sick from the treatment or just very tired. Or maybe your parent will feel okay and want your company. Try talking if your mom or dad feels up to it. Let your parent know how much you love them. Try saying something like this:

- "I love you."

- "Can I get you anything?"

- "Am I doing the right thing?"

- "How about some company?"

Keeping Family And Friends In The Loop

Is it getting to be too much to answer the phone and tell people how your mom or dad is doing? That can be a lot for anyone. Ask others to help you share news of how your parent is doing and what help your family needs. Maybe a relative or family friend can be the contact person. Some families use telephone chains. Others use e-mail, a blog, or a social media site.

Growing Stronger As A Family

Some families can grow apart for a while when a parent has cancer. But there are ways to help your family grow stronger and closer. Teens who saw their families grow closer say that it happened because people in their family did the following:

- **Tried** to put themselves in the other person's shoes and thought about how they would feel if they were the other person.

- **Understood** that even though people reacted differently to situations, they were all hurting. Some cried a lot. Others showed little emotion. Some used humor to get by.

- **Learned** to respect and talk about differences. The more they asked about how others were feeling, the more they could help each other.

Asking Others For Help

You and your family may need support from others. It can be hard to ask. Yet most of the time people really want to help you and your family.

People who your mom, dad, or you may ask for help include:

- Aunts, uncles, and grandparents

- Family friends

- Neighbors

- Teachers or coaches

- School nurses or guidance counselors

- People from your religious community

- Your friends or their parents

Your Relationship With Your Parents

Your mom or dad may ask you to take on more responsibility than other kids your age. You might resent it at first. Then again, you may learn a lot from the experience and grow to appreciate the trust your parents have in you.

Taking Care Of Yourself

It's important to "stay fit"—both inside and out. Here are some tips to help you keep on track during this experience.

Dealing With Stress

Stress can make you forgetful, frustrated, and more likely to catch a cold or the flu. Here are some tips that have helped other teens manage stress. Do one or two of these things each week to take care of your mind and body.

Stay Connected

- Spend some time at a friend's house.

- Stay involved with sports or clubs.

Relax And Get Enough Sleep

- Take breaks. You'll have more energy and be in a better frame of mind.

- Get at least eight hours of sleep each night.

- Pray or meditate.

- Make or listen to music.

How can people help your family?

- Go grocery shopping or run errands
- Make meals
- Mow the lawn
- Do chores around the house
- Keep your parent company
- Give rides to school, practice, or appointments
- Help with homework
- Invite you over for a meal or a day trip
- Talk with and listen to you

Help Others

- Join a walk against cancer.
- Plan a bake sale or other charity event to raise money to fight cancer.

Avoid Risky Behaviors

- Stay away from smoking, drinking, and taking drugs.

Put Your Creative Side To Work

- Keep a journal to write down your thoughts and experiences.
- Draw, paint, or take photographs.
- Read biographies to learn what helped others make it through challenging times.

Eat And Drink Well

- Drink plenty of water each day.
- In the evening, switch to caffeine-free drinks that won't keep you awake.
- Grab fresh fruit, whole-grain breads, and lean meats like chicken or turkey when you have a choice.
- Avoid sugary foods.

How You Can Help Your Parent

- Spend time with your parent. Watch a movie together. Read the paper to your parent. Ask for help with your homework. Give hugs. Say, "I love you." Or just hang out in silence.

- Lend a hand. Bring water or offer to make a snack or small meal.

- Try to be upbeat, but be "real," too. Being positive can be good for you and your whole family. But don't feel like you always have to act cheerful, especially if it's not how you really feel. It's okay to share your thoughts with your parent—and let them comfort you. Be yourself.

Get Help When You Feel Down And Out

Many teens feel low or down when their parent is sick. It's normal to feel sad or "blue" during difficult times. However, if these feelings last for two weeks or more and start to interfere with things you used to enjoy, you may be depressed. **The good news is that there is hope and there is help**. Often, talking with a counselor can help. Below are some signs that you may need to see a counselor.

Are you:

- Feeling helpless and hopeless? Thinking that life has no meaning?
- Losing interest in being with family or friends?
- Finding that everything or everyone seems to get on your nerves?
- Feeling really angry a lot of the time?
- Thinking of hurting yourself?

Do you find that you are:

- Losing interest in the activities you used to enjoy?
- Eating too little or a lot more than usual?
- Crying easily or many times each day?
- Using drugs or alcohol to help you forget?
- Sleeping more than you used to? Less than you used to?
- Feeling tired a lot?

If you answered "yes" to any of these questions, it's important to talk to someone you trust.

- Be patient. You are all under stress. If you find you are losing your cool, listen to music, read, or go outside to shoot hoops or go for a run.

- Share a laugh. You've probably heard that laughter is good medicine. Watch a comedy on TV with your parent or tell jokes if that's your thing. Also, remember that you're not responsible for making everyone happy. You can only do so much.

- Buy your parent a new scarf or hat. Your parent might enjoy a new hat or scarf if he or she has lost their hair during treatment.

- Keep your parent in the loop. Tell your parent what you did today. Try to share what is going on in your life. Ask your parent how his or her day was.

- Talk about family history. Ask your parent about the past. Look through pictures or photo albums. Talk about what you're both most proud of, your best memories, and how you both have met challenges. Write, or make drawings, about what you and your parent share with each other.

- Keep a journal together. Write thoughts or poems, draw, or put photos in a notebook that the two of you share. This can help you share your feelings when it might be hard to speak them aloud.

What if treatment doesn't help?

If treatment doesn't help your parent, you and your family will face even more challenges. Hearing that your parent might die is very difficult. You may feel many of the same emotions you felt when you first learned that your mom or dad had cancer. No book can give you all the answers or tell you exactly how you will feel. But when the future is so uncertain, teens say of these actions may help:

- Make the most of the time you have. Do special things as a family. At home, make time for your mom or dad. Call and visit as much as you can if your parent is in the hospital. Write notes and draw pictures. Say "I love you" often. If possible, try to have some special times together. If you have not gotten along in the past, you may want to let your parent know you love him or her.

- Stay on track. When people get bad news, they often feel like they're living outside of themselves—that life is moving along without them. That's why it's important to keep a schedule. Get up at the same time each day. Go to school. Meet with friends.

- Get help when you feel alone. Make sure you find people who can help you. In addition to your family, it may help to talk to a social worker, counselor, or people in a support group.

- Help with younger brothers and sisters. Play with your brothers and sisters to give your parent a break. Pull out games or read a book with your siblings. This will help you stay close and also give your parent time to rest.

After Treatment

When your parent is finally done with treatment, you may feel a whole range of emotions. Part of you is glad it is over. Another part of you may miss the freedom or new responsibilities you had while your parent was getting treatment. You may feel confused that your parent still looks sick and is weaker than you expected. You may be afraid the cancer will come back. You may look at life differently now. All these feelings are normal. If you and your family are still feeling that life after treatment is harder than you thought it might be, you might want to talk to a counselor to get guidance through this time.

Chapter 49

When Your Brother
Or Sister Is Seriously Ill

Siblings can be many things: friends, allies, role models—and let's face it, sometimes they can just be annoying.

But when your sibling has a serious illness, it adds another dimension to your relationship—and to your life. You may find yourself juggling some pretty intense and confusing emotions. You're not alone in feeling this way, and it's important to take care of yourself during this stressful time.

"How Could I Be Feeling This?"

The teen years are a time of growing independence and changing relationships with parents. Having a sibling with a serious illness adds even more loops and layers to the emotional roller coaster.

At times, you may feel worried about your sibling and about your parents and other caregivers. At other times, you'll probably feel angry, jealous, stressed out, or abandoned—and you may feel guilty about having these emotions, even though they're perfectly natural.

If your sibling's illness or treatments have obvious side effects like hair loss or behavioral changes, you may even be embarrassed about the way he/she looks or acts.

These emotions (and the many others you'll feel) are perfectly natural. They don't make you a terrible brother, sister, or person—just a normal human being.

About This Chapter: "When A Sibling Is Seriously Ill," April 2012, reprinted with permission from www.kidshealth .org. This information was provided by KidsHealth®, one of the largest resources online for medically reviewed health information written for parents, kids, and teens. For more articles like this, visit www.KidsHealth.org, or www.TeensHealth.org. Copyright © 1995-2013 The Nemours Foundation. All rights reserved.

What You Can Do

Find Support: If you find yourself getting swept away by negative feelings, try to be understanding of yourself and what you are going through. Accept that your feelings are natural and see if you can find support to help you avoid taking your fears and feelings out on yourself or your family. (And if you do slip up and lose your temper, forgive yourself, apologize, and move on. Everyone has trouble making sense of emotions sometimes, even adults.)

Talk to a parent or an adult you trust, and consider joining a support group—many hospitals and medical facilities have sibling support groups.

Write It Out: Try keeping a journal of your feelings and thoughts, or compose songs or poetry about how you feel. Let yourself be totally honest and don't judge yourself for what you feel. If you are not much for handwriting, you can always create a password-protected document or (if you're not a writer at all), use art or karate or some other form of self-expression. Think of it as a safe way to vent and work through your feelings and release anger and stress safely.

Take Time For Yourself: Don't forget to take time for yourself to have fun, relax, and spend time with people who care about you. It's great to help the family—they really need you right now. But you don't need to be on call 24/7. Be sure to make time for yourself too.

Common Reactions To A Sibling's Illness

Here are some of the strong, sometimes conflicting, reactions most teens have to a sibling's illness:

- Worry that a sister or brother will die or become permanently disabled
- Fear of "catching" the sibling's disease
- Guilt about being healthy and able to enjoy activities that your brother or sister can't
- Worry about not being able to go on vacation or play on a travel team
- Anger because parents are devoting most of their time and energy to your sibling
- Worry that no one in the family cares about you or feeling neglected because family members spend so much time focused on the sibling who is ill
- Resentment when your brother or sister doesn't have to help out or do chores
- Resentment that the family has less money to spend because the sibling is sick
- Wishing that things could be the way they were before the illness
- Guilt about being mean to the sibling in the past
- General worry or anxiety about an uncertain future

Helping Your Family—And Yourself

Because of your age, you can be a big help to your family—you can cook, do household chores, run errands, babysit, and help out in ways little kids can't. Doing these things can help you feel good about yourself: you can really make a difference. In fact, many teens whose siblings battled a serious illness say they emerged feeling stronger for it.

Taking an active role as a caretaker can be character-building. It can help you gain maturity, self-esteem, an increased awareness of and empathy for others in similar situations, and make you feel closer to your family.

Being able to help also lets you feel more in control when things get crazy. But being able to help can have downsides if you feel like parents depend on you too much or take your help for granted.

Sometimes the expectations get too great and your family responsibilities start to get in the way of your well-being or schoolwork. That's when it's time to speak up so you don't get trapped in a cycle of resentment and guilt. If you're not ready to talk directly to your parents, talk to the social worker at the hospital, your school counselor, the parent of a friend, or your coach.

If you start to feel overwhelmed by everything you're expected to do (or the things you think you should do), talk to your parents and try to let them know what you're feeling. Tell them you want to help, but you're worried about school and other responsibilities. Work together to find ways to compromise so you can still help out but also stay connected to friends, sports, and other activities that are important to you. If you can't talk to your parents, talk to a trusted adult about what you can do.

It can help to remember that, even if parents and siblings are too busy and stressed to acknowledge it right now, your help and support mean a lot to them.

Other Ways To Cope

Even if you feel OK, any family living with a child with an illness is under stress. Here are some ways to help you cope:

Stay Informed: Knowing the facts about your sibling's illness and what your brother or sister is going through can help you avoid unnecessary fears. It can also help you get a handle on what's happening. Ask questions of your sibling, parents, and the medical staff. Your parents might not be sure about how much they can open up to you, so help them understand that you want to hear and be heard.

It's common to be concerned about catching a disease. Most childhood illnesses like cancer, sickle cell disease, diabetes, epilepsy, and kidney disease are not contagious. If you are concerned about carrying a genetic risk for an illness, ask your parents if you can talk to a genetics specialist.

Designate A "Go-To" Adult: Find an adult (maybe a teacher, aunt, or uncle) to lean on for support and advice when you need something and your parents aren't available. Even though you're no longer a kid, everyone needs someone to turn to. Having an adult to talk to can help you process what you're experiencing.

Stay Positive: Remember, just like your sibling, you deserve time to relax, have fun, and be silly. So spend time with people who care about you and do things that are relaxing and fun. Sometimes, just hanging out with your brother or sister and watching a movie or playing a board game can make you feel OK again. Do what you need to do to take care of yourself both inside and outside your family.

Chapter 50

How Can I Help If My Friend Has Cancer?

Your friend has been diagnosed with cancer but you're the one freaking out: What can I do? How should I act? Is it OK to talk about it? What's "normal" now?

It's hard to know how to respond when someone you love—someone your own age—is diagnosed with cancer. It can be frightening, confusing, and may bring on some heavy thoughts about life and death. You might even struggle with the temptation to pull back from your friendship so you can avoid the uncomfortable feelings you have. But your friend needs you now more than ever. So what should you do?

It's normal to have to difficult feelings; don't try to brush them off. Try to think a bit about what you're feeling. You'll expect to feel sadness, of course, and fear, and maybe anger. But it's also natural to feel some surprising emotions like disappointment or embarrassment.

Of course you don't want to burden your friend with your feelings. But you need support, too. So try to find someone you can turn to—like a parent or school counselor. Once you have a way of dealing with your own feelings, it will be easier not to let your emotions or fears get in the way of being a good friend.

Here are some ways you can help.

About This Chapter: "My Friend Has Cancer. How Can I Help?" November 2011, reprinted with permission from www.kidshealth.org. This information was provided by KidsHealth®, one of the largest resources online for medically reviewed health information written for parents, kids, and teens. For more articles like this, visit www.KidsHealth.org, or www.TeensHealth.org. Copyright © 1995-2013 The Nemours Foundation. All rights reserved.

Be Prepared

You probably know that your friend could lose hair as a side effect of cancer treatment. But you may also notice emotional and physical changes in your friend. Some things that you may see happen include:

Vomiting And Nausea: Try not to be hurt if the double-chocolate brownies you baked with such love sit untouched on the plate. Your friend may not feel like eating—at home or out. In fact, someone with cancer may not feel like going out at all if he or she is worried about throwing up in public. You might want to reassure your friend that you know this is a possibility and that you realize it's a side effect of cancer treatment.

Weakness, Fatigue, And Lack Of Endurance: Cancer treatments can make even the smallest things a big struggle—like walking up stairs or carrying schoolbooks. Your friend may suddenly become too tired to talk on the phone or be unable to walk around the mall. Let your friend take things at his or her own pace, though. Don't automatically assume people with cancer won't want to go out or that they should stay home. Let your friend make the call, but be understanding if the exertion proves too much.

Embarrassment: Your friend may be even more self-conscious about having cancer because he or she can't do what other people do or look the way they look.

But your friend's not the only one who may feel awkward. Be prepared for your own feelings, too: Some people can feel uncomfortable about being seen with a friend who has no hair or looks physically different. We all feel temporary embarrassment at times—who hasn't cringed at something a friend does or wears? The good news is, we get over it.

Difficulty Keeping Up In School: Your friend may fall behind in school. Cancer treatments can sap a lot of energy and teens getting chemotherapy or radiation may struggle academically. People can also feel disconnected and left out of things when they miss school a lot.

Emotional Support

So what can you do to help your friend? Here are some ideas.

Be There: OK, so this is obvious, but it's also critically important. Teens with cancer often feel isolated and alone, especially if they're in the hospital or away from school for long stretches of time. Visit as often as you can. Fight the urge to stay away because you feel awkward or wish this weren't happening. Even if you aren't sure what to say to your friend, just being there to show your support will mean so much. If distance or your schedule makes it hard to be there in person, stay in touch by sending notes and cards and by emailing, IMing, phoning, or texting.

You can also offer to drive other friends to the hospital or set up an email list or an online social network group so your friend can stay connected.

Talk About It—And Listen: Friends going through tough times like to talk about it. Listen, ask questions, and do some basic research on your own so you can understand more about the type of cancer and what your friend might be feeling. Don't be afraid to ask questions of your friend's family, the doctors, and other cancer patients.

Be Patient: People with cancer, understandably, are often sad, anxious, and afraid. On top of that, some treatments have side effects like fatigue or mood swings. If you show up to visit and your friend seems distant, angry, or less than enthused, try not to take it personally. Don't give up; your friend is going through a lot. Come back again tomorrow and chances are things will be better.

Keep It Real—But Keep It Positive: It can help to talk about the future and to make plans in a realistic, compassionate way. Don't shrug off your friend's fears or concerns about death, but do try to offer realistic specific examples of other people—famous people, people you know—who have survived this type of cancer. (No examples come to mind? Do a web search!)

Practical Support

"If there's anything I can do…" is a nice thing to say. But families of teens with cancer often say that the more specific the offer, the better.

Here are a few things you can offer to do:

Be The Point Person: Help your friend's family spend less time updating people by phone or email—offer to relay messages to friends, teachers, and others on a regular basis. Make sure you have the phone numbers and email addresses you need, and then create a list so you can text or email everyone at once when there is news to report.

Go A Little Nutty: Don't be afraid to be silly. Humor can be an excellent distraction, so consider showing up with joke books, Mad Libs (remember those?), Silly String, comedy DVDs, weird little toys—anything you think your friend would like. If your friend is feeling low on energy, which is common during treatment, bring in the fun and turn up the silliness.

Make A Care Package: Talk with your friend's parents about what foods your friend can and can't have—and what foods might be favorites right now (when people are sick, their tastes can change). Or put together some fun, escapist stuff for your friend to do while alone, perhaps fast-read novels or games like Sudoku. Wrap up your package and bring it to the hospital or your friend's home.

Step In With Siblings: If your friend has siblings, spend some time with them. They probably feel a lot of the same things you do, so you might be able to help each other through it.

Help Out With Schoolwork: Offer to help your friend with homework—everything from passing along assignments to tutoring your friend or working together if it's appropriate. Even something as simple as taking really good notes (or asking someone else to do so if your friend is not in your class) can be a huge help.

Create A Blog: Have friends and family members contribute to a blog—or, offline, fill a small notebook—with funny or meaningful stories, quotes, and trivia from your friendship. Be careful not to give it a tone of "these were the last good times," but instead let it be a fun reminder of how much your friend means to everyone and how eager you are for his/her recovery so you can keep making memories! Consider adding pictures and making it look like a celebrity magazine about your friend. Give it as a gift so your friend can read it when feeling down.

Take Care Of Yourself: Your friend's cancer will take a toll on you, too, so try to be aware of your own emotional needs. Consider keeping a journal as well as talking with a trusted adult about the impact this has on you.

Remember!

The bottom line: The most important thing is to be there for your friend, in whatever way feels natural.

Part Six
If You Need More Information

Chapter 51

Additional Reading About Cancer

Books

AfterShock: What to Do When the Doctor Gives You—Or Someone You Love—a Devastating Diagnosis

By Jessie Gruman (Walker & Company, 2007)

American Cancer Society Complete Guide to Nutrition for Cancer Survivors, Second Edition

By Barbara Grant and others (American Cancer Society, 2010)

Cancer Etiquette: What to Say, What to Do When Someone You Know or Love Has Cancer

By Rosanne Kalick (Lion Books, 2005)

Cancer: 50 Essential Things to Do: 2013 Edition

By Greg Anderson (Plume, 2012)

Cancer in the Family: Helping Children Cope with a Parent's Illness

By Sue P. Heiny and others (American Cancer Society, 2001)

Cancer Sourcebook, Sixth Edition

Edited by Karen Bellenir (Omnigraphics, 2011)

About This Chapter: There are a myriad of books and other publications about cancer. The list provided in this chapter was compiled from the recommendations of many sources deemed reliable. It is intended as a starting point for further research. Inclusion does not constitute endorsement and there is no implication associated with omission. Books are listed alphabetically by title.

Cancer Survivorship Sourcebook
Edited by Karen Bellenir (Omnigraphics, 2007)

Cancer Survivor's Companion: Practical Ways to Cope with Your Feelings After Cancer
By Frances Goodhart and Lucy Atkins (Platkus Books, 2013)

Chemotherapy and Radiation for Dummies
By Alan P. Lyss, Humberto Fagundes, and Patricia Corrigan (Wiley 2005)

Chemotherapy Survival Guide: Everything You Need to Know to Get Through Treatment
By Judith McKay and Tammy Schacher (New Harbinger Publications, 2009)

Chicken Soup for the Soul: The Cancer Book: 101 Stories of Courage, Support & Love
By Jack Canfield and others (Chicken Soup for the Soul Publishing, 2009)

Childhood Cancer: A Parent's Guide to Solid Tumor Cancers, Second Edition
By Honna Janes-Hodder and Nancy Keene (Patient Centered Guides, 2002)

Complete Guide to Complementary Therapies in Cancer Care: Essential Information for Patients, Survivors, and Health Professionals
By Barrie R. Cassileth (World Scientific Publishing, 2011)

Everyone's Guide to Cancer Therapy: How Cancer Is Diagnosed, Treated, and Managed Day to Day, Fifth Edition
By Andrew Ko, Ernest Rosenbaum, and Malin Dollinger (Somerville House, 2008)

Everything Changes: The Insider's Guide to Cancer in Your 20s and 30s
By Kairol Rosenthal (Wiley, 2009)

Hope in the Face of Cancer: A Survival Guide for the Journey You Did Not Choose
By Amy Givler (Harvest House, 2003)

Johns Hopkins Patients' Guide to Leukemia
By Candis Morrison and Charles L. Hesdorffer (Jones and Bartlett Learning, 2010)

Last Lecture
By Randy Pausch with Jeffrey Zaslow (Hyperion, 2008)

Perseverance: True Voices of Cancer Survivors
By Carolyn Rubenstein (Forge, 2009)

Publications Available From The NCI

The National Cancer Institute Publications Locator provides free NCI educational and support publications about cancer for patients and their families, health care providers, and the public through its website at https://pubs.cancer.gov/ncipl/annc.aspx.

The following is a brief list of a few of the available general-interest publications available from the NCI:

Chemotherapy and You: Support for People With Cancer
http://www.cancer.gov/cancertopics/coping/chemotherapy-and-you

Dictionary of Cancer Terms
http://www.cancer.gov/dictionary

Eating Hints: Before, During, and After Cancer Treatment
http://www.cancer.gov/cancertopics/coping/eatinghints

NCI Cancer Bulletin
http://www.cancer.gov/ncicancerbulletin/archive

Pain Control: Support for People With Cancer
http://www.cancer.gov/cancertopics/coping/paincontrol

Radiation Therapy and You: Support for People With Cancer
http://www.cancer.gov/cancertopics/coping/radiation-therapy-and-you

Taking Time: Support for People With Cancer
http://www.cancer.gov/cancertopics/takingtime

What You Need To Know About™ Cancer
http://www.cancer.gov/cancertopics/wyntk/cancer

Chapter 52

Web-Based Resources And Support Groups

American Brain Tumor Association

Website: http://www.abta.org

E-mail: info@abta.org

Toll-Free: 800-886-2282

(800-886-ABTA)

Phone: 773-577-8750

Activities: Supports research and offers information to brain tumor patients and their families.

American Cancer Society

Website: http://www.cancer.org

Toll-Free: 800-227-2345

Phone: 404-320-3333

TTY: 866-228-4327

Activities: Provides services and programs for cancer patients and their families, supports research, and offers cancer-related information.

American Institute for Cancer Research

Website: http://www.aicr.org

E-mail: aicrweb@aicr.org

Toll-Free: 800-843-8114

Phone: 202-328-7744

Activities: Provides information about cancer prevention and nutrition concerns.

American Psychosocial Oncology Society

Website: http://www.apos-society.org

E-mail: info@apos-society.org

Toll-Free: 866-276-7443

(866-APOS-4-HELP)

Activities: Works to help people with cancer find counseling services in their own communities.

American Society of Clinical Oncology—Cancer.Net

Website: http://www.cancer.net/coping/
age-specific-information/cancer-teens
E-mail: contactus@cancer.net
Toll-Free: 888-651-3038
Phone: 571-483-1780

Activities: Cancer.Net provides oncologist-approved information on cancer specific to teens.

CancerCare

Website: http://www.cancercare.org
Toll-Free: 8008134673
Phone: 2127128400

Activities: Provides free professional counseling, educational programs, practical help, and financial assistance to people affected by cancer.

Cancer Financial Assistance Coalition

Website: http://www.cancerfac.org
E-mail: contact@cancerfac.org

Activities: Coalition of 14 organizations provides database to help cancer patients and caregivers manage their financial challenges.

Cancer Support Community—Group Loop

Website: http://www.grouploop.org
Toll-Free: 888-793-9355
Phone: 202-659-9709

Activities: Provides online site for teens to find support and education while dealing with a cancer diagnosis.

CaringBridge

Website: http://www.caringbridge.org
Phone: 651-789-2300

Activities: Offers personal websites to help patients and family stay connected to others during illness, treatment, and recovery.

Children's Brain Tumor Foundation

Website: http://www.cbtf.org
E-mail: info@cbtf.org
Toll-Free: 866-228-4673
Phone: 212-448-9494

Activities: Works to improve treatment, quality of life, and long-term outlook for children with brain and spinal cord tumors.

CureSearch

Website: http://www.curesearch.org
E-mail: info@curesearch.org
Toll-Free: 800-458-6223

Activities: Supports research and provides treatment information and support resources to patients, families, and health professionals.

Fertile Hope

Website: http://www.fertilehope.org
Toll-Free: 855-220-7777
(LIVESTRONG Navigation Services)

Activities: Helps patients cope with the risk of infertility associated with cancer treatments.

FORCE: Facing Our Risk of Cancer Empowered

Website: http://www.facingourrisk.org
E-mail: info@facingourrisk.org
Toll-Free/Helpline: 866-288-RISK
(866-288-7475)

Activities: A resource for people affected by hereditary and ovarian cancers.

4th Angel Mentoring Program

Website: http://www.4thangel.org
E-mail: 4thAngel@ccf.org
Toll-Free: 866-520-3197

Activities: Pairs cancer patients or caregivers with trained mentors to provide emotional support.

I'm Too Young for This! Cancer Foundation

Website: http://stupidcancer.org
E-mail: contact@stupidcancer.org
Toll-Free: 877-735-4673

Activities: Raises awareness that cancer affects young adults and works to ensure that they receive age-appropriate resources.

Joe's House

Website: http://www.joeshouse.org
E-mail: info@joeshouse.org
Toll-Free: 877-563-7468
Activities: Helps cancer patients and their families find lodging near treatment centers.

Leukemia & Lymphoma Society

Website: http://www.lls.org
Toll-Free: 800-955-4572
Phone: 914-949-5213
Copay Assistance Program: 877-557-2672

Activities: Supports research to find a cure for blood cancers and works to help patients and their families.

LIVESTRONG Foundation

Website: http://www.livestrong.org
General: 877-236-8820
Cancer Navigation: 855-220-7777

Activities: Offers support and financial assistance to cancer survivors.

Look Good. Feel Better for Teens

Website: http://lookgoodfeelbetter.org/
programs/programs-for-teens
Toll-Free: 800-395-5665
(800-395-LOOK)

Activities: Seeks to meet the appearance-related and social needs of teens (aged 13–17) with cancer, a program of the American Cancer Society.

Lymphoma Foundation of America

Website: http://www.lymphomahelp.org
E-mail: LFA@lymphomahelp.org
Toll-Free: 800-385-1060 (Hotline)
Phone: 734-222-1100

Activities: Offers counseling and support for lymphoma survivors.

Lynch Syndrome International

Website: http://www.lynchcancers.com
E-mail: info@lynchcancers.org
Phone: 707-689-5089

Activities: Provides support for individuals afflicted with the hereditary condition Lynch syndrome.

Max Foundation

Website:
http://www.themaxfoundation.org
Toll-Free: 888-462-9368
Phone: 425-778-8660

Activities: Helps underserved people with rare cancers and blood cancers get access to programs and services.

Melissa's Living Legacy Teen Cancer Foundation

Website: http:teenslivingwithcancer.org
E-mail: info@teenslivingwithcancer.org

Activities: Provides support and information to teens with cancer.

National Bone Marrow Transplant Link

Website: http://www.nbmtlink.org
E-mail: info@nbmtlink.org
Toll-Free: 800-546-5268
Phone: 248-358-1886

Activities: Serves stem cell transplant patients.

National Cancer Institute

Website: http://www.cancer.gov
Toll-Free: 800-422-6237
(800-4-CANCER)
TTY: 800-332-8615

Activities: The federal government's principal agency for cancer research.

National Children's Cancer Society

Website: http://www.thenccs.org
Toll-Free: 800-532-6459
(800-5-FAMILY)
Phone: 314-241-1600

Activities: Works to improve the lives of children with cancer and provides assistance to families.

National Hospice and Palliative Care Organization (NHPCO)

Website: http://www.nhpco.org
E-mail: nhpco_info@nhpco.org
Phone: 703-837-1500

Activities: A professional organization for those who seek to improve care at the end of life.

National Patient Travel Center

Website: http://www.patienttravel.org
Email:
info@nationalpatienttravelcenter.org
Toll-Free: 800-296-1217

Activities: Helps patients find medical air transportation.

Patient Advocate Foundation

Website: http://www.patientadvocate.org
Email: help@patientadvocate.org
Toll-Free: 800-532-5274

Activities: Provides professional case management services to help patients maintain their financial stability and safeguard their access to health care, insurance, and employment.

Prevent Cancer Foundation

Website: http://preventcancer.org
E-mail: pcf@preventcancer.org
Toll-Free: 800-227-2732
Phone: 703-836-4412

Activities: Supports cancer prevention research and works to educate the public.

R.A. Bloch Cancer Foundation, Inc.

Website: http://blochcancer.org
E-mail: hotline@blochcancer.org
Toll-Free: 800-433-0464
Phone: 816-854-5050

Activities: Matches cancer patients with trained volunteers who have been treated for the same kind of cancer.

Sisters Network® Inc.

Website: http://www.sistersnetworkinc.org
E-mail: infonet@sistersnetworkinc.org
Toll-Free: 866-781-1808
Phone: 713-781-0255

Activities: Works to help meet the needs of African American breast cancer survivors.

Skin Cancer Foundation

Website: http://www.skincancer.org
Toll-Free: 800-754-6490
Phone: 212-725-5176

Activities: Promotes prevention, early detection, and effective treatment of skin cancer.

St. Jude Children's Research Hospital—Cure4Kids

Website: https://www.cure4kids.org

Activities: Educates health professionals, scientists, parents, educators, and kids on cancer and other serious illnesses.

Starlight Children's Foundation

Website: http://www.starlight.org
E-mail: info@starlight.org
Phone: 310-479-1212

Activities: Builds playrooms and teen lounges in hospitals and works to improve the quality of life for children with serious medical concerns.

Thyroid Cancer Survivors' Association, Inc.

Website: http://www.thyca.org
E-mail: thyca@thyca.org
Toll-Free: 877-588-7904

Activities: Offers support and other services to thyroid cancer survivors, family members, and others.

Young Survival Coalition

Website: http://www.youngsurvival.org

E-mail: info@youngsurvival.org

Toll-Free: 877-972-1011

Phone: 646-257-3000

Activities: Provides resources, connections, and outreach to young women who are diagnosed with breast cancer.

Chapter 53

How To Find Cancer Clinical Trials

Who sponsors clinical trials?

Government agencies, such as the National Cancer Institute (NCI) and other parts of the National Institutes of Health (NIH), the Department of Defense, and the Department of Veterans Affairs, sponsor and conduct clinical trials. In addition, organizations or individuals, including physicians, academic medical centers, foundations, volunteer groups, and biotechnology and pharmaceutical companies, also sponsor cancer clinical trials.

NCI sponsors a large number of clinical trials each year, and it has developed a variety of programs to make cancer clinical trials widely available in the United States and elsewhere. These programs include the following:

The Clinical Trials Cooperative Group Program brings researchers, cancer centers, and doctors together into cooperative research groups. These groups work with NCI to identify important questions in cancer research and to design and conduct clinical trials that involve patients at multiple locations to answer those questions. Cooperative groups are located throughout the United States and in Canada and Europe. For more information go to http://dctd.cancer.gov/ProgramPages/ctep/major_ctcgp.htm.

The Office of Cancer Centers provides support to research-oriented institutions that have been recognized as NCI-designated cancer centers because of their scientific excellence.

About This Chapter: This chapter begins with text excerpted from "Cancer Clinical Trials," National Cancer Institute (NCI), February 22, 2013. Available at: www.cancer.gov. Information listed under "Other Resources For Finding Clinical Trials" was compiled from various sources deemed reliable. Website and contact information was updated by the editor in May 2013.

The **Community Clinical Oncology Program (CCOP)** makes clinical trials available in a large number of communities across the United States. Local hospitals throughout the country affiliate with an NCI-designated cancer center or Clinical Trials Cooperative Group, which makes it easier for doctors at those hospitals to offer their patients participation in an NCI-sponsored clinical trial. As a result, patients do not have to travel long distances or leave loved ones to take part in an NCI-sponsored trial. The Minority-Based Community Clinical Oncology Program focuses on encouraging minority populations to take part in cancer clinical trials. For more information go the CCOP webpage at http://ccop.cancer.gov.

The **NCI Community Cancer Centers Program (NCCCP)** consists of 21 community hospitals in 16 states that support cancer research and deliver advanced cancer care. One of the goals of the NCCCP is to increase patient participation in clinical trials, with a focus on reaching underserved populations, including minorities, the elderly, and others who are typically underrepresented in clinical trials. For more information go the NCCCP webpage at http://ncccp.cancer.gov.

The **Specialized Programs of Research Excellence (SPOREs)** bring together scientists and researchers to design and implement research programs, including clinical trials, to improve the prevention, detection, diagnosis, and treatment of specific types of cancer.

The **National Institutes of Health Clinical Center,** a research hospital located in Bethesda, Maryland, is part of the NIH. Trials at the Clinical Center are conducted by the components of NIH, including NCI. The NCI fact sheet "Cancer Clinical Trials at the NIH Clinical Center" has more information. This fact sheet is available at http://www.cancer.gov/cancertopics/factsheet/NCI/clinical-center.

Where can people find more information about clinical trials?

In addition to the resources described above, people interested in taking part in a clinical trial should talk with their health care provider. Information about cancer clinical trials is also available from NCI's Cancer Information Service (800-4-CANCER) or by instant messaging at https://livehelp.cancer.gov. CIS information specialists use NCI's website to identify and provide detailed information about clinical trials that are currently accepting patients. NCI's website contains updated information about NCI-sponsored clinical trials and many other clinical trials conducted by independent investigators at hospitals and medical centers in the United States and around the world, as well as trials sponsored by pharmaceutical companies.

People also have the option of searching for clinical trials on their own by visiting the clinical trials search form http://www.cancer.gov/clinicaltrials/search. Another resource is NLM's ClinicalTrials.gov, which lists clinical trials for a wide range of diseases and conditions, including cancer, at http://www.clinicaltrials.gov.

Other Resources For Finding Clinical Trials

American Cancer Society
Clinical Trial Matching Service 800-303-5691
http://www.cancer.org/treatment/treatmentsandsideeffects/clinicaltrials/app/clinical-trials
-matching-service

CancerConsultants.com
http://news.cancerconnect.com/clinical-trials

Cancer Research UK
http://www.cancerresearchuk.org/cancer-help/trials

CenterWatch
http://www.centerwatch.com/clinical-trials/listings

Clinical Trials and Noteworthy Treatments for Brain Tumors
http://www.virtualtrials.com

CureSearch: Children's Oncology Group
http://www.curesearch.org

Current Controlled Trials (International)
http://www.controlled-trials.com

EmergingMed
http://www.emergingmed.com

IFPMA: International Federation of Pharmaceutical Manufacturers & Associations
http://clinicaltrials.ifpma.org/clinicaltrials

TrialCheck
https://www.eviticlinicaltrials.com/services

Index

Index

Page numbers that appear in *Italics* refer to tables or illustrations. Page numbers that have a small 'n' after the page number refer to citation information shown as Notes. Page numbers that appear in **Bold** refer to information contained in boxes within the chapters.

A

AAP (American Academy of Pediatrics), cancer center standards 207–8

ABCDE features, melanoma 160, **162**, 197–98

"Abnormal Pap Tests" (Boston Children's Hospital) 68n

absolute neutrophil count (ANC), described 227, 228

achondroplasia, genetic origin 17

actinic keratosis, described 159

acupuncture
cancer symptoms 269, **299**
safety **270**

acute leukemia, described 133

acute lymphoblastic leukemia (ALL)
clinical trials **277**
described 133, 135–39

acute myeloid leukemia (AML), described 133, 140–44

acute pain, described 291

acute promyelocytic leukemia (APL), described 140, 144

adenomas, colon 112, **114**

adjuvant therapy
leukemia 143
testicular cancer 185

adolescents, clinical trials **276–77**

adult, designating go-to 366

advanced practice nurse 215

AGC (atypical glandular cells), Pap test results 70

age, cancer risk 14

Agency for Toxic Substances and Disease Registry (CDC), website address 25

alcohol use
cancer risk 14
cancer survivor 312–13, 315

alkaline phosphatase, bone cancer 82

alkylating agents
fertility problems 344
late effects 334, 338, 339

ALL *see* acute lymphoblastic leukemia

allogenic transplants,
stem cell 257, **258**, 258–59, 262

all-trans retinoic acid (ATRA) 144

AMA (American Medical Association), contact information 310

American Academy of Dermatology,
sun exposure recommendations 36

American Academy of Pediatrics (AAP),
cancer center standards 207–8

American Brain Tumor Association,
contact information 377

American Cancer Society
clinical trials 385
contact information 316, 377

American Counseling Association,
contact information **316**

American Institute for Cancer Research,
contact information 311, 377

American Medical Association (AMA),
contact information 310

American Psychosocial Oncology
Society, contact information 377

American Society of Clinical Oncology
cancer and friendships publication 319n
contact information 378

American Society of Pediatric
Hematology/Oncology (ASPHO),
cancer center standards 207–8

American Thyroid Association,
thyroid cancer publication 187n

amifostine 247

AML (acute myeloid leukemia),
described 133, 140–44

amputation
bone cancer **82**
soft tissue sarcoma 176

anabolic steroids
versus cortisol-type steroids 235
health risks 62–63

analgesics
cancer pain 291–92, 294–95
injecting around spine 296–97

anaplastic thyroid cancer,
described 189

ANC (absolute neutrophil count),
described 227, 228

Anderson Cancer Center
see University of Texas MD
Anderson Cancer Center

anemia
chemotherapy 226
fatigue 284, 285
sickle cell 17
treatment 288

anesthesia, types 252

anesthesiologist 214, 252

angiogram, bone cancer 81

angiomas, genital area 199

Ann Arbor staging system, described 219

anthracyclines, late effects 330

antibodies, monoclonal
see monoclonal antibodies

antiestrogens 178

antioxidants 267, 269

anxiety
cancer survivor 314–15, 332
fatigue **287**
parent with cancer 354

apheresis, peripheral blood stem cell 259, **261**

APL (acute promyelocytic leukemia),
described 140, 144

arsenic *24*

arsenic trioxide 144

ASCUS (atypical squamous
cells of undetermined significance),
Pap test results 69–70

ASPHO (American Society of
Pediatric Hematology/Oncology),
cancer center standards 207–8

astrocytomas, described 90

ATRA (all-trans retinoic acid) 144

attending physician 213

attention fatigue, described 287

autologous transplants,
stem cell 257, 260, 262–63

B

basal cells, described 155, 157

basal cell skin cancer
described 27, 156, 157
risk factors 159–60
staging 163, 165
symptoms 161

"Basic Information About Skin
    Cancer" (CDC) 27n, **28n**
"Basics on Genes and Genetic
    Disorders" (Nemours Foundation) 15n
basophils 227
behavioral risk factors, described 23
benign growths, skin 156
benign tumors
    breast 93
    defined 4
benzene *24*, 134
beta-carotene 267
bile duct cancer, environmental causes *22*
bile ducts, late effects 335
biological therapy
    colorectal cancer 117, 119
    fatigue 285
    melanoma 169–70
    palliative 296
biopsy
    bone cancer 81–82
    brain tumor 87
    breast cancer 96
    cervical cancer 103, 108
    colorectal cancer **116**
    colposcopy with 71–72
    described **254**
    Hodgkin lymphoma 148, 149
    leukemia 136, 143
    skin cancer 162, 163, 165
    soft tissue sarcoma 175, 176
    testicular cancer 183
birth control pills, cancer risk 59–62
bladder cancer, environmental causes *22*
R.A. Bloch Cancer Foundation,
    contact information 381
blood cells
    chemotherapy effects 119, 169
    development 131–32, *132*, 257
blood chemistry studies, leukemia 136–37
blood disorders, leukemia risk 134
blood transfusions
    anemia 226, 288
    leukemia **144**

blood vessels
    late effects 330
    tumors **174**
bone cancer
    described 79–84
    prosthetics **82**
"Bone Cancer" (NCI) 79n
bone marrow
    blood cell development 131–32, *132*, 257
    donating **261**, **263**, 264
    harvesting 259, 261
    lymph system 146, *146*
bone marrow aspiration and biopsy
    Hodgkin lymphoma 149
    leukemia 136
bone marrow transplantation
    described 9, 257–64
    neuroblastoma 172
"Bone Marrow Transplantation
    and Peripheral Blood Stem
    Cell Transplantation" (NCI) 257n
bone pain, described 293
bones
    late effects 338
    strengthening painful 298–99
bone scan
    bone cancer 81
    breast cancer 96
bone tumors, soft tissue sarcoma **174**
Boston Children's Hospital, Center for Young
    Women's Health, Pap test publication 68n
botanical supplements
    cancer symptoms/treatment **268**, 268–69
    safety **270**
Bowen disease
    described 165
    treatment 168, 169
boyfriends, cancer and **321**
boys
    breast lumps **76**
    HPV vaccine 54, **55**
brachytherapy
    colorectal cancer 119
    described 239, 244–45, 247

brain
    late effects 331, **332**
    major parts **86**
brain stem, described **86**
brainstem gliomas, described 90
brain tumors
    described 85–92
    environmental causes *22*
    medical team **88**
    mobile phones 12
"Brain Tumors" (Nemours Foundation) 85n, **88n**
BRCA1 or BRCA2 gene, mutations 61
breast cancer
    described 93–99
    environmental causes *22*
    in men **94**
    mobile phones 12, 13
    obesity 49, 50
    oral contraceptives 59, 60
    in teens 75
breasts
    anatomy 93, *95*
    development 73
    lumps and bumps 75–76, **76**
breast self-exam (BSE)
    cancer screening **74**
    how to perform 73–76
bronchial cancer, environmental causes *22*
bumps
    breast 75–76, **76**
    genital area 197–99
"Bumps and Lumps: When Do They Require
    Medical Attention?" (Mullen and Shile) 197n

C

California Environmental
    Health Tracking Program,
    cancer and environment publication 21n
cancer
    defined 3
    myths 11–14
    origins 3–4, *5*, 7–8
    questions 201–5
    statistics 4, **8**, 50–51

cancer, *continued*
    types **4**, 5
    in young people 7–10
"Cancer And Complementary
    Health Practices" (NCCAM) 265n
"Cancer and Obesity" (Obesity Society) 49n
"Cancer and the Environment"
    (California Environmental
    Health Tracking Program) 21n
"Cancer and Your Friends"
    (American Society of
    Clinical Oncology) 319n
CancerCare, contact information 316, 378
cancer cells
    breast 93–94
    formation and growth 3, *5*, 7
    radiation effects 239, **240**
    skin 156
    spread 106
"Cancer Clinical Trials" (NCI) 273n, 383n
CancerConsultants.com, clinical trials 385
Cancer Financial Assistance Coalition,
    contact information 378
Cancer.Net *see* American
    Society of Clinical Oncology
"Cancer of the Thyroid" (American
    Thyroid Association) 187n
cancer pain
    treatment 289, 294–300
    types and causes 291–94
cancer prevention
    clinical trials 273–74
    complementary health practices 267–68
    girls 65–72
    skin cancer 30–31, 313–14
"Cancer Prevention for Girls:
    Why See a Gynecologist"
    (Office of Women's Health) 65n
Cancer Research UK
    cancer pain publications 291n, **292n**, **299n**
    clinical trials 385
cancer staging
    breast cancer 96–98
    cervical cancer 104–7
    colorectal cancer 115, **116**

cancer staging, *continued*
    described 217–21, **221**
    extracranial germ cell tumor 126–28
    lymphoma 149–51, **150**, 153, **154**
    neuroblastoma 171
    skin cancer 163, 165
    soft tissue sarcoma 175–76
"Cancer Staging" (NCI) 217n
Cancer Support Community
  —Group Loop, contact information 378
cancer treatment
    body changes 301–3
    clinical trials 273
    emotional challenges after 314–17
    healthy living after 310–14
    late effects *see* late effects
    medical considerations after 305–10
    methods 8–10
"Can I Have Children
  After Cancer Treatment?"
  (Nemours Foundation) 343n
cannabinoids **268**
Cannabis and Cannabinoids (PDQ):
  Patient version (NCI) **268n**
carboplatin, late effects 340, 341, 342
carcinoma, defined **4**
"Care For Children And
  Adolescents With Cancer" (NCI) 207n
CaringBridge, contact information 378
carriers, defined 17
cartilage tumors, examples **174**
CAT scan
  see computed tomography scan
CDC
  see Centers for Disease
  Control and Prevention
celiac nerve block, described 297
cell phones, cancer risk 12, 13
cells
    chemotherapy effects 119, 169
    normal *versus* cancer 3, *5*, 7, 93, 156
cementoplasty, percutaneous 298–99
Center for Young Women's Health,
  Boston Children's Hospital,
  Pap test publication 68n

Centers for Disease Control and Prevention (CDC)
  Agency for Toxic Substances
      and Disease Registry 25
  contact information 311
  publications
    human papillomavirus 53n, **55n**
    smoking and tobacco use 39n
    tanning and
        skin cancer 27n, **28n**, **29n**, **34n**
CenterWatch, clinical trials 385
central nervous system
  components **86**
  late effects 331, **332**
central nervous system cancers
  defined **4**
  environmental causes *22*
central venous lines
  chemotherapy 224
  surgery **254**
cerebellum, described **86**
cerebrum, described **86**
Cervarix 54, 55, **55**
cervical cancer
  described 101–10
  HPV and 53–54, 55, **55**, 57, 101–2, **102**
  oral contraceptives 59, 61–62
  Pap test results 70
  signs **103**
Cervical Cancer Treatment (PDQ):
  Patient version (NCI) 101n
chaplains 216
chemicals
  carcinogenic 21, *24–25*
  tobacco smoke **40**, 43
chemotherapy
  bone cancer 83
  bone marrow/peripheral blood cell
      transplant 257, **258**, 262–63
  brain tumor 89
  breast cancer 99
  cervical cancer 109
  colorectal cancer 116, 117, 118–19
  described 8, 9, 223–25
  extracranial germ cell tumors 128
  fatigue 284

chemotherapy, *continued*
 fertility problems 344
 hair loss 12
 leukemia 134, 138, 143
 lymphoma 151, 152, 154
 medications *232–33*, 234
 neuroblastoma 172
 pain 291
 palliative 296
 questions 203
 radiation therapy and **246**
 side effects 119, 169, 225–34, 301–3
 skin cancer 168–69
 soft tissue sarcoma 177
 surgery and **254**
 testicular cancer 185
 thyroid cancer 191
"Chemotherapy in Children"
 (CureSearch) 223n
Child Extracranial Germ Cell
 Tumors Treatment (PDQ):
 Patient version (NCI) 123n
Childhood Acute Lymphoblastic
 Leukemia Treatment (PDQ):
 Patient version (NCI) 131n, **139n**
Childhood Acute Myeloid Leukemia/Other
 Myeloid Malignancies Treatment (PDQ):
 Patient version (NCI) 131n, **141n, 144n**
Childhood Brain and Spinal Cord
 Tumors Treatment Overview (PDQ):
 Patient version (NCI) **86n**
"Childhood Cancer" (Nemours Foundation) 7n
Childhood Hodgkin Lymphoma
 Treatment (PDQ): Patient version (NCI) 145n
Childhood Non-Hodgkin Lymphoma
 Treatment (PDQ): Patient version (NCI) 145n
Childhood Rhabdomyosarcoma
 Treatment (PDQ): Patient version (NCI) 173n
Childhood Soft Tissue Sarcoma
 Treatment (PDQ): Patient version (NCI) 173n
child life specialist 216
Children's Brain Tumor Foundation,
 contact information 378
children's cancer centers, specialized 207–11

Children's Oncology Group (COG; NCI)
 cancer staging 220
 contact information 207, 211
chloroma, described 140, 142
chondrosarcoma, described 80
choriocarcinomas, described 124
chromosomes, described 15–16
chronic lymphocytic leukemia (CLL),
 described 133
chronic myeloid leukemia (CML),
 described 133, 140–44, **141**
chronic pain, described 291–92
cisplatin, late effects 340, 341, 342
classical Hodgkin lymphoma, defined **147**
clinical psychologist 216
clinical trials
 adolescents and young adults **276–77**
 bone cancer 84
 bone marrow/peripheral blood
  cell transplant 262, 264
 cervical cancer 108
 chemotherapy 224–25
 children's cancer centers 208–10
 complementary health practices 267–70
 described 273–79
 germ cell tumor 128, 129
 leukemia 144
 phases 209, 278–79
 questions 202, 203
 radiation therapy 248–49
 resources 383–85
 soft tissue sarcoma 178
 testicular cancer 186
Clinical Trials and Noteworthy Treatments
 for Brain Tumors, website address 385
Clinical Trials Cooperative
 Group Program (NCI) 383
"Clinical Trials Offer A Path To Better Care
 For AYAs With Cancer" (Reynolds) **277n**
CLL (chronic lymphocytic leukemia),
 described 133
clothing, UV protection 31
CML (chronic myeloid leukemia),
 described 133, 140–44, **141**
college, planning 326–28

colonoscopy, colorectal cancer 112, 117

color blindness, described 17

colorectal cancer

    calcium 267

    described 111–21

    familial **114**

    grilled meat 45, 46

    obesity 49, 50, 51

    staging **116**

colostomy, colorectal cancer 118, 121

colposcopy, described 71–72, 103

Community Clinical Oncology Program
    (CCOP; NCI) 384

complementary health practices

    cancer pain **299**, 300

    described 265–71

    medical marijuana **268**

    safety **270**

complete blood count (CBC)

    with differential, leukemia 136

computed tomography scan

    (CAT scan; CT scan)

    bone cancer 81

    breast cancer 96

    cervical cancer 105

    Hodgkin lymphoma 149

    leukemia risk 134

    soft tissue sarcoma 176

"Congressional Report Exposes Tanning
    Industry's Misleading Message to Teens"
    (Skin Cancer Foundation) **33n**

conization, cervical cancer 108

connective tissue tumors, examples **174**

contraceptives, cancer risk 59–62

Cooke, David A. 79n, 111n, **114n**,
    116n, 131n, 207n

cord blood banks, described 260, 264

cortisol *see* steroids

cosmetics, SPF factor **29**

counseling

    cancer survivor **316**, 317, 346

    fatigue 290

    genetic **19**

    parent with cancer **359**

craniopharyngiomas, described 91

cryosurgery

    bone cancer 83

    cervical cancer 109

    skin cancer 167

CT scan *see* computed tomography scan

CureSearch

    chemotherapy publication 223n, *233n*

    clinical trials 385

    contact information 378

Current Controlled Trials
    (International), clinical trials 385

Cushing syndrome, symptoms 237

cyclophosphamide 344

cystic fibrosis, genetic origin 17

cystoscopy, cervical cancer 105

cysts, genital area 199

cytogenetic analysis, leukemia 136

Cytomel (liothyronine) 190

Cytoxan (cyclophosphamide) 344

D

DDT *24*

dental care, cancer survivor **334**

deoxyribonucleic acid (DNA)

    damage 3, 21, **240**

    described 15–16

    HPV test 103

depression

    cancer survivor **316**, 332

    fatigue **287**

    parent with cancer 354, **359**

    treatment 289

dermatologist 162

dermis, described 155

diabetes mellitus, cancer survivor 335

diagnostic trials, described 274

diarrhea, chemotherapy 228–29

diet and nutrition

    anemia 288

    cancer risk 12, 14

    cancer survivor 311, **312**, 315

    chemotherapy side effects 228–34

    fatigue 285

    vitamin D intake 35, 36–37

dietary supplements, cancer prevention/
    treatment 266, **266**, 267–69, **270**
differential
        leukemia 136
        neutropenia 227
digestive system
        chemotherapy effects 119, 169
        late effects 334
        structure and function 111
dioxin *24*
DNA *see* deoxyribonucleic acid
doctor(s)
        health care team 213–15
        questions to ask 201–5
Down syndrome, genetic origin 17
dronabinol **268**
"Drug Facts: Anabolic Steroids"
    (NIDA) 59n
dry mouth, chemotherapy 229, 230–31
ductal carcinoma, breast 94
dysplasia, cervical 101
dysplastic nevus, described **159**, *161*

E

ears, late effects 340
education
        cancer and 323–28
        friend with cancer 368, 370
        late effects and **332**
electrical nerve stimulation, cancer pain 299
electricity pylons, cancer risk 12
electrodesiccation and curettage,
    skin cancer 167
eligibility criteria, clinical trial 275
embryonic stem cells, described 257
EmergingMed, clinical trials 385
emotional issues
        cancer survivor 314–17
        fatigue **287**
        fertility problems 345–46
        friend with cancer 367, 368–69
        late effects 332–33
        parent with cancer 350–52, 354, **359**
        sibling with illness 363, **364**

endocervical curettage,
    cervical cancer 103
endometrial cancer
        obesity 49
        oral contraceptives 59, 61
energy, increasing 289–90
enterostomal therapist 121
environment
        cancer and 21–26, *22*
        genes, heredity, and 16
        specific concerns *24–25*, 25
eosinophils 227
ependymomas, described 90
epidermis, described 155
epidural anesthesia, described 296
epigenetic modifications, described 21
esophageal cancer
        obesity 49
        smokeless tobacco **44**
estrogen 59
Ethyol (amifostine) 247
Ewing sarcoma family of tumors (ESFTs)
        clinical trials **277**
        described 80
excisional biopsy, skin 162, 165
excisional skin surgery, described 166
exercise
        cancer survivor 311–12, 315
        fatigue relief 289
external-beam radiation therapy,
    described 239, 242–44, 247
extracranial germ cell tumors
        described 123–29
        risk factors **125**
extragonadal germ cell tumors,
    described 124–25, 127
eyes, late effects 340–41

F

familial adenomatous polyposis (FAP),
    described **114**
family
        parent with cancer 354–57
        ways to help **358**, 365

family history
    cancer risk assessment **18–19**
    leukemia 134
    skin cancer 158
FAP (familial adenomatous
    polyposis), described **114**
fatigue, cancer-related 283–90, 368
Fatigue (PDQ): Patient version (NCI) 283n
fat tissue tumors, example **174**
FDA *see* US Food and Drug Administration
feelings *see* emotional issues
Fertile Hope, contact information 378
fertility
    after cancer treatment 339, 343–46
    preserving 339, 345
    questions **345**
    after testicular cancer **184**, 186
fever, chemotherapy 229
fibrocystic breast changes, described 75
fibrohistiocytic tumors, examples **174**
fibrous tissue tumors, examples **174**
fish, grilling 45, 46
fluorouracil (5-FU), skin cancer 168
follicular thyroid cancer, described 189
follow-up care
    late effects **331**
    oncology 307, 310
Food and Drug Administration
    see US Food and Drug Administration
food coloring, cancer risk 13
FORCE: Facing Our Risk of Cancer
    Empowered, contact information 379
4th Angel Mentoring Program,
    contact information 379
friend(s)
    with cancer 367
    cancer and your 319–21, **321**
    staying connected 324, 356, 357
fruits, grilling 46–47

G

gallbladder cancer, obesity 49
Gardasil 54, 55, **55**, 57
general anesthesia, surgery 252, 253

genes
    cancer 11
    changing 20
    colorectal cancer risk 111, 112, 113, **114**
    described 15–16
gene therapy, described 20
genetic counselor **19**
genetic disorders, described 16–17
genetic mutations, cancer and 3, *5*, 11, 16–17
Genetics of Colorectal Cancer (PDQ):
    Health professional version (NCI) **114n**
genetic testing
    described 17
    determining need **18–19**
genital area, bumps and lumps 197–99
genital warts
    described 198
    HPV and 54, 55, **55**, 57
germ cells, testicular 181
germ cell tumors
    brain 91
    extracranial 123–29
    testicular **182**
germinomas, described 91, 124
girlfriends, cancer and **321**
girls
    cancer prevention 65–72
    HPV vaccines 54, **55**
Gleevec (imatinib mesylate) 139, 143
gliomas, brainstem 90
gonadal germ cell tumors
    described 124, **125**, 125–27
    testicular **182**
graft-versus-host disease,
    post-transplant **258**, 259, 262
graft-versus-tumor effect,
    post-transplant **258**, 262
gray (Gy), defined **241**
green tea, cancer prevention 268
grilling, safer 45–47
growth hormone, low level 336, 337
Gwynne, Tony **44**
Gy (gray), defined **241**
gynecologist, reasons to visit 65–68
gynecomastia, described **76**

H

hair loss, cancer treatment 12, 119, 169, 229, 301–2

hairy cell leukemia, described 133

hats, UV protection 31

HCAs (heterocyclic amines), grilling 46

health care team

    brain tumor care **88**

    children's cancer center 208

    leukemia care **139**

    members 213–16

"Healthier Ways to Grill Meat"
(Nathan-Garner) 45n

health insurance coverage

    bone marrow/peripheral blood
        cell transplant 263–64

    children's cancer centers 210

    HPV vaccination 57–58

Healthy People 2020, indoor tanning goals 34

hearing loss, cancer survivor 340

heart, late effects 330

heart disease, smoking and 41–42

hematocrit, anemia 226

hematopoietic stem cells,
described 131–32, *132*, 257

hemoglobin, anemia 226

hemophilia, described 17

heredity, genes and 16

herpes, genital blisters 198

HER2 test, breast cancer 95

heterocyclic amines (HCAs), grilling 46

HLA (human leukocyte-associated) antigens,
matching 258–59, 264

Hodgkin lymphoma

    described 145–52

    types **147**

homebound tutoring and schooling 323–24

hormonal drugs, cancer risk 59–63

hormone receptor tests, breast cancer 95

hormone therapy

    breast cancer 95, 99

    palliative 296

    soft tissue sarcoma 178

"How to Perform a Breast Self-Examination"
(Nemours Foundation) 73n

HPV *see* human papillomavirus

"HPV Vaccine for Preteens and Teens"
(CDC) 53n, **55n**

"HPV Vaccine—Questions and Answers"
(CDC) 53n

HSIL (high grade squamous
intraepithelial lesion), Pap test results 70

HTLV-1 infection, leukemia risk 134

Human Genome Project, described 20

human leukocyte-associated (HLA) antigens,
matching 258–59, 264

human papillomavirus (HPV)

    cancer risk 53–58

    cervical cancer 61–62, 101–2, **102**

    genital warts 198

    oral contraceptives 61–62

    skin cancer 160

    tests 70, 103

    transmission 13

    vaccines 53, 54–58, **55**, **68**, 198

human T-cell leukemia virus type 1
(HTLV-1), leukemia risk 134

Huntington disease, genetic origin 17

hydrocephalus, brain tumors 87

hypnosis, cancer symptoms 269

hysterectomy, cervical cancer 108–9

I

ifosfamide, late effects 341, 342

IFPMA (International Federation
of Pharmaceutical Manufacturers
& Associations), clinical trials 385

image-guided radiation therapy (IGRT),
described 243

"I'm A Guy. Why Do I Have A Lump In
My Breast?" (Nemours Foundation) **76n**

imatinib mesylate 139, 143

imiquimod 168

immune system, damaged 22

immunophenotyping

    Hodgkin lymphoma 148

    leukemia 136

implant radiation
see brachytherapy

I'm Too Young for This! Cancer Foundation,
  contact information 379
incident pain, defined 292
incisional biopsy, skin 162
indoor tanning
  congressional report **32–33**
  dangers 29, 31–32, 158, 313
  facts **34**
  myths 32–34
  policies 34
"Indoor Tanning" (CDC) 27n, **34n**
infections
  genital area 198, 199
  leukopenia 228
inflammatory breast cancer, described 98
informed consent, clinical trial 276–78
Institutional Review Board (IRB) 275–76
insulin resistance, cancer survivor 335
intensity-modulated
  radiation therapy (IMRT), described 243
interferon 169
interleukin-2 169
internal radiation *see* brachytherapy
International Federation of
  Pharmaceutical Manufacturers
  & Associations (IFPMA),
  clinical trials 385
intraoperative radiation therapy (IORT),
  colorectal cancer 120
intrathecal anesthesia, described 296, 297
intrathecal chemotherapy, defined 9
intravenous chemotherapy, defined 9
IRB (Institutional Review Board) 275–76
"Is Some Sun Good?"
  (Sun Safety for Kids) 35n

J

jaws, late effects 333–34
jewelry, preoperative removal **253**
Joe's House, contact information 379
joints, late effects 338
journal, keeping 364
juvenile myelomonocytic leukemia,
  described 140–44, **141**

K

"Keeping Your Past in the Rear View Mirror"
  (National Children's Cancer Society) 305n
Kelly, Jeanne *5n*
kidney cancer
  environmental causes *22*
  obesity 49, 50, 51
kidneys, late effects 341
kissing, cancer risk 14
kyphoplasty, described 298–99

L

lactose intolerance, diet 228
laparoscopy
  cervical cancer 105
  colorectal cancer 117–18
  Hodgkin lymphoma 148
laser surgery, cervical cancer 109
late effects
  brain tumors 91–92
  described **306**, 329–42
  fatigue 290
  fertility 343–46
  follow-up care **331**
  radiation therapy 247, 248
  risk reduction 305
Late Effects Assessment Tool 305, 308
Late Effects of Treatment For Childhood
  Cancer (PDQ): Patient version (NCI) 329n
LEEP (loop electrosurgical excision procedure),
  cervical cancer 109
lenalidomide 144
leukapheresis, leukemia **144**
leukemia
  acute lymphoblastic 135–39
  acute myeloid 140–44
  clinical trials **277**
  described **4**, 131–35
  environmental causes *22*
  graft-versus-tumor effect **258**, 262
  myths 14
  supportive care **144**
  treatment team **139**

leukemia cutis, described 142

Leukemia & Lymphoma Society,
   contact information 379

levothyroxine 190, 191–92

lifestyle choices
      cancer risk 6, **18**
      cancer survivor 310–14, 315, **342**

limb-sparing surgery
      bone cancer **82**, 83
      soft tissue sarcoma 176

liothyronine 190

liver, late effects 335, **335**

liver cancer
      environmental causes *22*
      oral contraceptives 59, 62

liver transplant, soft tissue sarcoma 178

LIVESTRONG Foundation,
   contact information 379

lobular carcinoma, breast 94

local anesthesia, surgery 252

local therapy, defined 117

Look Good. Feel Better for Teens,
   contact information 379

loop electrosurgical
   excision procedure (LEEP),
   cervical cancer 109

LSIL (low grade squamous
   intraepithelial lesion), Pap test results 70

Lu, Karen **18, 19**

lumbar puncture, leukemia 143

lumpectomy, breast cancer 99

lumps
      breast 75–76, **76**
      genital area 197–99

lung cancer
      beta-carotene 267
      environmental causes *22*
      obesity 50
      secondhand smoke **42**, 311

lungs
      late effects 339–40
      smoking effects 42

lymph, described 145

lymphadenectomy, soft tissue sarcoma 176

lymph node biopsy
      breast cancer 96
      soft tissue sarcoma 176

lymph nodes
      cancer spread 157
      cancer staging 218–19
      described 145, *146*

lymphocytes 227

lymphoid stem cells,
   development 132, *132*, 135

lymphoma
      defined **4**
      Hodgkin 145–52, **147**
      non-Hodgkin *22*, 152–54

Lymphoma Foundation of America,
   contact information 379

lymph system, anatomy 145–46, *146*

lymph vessels
      described 145, *146*
      tumors **174**

Lynch Syndrome International,
   contact information 380

M

magnetic resonance imaging (MRI)
      bone cancer 81
      breast cancer 96
      Hodgkin lymphoma 149
      soft tissue sarcoma 175

malignant growths, skin 156

malignant tumors
      breast 94
      defined 4
      germ cell 124

Marfan syndrome, genetic origin 17

marijuana, medical **268**

massage therapy
      cancer symptoms 269, 300
      safety **270**

mastectomy, breast cancer 99

masturbation, cancer risk 14

Max Foundation, contact information 380

MD Anderson Cancer Center *see* University
   of Texas MD Anderson Cancer Center

meat
  cancer risk 12
  safer grilling 45–46
mediastinoscopy, Hodgkin lymphoma 148
medical appointments, cancer survivor 307–8
medical history, recordkeeping 306–7
medical marijuana, cancer treatment **268**
medical team *see* health care team
medications
  chemotherapy *232–33*, 234
  fatigue side effect 287
  painkillers 291–92, 294–95, 296–97
  questions 204
  skin cancer risk 158
meditation, cancer symptoms 269
medullary thyroid cancer, described 189
medulloblastomas, described 90
melanin 29
melanocytes, described 155, 156
melanoma
  asymmetrical **159**
  described 27, 156, 157
  incidence **158**
  indoor tanning 32, **33**
  prevention 313
  staging 163, 165
  symptoms 160, *160*, *161*, **162**, 197–98
  treatment 168–70
Melissa's Living Legacy Teen Cancer Foundation
  contact information 380
  publications
    cancer care hospital team 213n
    neuroblastoma 171n
    prosthetics **82n**
    surgery **254n**
mesothelioma, environmental cause *22*
metabolic syndrome, late effects 337
metallic compounds *24*
metastasis
  bone cancer 79, 83
  brain tumor 86
  cancer staging 219
  defined 4, 7, 157
  methods 106

metastasis, *continued*
  neuroblastoma 171
  skin cancer 157, 163
  thyroid cancer 191
methotrexate, late effects 338, 342
minipill, described 59
mini-transplant, stem cell 262
mobile phones, cancer risk 12, 13
modified radical hysterectomy,
  cervical cancer 108–9
Mohs surgery, skin cancer 167
moles
  checking 313, 314
  described 156
  melanoma risk **159**, 160, *160*, *161*, **162**
mollusca, genital area 199
monoclonal antibodies
  colorectal cancer 119
  lymphoma 151–52
  radiation therapy 245
monocytes 227
Monsel's solution, colposcopy 72
mouth cancer, smokeless tobacco **44**
mouth care, general 229
mouth sores, care 229–30
MRI *see* magnetic resonance imaging
Mullen, Renata 197n
myelodysplastic syndromes, described **141**
myeloid malignancies, described 140–44, **141**
myeloid stem cells, development 131, *132*, 140
myeloma, defined **4**
"My Friend Has Cancer. How Can I Help?"
  (Nemours Foundation) 367n
"Myth Buster" (Teenage Cancer Trust) 11n
myths
  cancer 11–14
  indoor tanning 32–34

N

nabilone **268**
nails, cancer treatment effects 303
Nathan-Garner, Laura **19n**, 45n
National Association of Social Workers,
  contact information **316**

National Bone Marrow Transplant Link,
   contact information 380
National Cancer Institute (NCI)
      Cancer Information Service 84, 211,
            221, 263, 264, 384
      cancer staging 220, **221**
      children's cancer centers 207–8, 210, 211
      clinical trials 274, 383–84
            bone cancer 84
            bone marrow/peripheral blood
                  cell transplant 264
            complementary health
                  practices 267, 270
            leukemia 144
            soft tissue sarcoma 178
            testicular cancer 186
      contact information 6, 311, 380
      publications
            bone cancer 79n
            bone marrow and stem cell
                  transplantation 257n
            brain and spinal cord tumors **86n**
            breast cancer 93n
            cancer information 3n, 375
            cancer staging 217n
            cervical cancer 101n
            children's cancer centers 207n
            clinical trials 273n, **277n**, 383n
            colorectal cancer 111n, **114n**, **116n**
            complementary health practices 271
            fatigue 283n
            germ cell tumors 123n
            late effects 329n
            leukemia 131n, **139n**, **141n**, **144n**
            lymphoma 145n
            medical marijuana **268n**
            melanoma and other
                  skin cancers 155n, *160n*, *161n*
            oral contraceptives 59n
            parent with cancer 349n
            questions to ask doctor 201n
            radiation therapy 239n
            secondhand smoke **42n**
            soft tissue sarcomas 173n
            testicular cancer 181n
National Center for Complementary
   and Alternative Medicine (NCCAM)
      complementary health therapy
            publications 265n, 271
      research 270
National Children's Cancer Society
   contact information 380
   publications
            cancer and education 323n
            after cancer treatment 305n
National Hospice and Palliative Care Organization
   (NHPCO), contact information 380
National Institute on Drug Abuse (NIDA),
   publications
            anabolic steroids 59n
            smokeless tobacco **44n**
National Institutes of Health (NIH)
   Clinical Center, clinical trials 210, 384
National Library of Medicine (NLM),
   clinical trials 384
National Marrow Donor Program,
   contact information **263**
National Patient Travel Center,
   contact information 380
National Suicide Prevention Lifeline **316**
nausea and vomiting,
   cancer treatment 231–34, **268**, 368
NCCAM *see* National Center for
   Complementary and Alternative Medicine
NCI *see* National Cancer Institute
NCI Community Cancer
   Centers Program (NCCCP) 384
Nemours Foundation, publications
            brain tumors 85n, **88n**
            breast lumps in guys **76n**
            breast self-exam 73n
            childhood cancer 7n
            fertility after cancer treatment 343n
            friend with cancer 367n
            genetics and cancer 15n
            sibling with serious illness 363n
            steroids and cancer treatment 235n
            surgery 251n
nerve blocks, types 297–98
nerve pain, described 293

neuroblastoma 171–72, **172**
"Neuroblastoma: Cancer Of
  The Nervous System" (Melissa's Living
  Legacy Teen Cancer Foundation) 171n
neuroendocrine system, late effects 336
neurologist, pediatric **88**
neuro-oncologist, pediatric **88**
Neuro-Oncology Branch (NCI),
  clinical trials 210
neurosurgeon, pediatric **88**, 88–89
neutropenia, chemotherapy 227–28
neutrophils, function 227
nevi *see* moles
nicotine 40, 41, 43
NIDA *see* National Institute on Drug Abuse
nitrates 25
NLM (National Library of Medicine),
  clinical trials 384
nodular lymphocyte-predominant
  Hodgkin lymphoma, defined **147**
non-Hodgkin lymphoma
    described 152–54
    environmental causes 22
nonseminomas, described 124, 126–27, **182**
nonsteroidal anti-inflammatory drugs,
  soft tissue sarcoma 178
note-taking, purposes **346**
nuclear disasters, thyroid cancer 188
nurses and nursing aides 215
nutrition *see* diet and nutrition
nutritionists 216

O

obesity
    cancer risk 13–14, 23–24, 49–51
    late effects **336**, 337
Obesity Society, obesity and cancer publication 49n
occupational risk factors, described 23
occupational therapists 216
Office of Cancer Centers (NCI), clinical trials 383
Office of Cancer Complementary and
  Alternative Medicine (NCI), website address 270
Office of Women's Health, cancer prevention
  publication 65n

Office on Smoking and Health,
  smoking and tobacco use 39n
oncology fellow 214
    see also pediatric oncologists
oral chemotherapy, defined 9
oral contraceptives, cancer risk 59–62
"Oral Contraceptives
  and Cancer Risk" (NCI) 59n
orchiectomy, testicular cancer 183, **184**, 185
organ damage, chemotherapy 234
organic compounds 25
oropharyngeal cancer, HPV and 54
orthopedic oncologist 82
osteosarcoma, described 79, 80
"Other Resources For Finding
  Clinical Trials" (NCI) 383n
"Other Ways of Treating Cancer Pain"
  (Cancer Research UK) 291n, **299n**
ovarian cancer, oral contraceptives 59, 60–61
ovarian germ cell tumors
    described 124, 125–26, 127
    risk factors **125**
ovaries, late effects 339

P

pain
    treatment 289, 294–300
    types and causes 291–94
painkillers
    cancer pain 291–92, 294–95
    injecting around spine 296–97
palliative cancer treatments, types 295–96
palliative radiation therapy,
    examples 240, 245
Palo Alto Medical Foundation,
  bumps and lumps publication 197n
pancreas, late effects 335
pancreatic cancer, smokeless tobacco **44**
papillary thyroid cancer, described 189
Pap tests
    abnormal 68–72
    cervical cancer 103
    described 67, 68
    repeat 70–71

parent
  with cancer 349–61
  visiting in hospital **353**
parotid cancer, smokeless tobacco **44**
pathological fracture, defined 298
pathologist 82
Patient Advocate Foundation,
  contact information 381
patient care technicians 215
PCBs (polychlorinated biphenyls) *25*
PDQ Cancer Information Summary (NCI) **86n,**
  101n, 111n, **114n,** 123n, 131n, 145n, 173n, 181n,
  221, 268n, 283n, 329n
PEComas (perivascular epithelioid cell tumors),
  examples **174**
pediatric oncologists
  children's cancer center 208
  germ cell tumor care 128
  leukemia care **139**
  primary 213
pediatric oncology, defined 8
Pediatric Oncology Branch (POB; NCI),
  clinical trials 210
pelvic exam
  cervical cancer 102–3
  described 67
pelvic exenteration, cervical cancer 109
pelvic inflammatory disease (PID), signs 66
percutaneous cementoplasty, described 298–99
peripheral blood stem cells
  described 257
  donating 259, **261,** 264
peripheral blood stem cell
  transplantation, described 257–64
peripheral nervous system tumors, example **174**
perivascular epithelioid cell tumors, examples **174**
petrochemical compounds *25*
PET scan *see* positron emission tomography
phantom pain, described 293–94
Philadelphia chromosome, acute
  lymphoblastic leukemia 136, 139
phlebotomists 216
photodynamic therapy, skin cancer 169
photon, defined 242

physical therapists 216
PID (pelvic inflammatory disease), signs 66
platelet count, low 226–27
platelets, development 131, *132,* 257
PNETs (primitive neuroectodermal
  tumors), described 90
polychlorinated biphenyls (PCBs) *25*
polycyclic aromatic compounds *25,* 46
polyps, colon 112, 113, **114**
positron emission tomography (PET scan)
  bone cancer 81
  breast cancer 97
  cervical cancer 105
  Hodgkin lymphoma 149
post-traumatic stress disorder (PTSD),
  cancer survivor 315–16, 332
potassium iodine 188
poultry, grilling 45, 46
power lines, cancer risk 12
pregnancy
  cancer and 12
  HPV vaccination 57
pretreatment surgical staging,
  cervical cancer 105
Prevent Cancer Foundation,
  contact information 381
"Preventing Tobacco Use Among Youth
  And Young Adults: We Can Make the Next
  Generation Tobacco Free" (CDC) 39n
"Prevention" (CDC) 27n, **29n**
primary cancer
  bone 79–80
  brain 86
  metastasis 106
primary care physician, finding 310
primitive neuroectodermal tumors (PNETs),
  described 90
progesterone 59
progestin 59, 60, 61
prostate cancer
  obesity 49
  vitamin E 267
"Prosthetics" (Melissa's Living
  Legacy Teen Cancer Foundation) **82n**
prosthetics, bone cancer **82**

protocols
    clinical trial 224–25, 275
    treatment 208
proton therapy, described 244
psychiatrists **214**
psychostimulants 289
PTSD (post-traumatic stress disorder),
  cancer survivor 315–16, 332
puberty, breast changes 73, **76**
Public Health Service,
  smoking and tobacco publication 39n
punch biopsy, skin 162

Q

"Questions for Your Doctor:
  Before the Orchiectomy" (Testicular
  Cancer Resource Center) **184n**
"Questions To Ask Your Doctor
  About Treatment" (NCI) 201n
"Questions To Ask Your Doctor When
  You Find Out You Have Cancer" (NCI) 201n
"Questions To Ask Your Doctor When
  You Have Finished Treatment" (NCI) 201n

R

R.A. Bloch Cancer Foundation,
  contact information 381
radiation exposure
    leukemia 134
    sources *24*
    thyroid cancer 188
radiation oncologist
    described 214
    treatment planning 240, **249**
radiation therapist, pediatric **88**
radiation therapy
    bone cancer 83
    bone marrow/peripheral blood cell
        transplants 257, **258**, 262
    brain tumor 89
    breast cancer 99
    cervical cancer 109
    colorectal cancer 116, 117, 119, 120

radiation therapy, *continued*
    described 8, 9–10, 239–49
    doses **241**, 245–46
    fatigue 284
    fertility problems 344
    leukemia 134, 138–39, **139**, 143
    lymphoma 151, 154
    neuroblastoma 172
    pain 291
    palliative 296
    questions 203
    side effects 247–48, 301–3
    soft tissue sarcoma 177
    testicular cancer 185
    thyroid cancer 191
    timing **246**, **254**
"Radiation Therapy for Cancer" (NCI) 239n
radical hysterectomy, cervical cancer 108–9
radical inguinal orchiectomy,
  testicular cancer 183, 185
radioactive iodine
    late effects 336
    systemic therapy 239, 245
    thyroid cancer 188, 190–91
radiofrequency ablation, palliative 296
radiologist 215
radioprotectors 247, 248–49
radiosensitizers 248–49
real-time imaging, radiation therapy 248–49
recombinant human TSH
  (rhTSH) 190–91, 192
rectal cancer
    described 111
    treatment 117, 120
    see also colorectal cancer
recurrent cancer
    cervical 108
    colorectal **116**, 121
    extragonadal germ cell 128
    fear 315
    lymphoma 151, 153
red blood cell count, low 226
red blood cells, development 131, *132*, 257
red meat, cancer risk 12, 45
Reed-Sternberg cells, Hodgkin lymphoma 148

referred pain, described 294
rehabilitation, colorectal cancer 120–21
rehabilitation medicine specialists, pediatric **88**
reproductive system, late effects 338–39
research team, clinical trial 275
    see also clinical trials
resident 214
respiratory therapists 216
retinoblastoma, osteosarcoma risk 80
Reynolds, Sharon **277n**
rhabdomyosarcoma, described 174, 178–80
"Risk Factors" (CDC) 27n

S

St. Jude Children's Research Hospital
   —Cure4Kids, contact information 381
salpingo-oophorectomy, bilateral 109
sarcomas
    defined **4**
    soft tissue 80, 173–80
scholarships, childhood cancer survivors 326
school *see* education
"School: Learning to Embrace
   Their New Educational Needs"
   (National Children's Cancer Society) 323n
screening
    breast cancer **74**
    clinical trials 274
    second cancer 342
Seattle Cancer Care Alliance,
   second opinion publication **204n**
Seattle Children's Hospital,
   cancer treatment effects publication 301n
secondary cancers
    brain 86
    formation 106
    late effects 342
    radiation exposure 248
    see also metastasis
secondhand smoke, cancer risk **42**, 311
"Secondhand Smoke and Cancer" (NCI) **42n**
second opinions
    breast cancer **98**
    getting 201–2, 203, **204**

seeds, radioactive isotope 244
"Seeking a Second Opinion"
   (Seattle Cancer Care Alliance) **204n**
segmental mastectomy, breast cancer 99
Seibel, Nita **276**
self-care
    friend with cancer 370
    parent with cancer 357–58
    sibling with illness 364
self-image, positive 345–46
seminomas, described 124, **182**
senses, late effects 340–41
sexuality, infertility and 346
sexually transmitted infections (STIs)
    genital bumps 198, 199
    tests **67**, 68
shade, UV protection 30, 313
shave biopsy, skin 162
Shaw, Peter **276**, **277**
Shile, Marlana Jean 197n
sibling(s)
    friend with cancer 370
    parent with cancer 355
    seriously ill 363–66
sickle cell anemia, genetic origin 17
sigmoidoscopy, colorectal cancer 112
silver nitrate, colposcopy 72
Sisters Network, contact information 381
skin
    cancer treatment effects 303
    layers 155
    self-exam 164
skin cancer
    basic information 27–28
    diagnosis 162
    environmental causes *22*
    genital area 197–98
    incidence **158**
    indoor tanning 31–34
    prevention 30–31, 313–14
    risk factors 12, 28–30, 157–60, **159**
    staging 163, 165
    symptoms *160*, 160–61, *161*, **162**
    treatment 165–70
    types 156–57

Skin Cancer Foundation
   contact information 381
   indoor tanning publication **33n**
skin graft, described 167
skin type
   skin cancer risk 12, 158
   tanning or burning 29–30
   vitamin D production 36
sleep-related fatigue
   activity-rest schedule 290
   described 287
smoking and tobacco use
   cancer risks 13, 25, 39–44
   disease and **40**
   leukemia 134
   quitting 43–44, **44**, 310–11
   secondhand smoke **42**, 311
   teens and young adults 39, **41**, **43**
smooth muscle tumors, example **174**
social issues, late effects 332–33
social norms,
   smoking and tobacco use 41
social worker 215, 263
soft tissue pain, described 293
soft tissue sarcomas
   described 80, 173–80
   signs **177**
   types **174**
specialist, finding 201–2, 203
Specialized Programs
   of Research Excellence
   (SPOREs; NCI) 384
speech therapists 216
sperm banking, testicular cancer 186, 345
SPF (sun protection factor), described **29**
spinal anesthesia, described 296–97
spinal cord
   late effects 331, **332**
   structure and function **86**
spinal cord tumors, described **86**
splanchnicectomy, described 297
spleen
   anatomy 146, *146*
   late effects 337–38
squamous cells, described 155, 157

squamous cell skin cancer
   described 27, 156, 157
   risk factors 159–60
   staging 163, 165
   symptoms 161
staff nurse 215
staging *see* cancer staging
Starlight Children's Foundation,
   contact information 381
stem cells,
   hematopoietic 131–32, *132*, 257
stem cell transplant
   leukemia 138–39, 143
   lymphoma 152, 154
   testicular cancer 185
stereotactic body
   radiation therapy, described 244
stereotactic radiosurgery, described 243
steroids
   anabolic 62–63, 235
   cancer treatment 235–38
   late effects 338
   side effects 236–37
   weight gain 303
"Steroids And Cancer Treatment"
   (Nemours Foundation) 235n
STIs *see* sexually transmitted
   infections
Stock, Wendy **277**
stoma, colorectal cancer 118, 121
stomach cancer, grilled meat 46
stomatitis, care 229–30
stool tests, colorectal cancer 112
Strasburg, Stephen **44**
stress
   cancer survivor 314–16, 332
   parent with cancer 357–58
students with disabilities,
   college planning 326
sulindac 178
summary staging system 220
sunburn
   skin cancer risk 157
   skin type 29–30

sun exposure
    cancer survivor 313–14
    protection **29**, 30–31
    skin cancer risk 157, 158–59
    ultraviolet light 27–28
    vitamin D production 35–37
sunglasses, UV protection 31, 313
sun protection factor (SPF), described **29**
Sun Safety for Kids, sunlight and vitamin D
   publication 35n
sunscreen, described **29**, 313
support
    cancer survivor **316**, 317, 346
    friend with cancer 368–70
    parent with cancer 356–57, **359**
    sibling with illness 364
supportive care
    clinical trials 273
    leukemia **144**
surgeon 214
surgery
    bone cancer **82**, 83
    brain tumor 87, 88–89
    breast cancer 99
    cervical cancer 105, 108–9
    colorectal cancer 116, 117–18, 120
    described 8, **254**
    extracranial germ cell tumor 128
    fatigue 285
    fertility problems 344
    Hodgkin lymphoma 152
    neuroblastoma 172
    questions 203
    radiation therapy timing **246**
    skin cancer 166–68
    soft tissue sarcoma 176–77
    testicular cancer **184**, 185
    thyroid cancer 190
    tumor debulking 296
    what to expect 251–55
"Surgery" (Melissa's Living Legacy
   Teen Cancer Foundation) **254n**
Surveillance, Epidemiology,
   and End Results (SEER) Program (NCI) 220

survival, cancer
    children and 10, **149**, **208**, **276**
    facts 11, 349
    obesity and 50
syngeneic transplants, stem cell 257, 258–59
syphilis, described 198, 199
systemic radiation therapy,
   described 239, 245, 247
systemic therapy, defined 117

T

talk therapy, fatigue 290
tamoxifen 290
tandem transplant, stem cell 262–63
tanning, cancer risk 27–34, 158
    see also indoor tanning
targeted therapy
    breast cancer 95, 99
    leukemia 139, 143
    lymphoma 151–52, 154
Tay-Sachs disease, genetic origin 17
Teenage Cancer Trust, publications
    cancer and friendships **321n**
    cancer myths 11n
Teens Living With Cancer
    see Melissa's Living Legacy Teen
    Cancer Foundation
teeth, late effects 333–34, **334**
TENS (transcutaneous
   electrical nerve stimulation),
   cancer pain 299
teratomas
    benign ovarian 124
    mature and immature 123
testicles
    described 181
    late effects 338
testicular cancer
    described 181–86
    testicular injury 13
Testicular Cancer Resource Center,
   orchiectomy publication **184n**
Testicular Cancer Treatment (PDQ):
   Patient version (NCI) 181n

testicular germ cell tumors
        described 124, 125, 126–27, **182**
        risk factors **125**
testosterone, synthetic 62
"Thinking About Complementary
    and Alternative Medicine"
    (NCCAM and NCI) 271
thoracoscopy, Hodgkin lymphoma 148
thorascopic sympathectomy, described 298
3-dimensional conformal radiation therapy
    (3D-CRT), described 242, 243
thrombocytopenia, chemotherapy 226–27
thymus, anatomy 145, *146*
Thyrogen (recombinant
    human TSH) 190–91, 192
thyroglobulin 192
thyroid cancer
        described 187–93
        environmental causes *22*
        obesity 49, 50
Thyroid Cancer Survivors' Association,
    contact information 381
thyroidectomy, thyroid cancer 190, 191
thyroid gland
        described **189**
        late effects 336
thyroid hormones, replacement 190–92
TNM staging system, described 218–20
tobacco industry, marketing strategies 40
        see also smoking and tobacco use
toilet seats, cancer risk 13
tomotherapy, described 243
tonsils, anatomy 146, *146*
total hysterectomy, cervical cancer 108
transcutaneous electrical nerve
    stimulation (TENS), cancer pain 299
transient myeloproliferative disorder,
    described 140, **141**, 143–44
TrialCheck, clinical trials 385
trihalomethanes *25*
triple-negative breast cancer,
    described 95–96
tumor marker test,
    testicular cancer 183

tumors
    benign or malignant 4, 79, 93–94
    debulking surgery 296
    defined 3
    primary, staging 218
    soft tissue **174**
    see also brain tumors; germ cell tumors
tutoring, homebound 323–24
"Types and Causes of Cancer Pain"
    (Cancer Research UK) 291n, **292n**
tyrosine kinase inhibitors 139, 143

U

ultrasound exam
        cervical cancer 105
        testicular cancer 182
ultraviolet (UV) light, types 27–28
        see also sun exposure
umbilical cord blood
        donation 264
        stem cell retrieval 257, 260
University of Texas MD
    Anderson Cancer Center, publications
        genetic testing **19n**
        safer grilling 45n
Unusual Cancers of Childhood (PDQ):
    Patient version (NCI) 111n
US Food and Drug Administration
        cannabinoid approvals **268**
        indoor tanning recommendations **33**
uterine cancer, obesity 50, 51
UV index, described **28**
        see also sun exposure

V

vaccines, HPV 53, 54–58, **55**, **68**, 198
Vaccines for Children (VFC) program 57–58
vegetables, grilling 46–47
vertebroplasty, described 298–99
View from Up Here: Your Guide to
    Surviving Childhood Cancer
    (National Children's Cancer Society) 305n
vinyl chloride *25*

viruses, cancer risk 21

vision problems, late effects 341

vitamin and mineral supplements

cancer prevention/treatment 266, 267, 269

safety **270**

vitamin D

blood test **36**

indoor tanning 33–34

sun exposure 35–37

W

watchful waiting

extracranial germ cell tumors 128

myeloid malignancies 144

soft tissue sarcoma 178

testicular cancer 185

weight

healthy 311

late effects **336**, 337

steroid therapy 303

see also obesity

"What about boyfriends and girlfriends?"
(Teenage Cancer Trust) **321n**

"What Can I Expect Will Happen
to My Body During Treatment?"
(Seattle Children's Hospital) 301n

"What Is Cancer?" (NCI) 3n

"What Painkillers Are" (Cancer Research UK) 291n

"What's It Like To Have Surgery?"
(Nemours Foundation) 251n

"What You Need To Know
About Breast Cancer" (NCI) 93n

"What You Need To Know About Cancer of
the Colon and Rectum" (NCI) 111n, **116n**

"What You Need to Know About Leukemia"
(NCI) 131n

"What You Need To Know
About Melanoma and Other
Skin Cancers" (NCI) 155n, *160n*, *161n*

"When A Sibling Is Seriously Ill"
(Nemours Foundation) 363n

"When Your Parent Has Cancer" (NCI) 349n

white blood cell count, low 227–28

white blood cells,
development 131–32, *132*, 257

"Who Needs Genetic Testing for Cancer?"
(Nathan-Garner) **19n**

Winslow, Terese *95n*, *132n*, *146n*

"With Announcement On Giving Up 'Dip,'
Washington National's Stephen Strasburg's
Pitches Hit Home" (NIDA) **44n**

X

X chromosome, described 15, 16, 17

x-rays

bone cancer 81

cervical cancer 105

leukemia 137

soft tissue sarcoma 175

see also radiation therapy

Y

Y chromosome, described 15, 16

yoga, cancer symptoms 269

yolk sac tumors, described 124

young adults, clinical trials **276–77**

Young Survival Coalition,
contact information 382

"Your Cancer Care Hospital Team"
(Melissa's Living Legacy Teen
Cancer Foundation) 213n